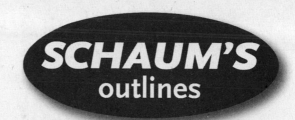

Pharmacology

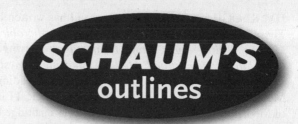

SCHAUM'S
outlines

Pharmacology

JAMES KEOGH, R.N.
Instructor, New York University

Schaum's Outline Series

Mc
Graw
Hill

New York   Chicago   San Francisco   Lisbon   London   Madrid
Mexico City   Milan   New Delhi   San Juan   Seoul
Singapore   Sydney   Toronto

JIM KEOGH is a registered nurse and has written books in the McGraw-Hill's Nursing Demystified series. These include: *Pharmacology Demystified, Microbiology Demystified, Medical-Surgical Nursing Demystified, Medical Billing and Coding Demystified, Nursing Laboratory and Diagnostic Tests Demystified, Dosage Calculations Demystified, Medical Charting Demystified, Pediatric Nursing Demystified, and Nurse Management Demystified*. His books can be found in leading university libraries including Yale University School of Medicine, University of Pennsylvania Biomedical Library, Columbia University, Brown University, University of Medicine and Dentistry of New Jersey, Cambridge University, and Oxford University. Jim Keogh, RN, A.A.S., MBA, is a former member of the faculty at Columbia University and is a member of the faculty of New York University.

Schaum's Outline of
PHARMACOLOGY

ISBN: 978-0-07-162362-9
MHID: 0-07-162362-0

Sponsoring Editor: Kimberly-Ann Eaton
Production Supervisor: Tama Harris McPhatter
Project Supervision: Print Matters, Inc.

Library of Congress Cataloging-in-Publication Data
Keogh, James Edward, 1948-
    Schaum's outline of pharmacology / James Keogh.
      p. ; cm. — (Schaum's outline series)
    Includes index.
    ISBN-13: 978-0-07-162362-9 (alk. paper)
    ISBN-10: 0-07-162362-0 (alk. paper)
1. Pharmacology—Outlines, syllabi, etc. I. Title.   II. Title: Outline of pharmacology.
      III. Series: Schaum's outline series.
    [DNLM: 1. Pharmaceutical Preparations—Examination Questions. 2.
    Pharmaceutical Preparations—Outlines. 3. Drug Therapy—Examination
    Questions. 4. Drug Therapy—Outlines. QV 18.2 K37s 2010]
    RM301.14.K46 2010
    615'.1—dc22   2009030257

This book is dedicated to Anne, Sandy, Joanne, Amber-Leigh Christine,
Shawn and Eric, without whose help and support
this book couldn't have been written.

Contents

CHAPTER 6. Route of Administration 46

CHAPTER 7. Dose Calculations 57

CHAPTER 8. Herbal Therapy 68

CHAPTER 9. Vitamins and Minerals 75

CHAPTER 10. Fluid and Electrolyte Therapy 88

CHAPTER 11. Nutritional Support Therapies 105

CHAPTER 12. Inflammation and Anti-Inflammatory Medication 114

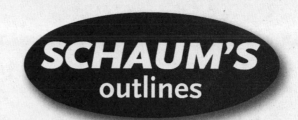

Pharmacology

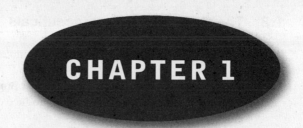

CHAPTER 1

What Is Pharmacology?

1.1 Definition

Pharmacology, derived from two Greek words: *Pharmakon* (the Greek word for drugs) and *logos* (the Greek word for science). It is the study of the effects of chemicals on living tissues. It focuses particularly on how chemicals help to:

- Prevent diseases
- Correct physiology of living tissues
- Cure or minimize diseases

Chemicals that have medicinal properties are referred to as *pharmaceuticals*. Pharmacology explores the safe and effective use of pharmaceuticals.

1.2 The Roots of Pharmacology

Ancient civilizations discovered that extracts from plants, animals, and minerals had medicinal effects on tissue. These discoveries became the foundation of empirical pharmacology. It was not until the late 1800s that developments in the sciences of physiology, organic chemistry, and biochemistry provided the scientific approach that is used in today's pharmacology.

Two separate disciplines developed. These are pharmacy and pharmacology. Pharmacy focuses on preparation and dispensing medication. Pharmacology is a blend of disciplines that collectively enable scientists to develop new medications that combat diseases. The branches of pharmacology are:

- Behavioral pharmacology: The study of how medication interacts with human behavior
- Biochemical pharmacology: The study of how medication interacts with the chemistry of the body
- Cardiovascular pharmacology: The study of how medication interacts with the cardiovascular system
- Chemotherapy: The study of how medication inhibits growth or kills selected cells
- Clinical pharmacology: The study of how medication affects the disease process and how medications interact with other medications
- Immunopharmacology: The study of how medication interacts with the body's immune response
- Molecular pharmacology: The study of how medication and hormones interact with cells
- Neuropharmacology: The study of how medication interacts with the neurologic system
- Pharmacokinetics: The study of how medications are absorbed, distributed, and eliminated from the body

1.3   The Sources of Pharmaceuticals

Pharmaceuticals are derived from one of four sources:

- Plants: Chemicals that provide medicinal properties are extracted from plants; for example, leaves from the foxglove plant are used to produce digitalis, which is used to treat congestive heart failure and cardiac arrhythmias.
- Animals: Animal byproducts, particularly hormones, are used to supplement human hormones. For example, estrogen can be recovered from the urine of a mare and insulin from the pancreas of pigs.
- Minerals: Trace elements of inorganic crystals are used to supplement minerals in humans. For example, iron is used to combat fatigue. Minerals are obtained from animals and plants.
- Synthetic Derivatives: Scientists are able to develop new medications, such as sulfonamides, by synthesizing (rearranging) chemical derivatives, resulting in new compounds.

1.4   Herbals

Herbals are nonwoody plants whose extracts are used for dietary supplements, but not for medication. Herbals are described according to their effects on tissue, such as increasing blood flow to the heart. Herbals are not usually described as cures for specific diseases. The Food and Drug Administration does not test or regulate herbals. Therefore there are no purity and strength standards for herbals, which make the effect of an herb unreliable. Herbals are sold over the counter. No prescription is required.

Unwanted side effects and undesirable interactions can occur when herbals are taken with prescription medication. For example, Coumadin, which is an anticoagulant, interacts with ginkgo, an herb that inhibits platelets, resulting in increased bleeding and stroke.

1.5   The United States Pharmacopeia National Formulary

The purity and strength of a medication influence the accuracy and reliability of the dose that is administered to the patient. *Purity* is the dilution or mixture of the medication with other materials that give the medication form so it can be given to the patient. The *strength* of a medication is its concentration or weight. The *dose* is the amount of the medication taken at one time and dosage is the amount taken over a period of time.

The United States Pharmacopeia National Formulary is a book that contains strength and purity standards for the manufacturing and control of medication. A medication that is listed in the United States Pharmacopeia National Formulary has the letters U.S.P. following its official name.

1.6   The 1938 Food, Drug, and Cosmetic Act

In the late 1930s, a pharmaceutical manufacturer distributed a sulfa medication to treat pediatric patients. The medication contained a highly toxic chemical similar to antifreeze that resulted in the death of hundreds of children. In response, the United States Congress passed the 1938 Food, Drug, and Cosmetic Act, which imposed strict regulations on the manufacturing of food, medication, and cosmetics. The 1938 Food, Drug, and Cosmetic Act requires that:

- Medication be proved safe before being sold
- The tolerance levels of medication be determined to assure patients are not poisoned
- Medication manufacturing facilities must pass government inspection
- Cosmetic and therapeutic devices be regulated

1.7 The 1952 Durham-Humphrey Amendment to the Food, Drug, and Cosmetic Act

Anyone could distribute medication so long as the medication was proved safe. This changed in 1952, when Congress determined that some medications were not safe unless the medication was directly supervised by a medical practitioner. These medications are those that are given by injection; depress the nervous system (hypnotics); dull the senses, relieve pain, and induce sleep (narcotics); are habit forming; and are still under investigation.

Congress passed the 1952 Durham-Humphrey Amendment to the 1938 Food, Drug, and Cosmetic Act that divided medications into two categories:

- Legend Medication: These are medications that must be prescribed and directly supervised by a medical practitioner and are known as a controlled substance. These include opioids, hypnotics, and potentially habit-forming or harmful medication. The medication label must read: "Caution: Federal law prohibits dispensing without a prescription."
- Over-the-Counter Medication: These are medications that do not need direct supervision by a medical practitioner. No prescription is required to purchase these medications.

1.8 The 1962 Kefauver-Harris Amendment to the Food, Drug, and Cosmetic Act

Manufacturers only had to prove that their medication is nontoxic to sell their medication. With the 1962 Kefauver-Harris Amendment to the 1938 Food, Drug, and Cosmetic Act, manufacturers also had to prove the effectiveness of the medication before it could be administered to patients. In addition, the 1962 Kefauver-Harris Amendment authorized the Food and Drug Administration, who oversees the pharmaceutical industry, to evaluate testing methods used by pharmaceutical manufacturers. This act also required the use of standard labeling on medication containers, specifically requiring that the label display contraindications for using the medication and possible adverse reactions that the medication might cause.

1.9 The 1970 Comprehensive Drug Abuse Prevention and Control Act

In an effort to contain widespread abuse of legend (prescription) medication, Congress passed the 1970 Comprehensive Drug Abuse Prevention and Control Act. This act categorized legend medication into five schedules based on the medication's potential for abuse. In addition, this act limited the number of refills for legend medication and required that practitioners use specially designated prescription pads when prescribing the medication.

These schedules are:

- Schedule I: Highest risk for abuse. May be available for investigational use only. Includes LSD, heroin, marijuana, and mescaline.
- Schedule II: High risk for abuse. Can lead to physical and psychological dependence. Can be used for medicinal purpose. Includes opioids, barbiturates, and stimulants.
- Schedule III: Moderate risk for abuse. Typically these medications are combined with other medication. Can be used for medicinal purpose. Includes opioids and barbiturates.
- Schedule IV: Low risk for abuse. Can lead to psychological dependency. Can be used for medicinal purpose. Includes chlordiazepoxide (Librium), benzodiazepines, and propoxyphene (Darvon).
- Schedule V: Least risk for abuse. Small amount combined with other medication. Can be used for medicinal purposes. Includes opioids.

1.10   Medication Names

Medication is given three names. These are:

- Chemical Name: Identifies the medication's chemical elements and compounds and used by scientists who work at the chemical level of the medication. For example, N-acetyl-*p*-aminophenol.
- Generic Name: The universally accepted name for the medication; appears on the medication label and in medication books such as the *Physicians' Desk Reference* (PDR); for example, acetaminophen.
- Brand Name: The trade name that manufacturers use to use market the medication. A medication can have multiple brand names; for example, Tylenol.

1.11   Medication Effects

Medication effects on tissue are classified as desirable and undesirable. A desirable effect occurs when the medication improves the patient's health. An undesirable effect occurs when the medication interferes with the patient's normal physiology. A medication can have both a desirable and an undesirable effect. The healthcare provider determines whether the desirable effects outweigh the undesirable effects before administering the medication to the patient. Additional medication may be given to reduce the undesirable effects of another medication.

A desirable effect is called the medication's therapeutic effect and is the reason for the healthcare provider to administer the medication. An undesirable effect is called either a side effect or an adverse side effect, depending on the consequence the undesirable effect has on the patient. A side effect is an undesirable effect that is relatively not harmful to the patient, such as drowsiness caused by an antihistamine. An adverse side effect is an undesirable consequence that is harmful to the patient, such as when healthy cells are destroyed along with cancerous cells during chemotherapy.

1.12   Medication Safety

The Food and Drug Administration requires that medication undergo rigorous testing before approving the medication. Testing includes the following animal studies to determine the medication's therapeutic index. A therapeutic index is a ratio between the median lethal dose and the median effective dose and indicates the safe dose to administer to the patient to achieve the therapeutic effect. These tests also provide scientists with information on how the medication is absorbed, distributed, metabolized, and excreted.

- Acute Toxicity Study: This is the initial test that determines the dose that is lethal to 50% of tested laboratory animals. The study reports symptoms experienced by the animals and the time symptoms appeared.
- Subchronic Toxicity Study: Two animal species are administered daily doses of the medication for 90 days. Animal test subjects are given physical examinations and laboratory tests during the 90 days to determine the medication's effect on organs.
- Chronic Toxicity Study: Two animal species are administered three dose levels—nontoxic, therapeutic, and toxic. The medication is usually administered over the life span of the test animal or the duration that the medication is intended to be given to humans. Animals are given physical exams and laboratory tests to determine the effect of the medication on organs and its potential carcinogenicity.

1.13   The Human Trial

Medications are tested in humans after animal studies are successfully completed. Testing in humans is called a human trial. There are four phases of a human trial, each of which requires approval from the Food and Drug Administration.

- Phase I: Initial Pharmacological Evaluation. Determines the safe dosage level for humans. The medication is given to volunteers at gradual doses. The first sign of toxicity is noted. Dosage levels below the toxic dose level are considered safe.
- Phase II: Limited Controlled Evaluation. Determines the therapeutic range for humans. Volunteers who have the disease or disorder are given the medication at gradual doses and are examined to determine the dose that provides the therapeutic effect.
- Phase III: Extended Clinical Evaluation. Determines the effects of the medication on a large group of patients who have the disease or disorder. If the medication proves effective, then the pharmaceutical manufacturer submits a New Drug Application (NDA) to the Food and Drug Administration for approval to market the medication.
- Phase IV: Post Marketing Surveillance Trial. Determines ongoing safety of the medication after the medication is being prescribed by healthcare providers.

1.14   Pregnancy Categories

Medications are tested to determine the medication's effect on a fetus. Based on these test results, medications are categorized according to their safety for being administered to patients during pregnancy. The pregnancy categories are:

- Category A: Adequate and well-controlled studies indicate no risk to the fetus in the first trimester of pregnancy or later.
- Category B: Animal reproduction studies indicate no risk to the fetus; however, there are no well-controlled studies in pregnant women.
- Category C: Animal reproduction studies have reported adverse effects on the fetus; however, there are no well-controlled studies in humans, but potential benefits may indicate use of the drug in pregnant women despite potential risks.
- Category D: Positive human fetal risk has been reported from investigational or marketing experience, or human studies. Considering potential benefit versus risk may, in selected cases, warrant the use of these drugs in pregnant women.
- Category X: Fetal abnormalities reported and positive evidence of fetal risk in humans is available from animal and/or human studies. The risks involved clearly outweigh the potential benefits. These drugs should not be administered to pregnant women.

Solved Problems

Source of Pharmaceuticals

1.1   Give an example of a plant whose medicinal properties are used for congestive heart failure.

Leaves from the foxglove plant are used to produce digitalis, which is used to treat congestive heart failure and cardiac arrhythmias.

1.2   What are herbals?

Herbals are nonwoody plants whose extracts are used for dietary supplements, but not for medication. Herbals are described according to their effect on tissue, such as increasing blood flow to the heart. These are not described as curing a disease.

Legal Environment of Medication

1.3   What is the objective of the 1938 Food, Drug, and Cosmetic Act?

Medication must be proved safe before being sold. A medication tolerance level must be determined to assure that patients are not poisoned. Medication manufacturing facilities must pass government inspection. Cosmetic and therapeutic devices are now regulated.

1.4   Why was the 1952 Durham-Humphrey Amendment of the Food, Drug, and Cosmetic Act passed?

The 1952 Durham-Humphrey Amendment of the Food, Drug, and Cosmetic Act was passed to categorize medication into those medications that require direct supervision by a medical practitioner, called Legend Medication, and those that did not require direct supervision, called over-the-counter medication.

1.5   What is another name given to legend medication?

Legend medications are also known as controlled substances.

1.6   Give examples of legend medications.

Legend medications are those that are given by injection; depress the nervous systems (hypnotics); dull the senses, relieve pain, and induce sleep (narcotics); are habit forming; and those still under investigation.

1.7   What is the purpose of the 1962 Kefauver-Harris Amendment to the Food, Drug, and Cosmetic Act?

The 1962 Kefauver-Harris Amendment to the Food, Drug, and Cosmetic Act required pharmaceutical manufacturers to prove the effectiveness of their medication before the medication could be administered to patients. This act also authorized the Food and Drug Administration to evaluate testing methods used by pharmaceutical manufacturers and required standard labeling of medication.

1.8   What is the purpose of the 1970 comprehensive Drug Abuse Prevention and Control Act?

The 1970 comprehensive Drug Abuse Prevention and Control Act categorized legend medication into five schedules based on the medication's potential for abuse.

1.9   What Schedule II medications are at high risk for abuse, and physical and psychological dependence?

Opioids, barbiturates, and stimulants that are not combined with other medication are at high risk for abuse, and physical and psychological dependence.

1.10 What Schedule I medications are at the highest risk for abuse and available only for investigational use?

LSD, heroin, marijuana, and mescaline are at the highest risk for abuse and available only for investigational use

Medication Names

1.11 How is a medication's chemical name used?

A medication's chemical name is used by scientists who work at the chemical level of the medication. The chemical name identifies the medication's chemical elements and compounds; for example, N-acetyl-*p*-aminophenol.

1.12 What is a medication's generic name?

A medication's generic name is the universally accepted name for the medication; it appears on the medication label and in medication books such as the *Physicians' Desk Reference* (PDR); for example, acetaminophen

1.13 What is a medication's brand name?

A medication's brand name is the trade name that manufacturers use to use market the medication; for example, Tylenol.

Medication Effects

1.14 What is a medication's therapeutic effect?

A medication's therapeutic effect is a desirable effect of the medication; it is the reason the healthcare provider administers the medication.

1.15 What is a medication's adverse side effect?

An adverse side effect is an undesirable effect of the medication that is harmful to the patient, such as when healthy cells are destroyed along with cancerous cells during chemotherapy.

1.16 What is a medication's side effect?

A medication's side effect is an undesirable effect that is relatively not harmful to the patient, such as drowsiness caused by an antihistamine.

Medication Safety

1.17 What is the purpose of a subchronic toxicity study?

A subchronic toxicity study is used to determine a medication's effect on organs. Two animal species are administered daily doses of the medication for 90 days. Animal test subjects are given physical examinations and laboratory tests during the 90 days to determine the medication's effect on organs.

1.18 What is the purpose of a chronic toxicity study?

A chronic toxicity study determines the effect of nontoxic, therapeutic, and toxic doses of a medication on organs and determines if a medication is potentially carcinogenic. Two animal species are administered three dose levels: nontoxic, therapeutic, and toxic. The medication is usually administered over the life span of the test animal or the duration that the medication is intended to be given to humans. Animals are given physical exams and laboratory tests to determine the effect of the medication on organs and if the medication is potentially carcinogenic.

1.19 What is the purpose of an acute toxicity study?

An acute toxicity study determines the medication's toxic symptoms and time when symptoms appear in animals. This is the initial test that determines the dose that is lethal to 50% of tested laboratory animals. The study reports symptoms experienced by the animals and the time symptoms appeared.

Human Trial

1.20 What is the purpose of Phase II Limited Controlled Evaluation of the human trial?

Phase II Limited Controlled Evaluation of the human trial determines the therapeutic range for humans. Volunteers who have the disease or disorder are given the medication at gradual doses and are examined to determine the dose that provides the therapeutic effect.

1.21 How do pharmaceutical manufacturers know the toxic dosage of a medication in the human trial?

Phase I, which is the Initial Pharmacological Evaluation, determines the safe dosage level by administering gradual doses to volunteers and noting the first sign of toxicity.

1.22 What is the purpose of the Post Marketing Surveillance trial?

The Post Marketing Surveillance trial determines ongoing safety of the medication after the medication is being prescribed by healthcare providers.

Pregnancy Categories

1.23 What is the purpose of a medication pregnancy category?

A medication pregnancy category indicates the medication's effect on a fetus and how safe the medication is to administer to a pregnant woman.

1.24 What does Pregnancy Category C indicate?

Pregnancy Category C indicates that animal reproduction studies have reported adverse effects on the fetus. There are no well-controlled studies in humans, but potential benefits may indicate use of the drug in pregnant women despite potential risks.

1.25 What does Pregnancy Category D indicate?

Pregnancy Category D indicates that positive human fetal risk has been reported from investigational or marketing experience, or human studies. Considering potential benefit versus risk may, in selected cases, warrant the use of these drugs in pregnant women.

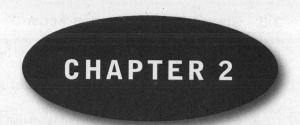

CHAPTER 2

Medication Actions and Interactions

2.1 Medication Actions

A medication action occurs between the medication molecules and molecules in the body, resulting in alteration of the body's physiological process. There are three ways medication alters the body's physiological process:

- Replacement: The medication replaces the body's molecules, such as estrogen replacement.
- Interruption: The medication interferes with the body's physiological process. For example, antihypertensive (high blood pressure) medication interferes with the physiological process that constricts blood vessels, causing a rise in blood pressure.
- Potentiation: The medication stimulates a physiological process, such as a diuretic that stimulates kidneys to excrete urine.

A medication action begins when the medication attaches to the receptor site (see Pharmacokinetics), resulting in the medication's therapeutic effect.

2.2 Multiple Medication Actions

A medication can have more than one action. These are:

- Desired Effect: The therapeutic effect
- Side Effect: An undesirable effect (sometimes the effect can be perceived as desirable, such as Benadryl's drowsiness effect) that does not harm the patient
- Adverse Effect: An undesirable effect that harms the patient

2.3   Strength of Medication Action

The strength of a medication action is determined by:

- Dose: The dose is how much of the medication is administered to the patient—the higher the dose, the stronger the medication action.
- Frequency: This is the number of times that medication is administered to the patient. An increased frequency usually strengthens the medication action.

2.4   Medication Activity

Drug activity is divided into three phases. These are:

- Pharmaceutical Phase: This is the form of the drug, such as a tablet or liquid.
- Pharmacokinetic Phase: This is the way the drug is absorbed, distributed, and eliminated.
- Pharmacodynamic Phase: This is the effect the drug has on the body.

2.5   The Pharmaceutical Phase

The pharmaceutical phase is the form of the medication such as a tablet, capsule, liquid, elixirs, or syrups. The medication form contains:

- Active Ingredient: The substance that causes the pharmaceutical response.
- Inactive Ingredient: Also called the excipient. This is a substance that does not cause the pharmaceutical response but helps delivers the medication. Inactive ingredients are used as fillers to give the medication shape and size and assist in the delivery of medication, such as the coating around tiny particles of a time-release capsule.

The form of the medication influences the time necessary for the medication to disintegrate and dissolve in the body. Disintegration is the breakdown of the medication form into particles. Dissolution is the dissolving of particles before the particles are absorbed.

The time for a medication to disintegrate and dissolve is called the rate limiting time. Table 2.1 shows the rate-limiting time for medication forms. Rate limiting time is higher if the medication is in acidic fluids rather than alkaline fluids.

TABLE 2.1 **Rate Limiting Time Rating for Drug Forms**

PREPARATION	ABSORPTION RATE (FASTEST TO SLOWEST)
Lipid soluble non-ionized Liquids, elixirs, syrups	1
Water soluble ionized Liquids, elixirs, syrups	2
Suspension solutions	3
Powders	4
Capsules	5
Tablets	6
Coated tablets	7
Enteric-coated tablets	8

2.6 Pharmacokinetics

Pharmacokinetics is the study of how a medication is:

- Absorbed: Through the skin, intestine, oral mucosa
- Distributed: Spread throughout the body
- Metabolized: Converted inside the body
- Excreted: Removed from the body through bile, urine, breath, or skin

About 80% of all medications are administered orally and flow through the gastrointestinal (GI) tract into the small intestines. The small intestines are the place where the membrane of the intestine absorbs medication particles and passes them into the bloodstream, where plasma circulates particles throughout the body. Plasma moves (distributes) molecules to the intended site of action and the molecules attach to the receptors' site, resulting in therapeutic effect. Cell membranes and tissues of body compartments can limit access to the site.

2.7 Medication Absorption

There are three ways in which drug particles are absorbed. These are:

- Passive diffusion: Medication particles move from a high to a low concentration, similar to how water flows downstream. No energy is expended because particles are moving along the natural flow.
- Active diffusion: Medication particles move against the natural flow. There is a higher concentration of plasma than there is of particles. Drug particles need enzyme or protein carriers to help particles move against the natural flow, such as to cross a membrane. Enzyme and protein carriers expend energy to move particles of the medication.
- Pinocytosis: Medication particles are engulfed by a cell and pulled across a membrane.

2.8 Absorption Rate

Absorption rate is the time necessary for a medication to be absorbed by the body and begins when the medication is administered to the patient.

The absorption rate is influenced by:

- Food: Hot, solid, fatty foods can slow absorption if eaten before medication is administered.
- Exercise: Slows absorption because circulation is diverted from the stomach to other areas of the body
- Stress and Pain: Can decrease absorption because of a change in circulation
- Circulation: Slows absorption if the medication is administered to a site that has poor circulation
- Route of Administration: Intravenously is nearly instantaneously absorbed. Intramuscular has slower absorption depending on the amount of blood vessels at the injection site. Subcutaneous tissue injection sites have a slower absorption rate than muscles. (Hint: Medication is absorbed faster in the deltoid [arm] muscle than the gluteal [backside] muscle because there are more blood vessels in the deltoid muscle.)
- Solubility: Medication particles dissolve in either lipid (fat) or water. Lipid soluble medication absorbs faster than water-soluble medication because membranes in the GI tract are composed of lipids and can directly transport particles into the bloodstream. Water-soluble medications must use an enzyme or protein carriers to be transported across the GI membrane and into the bloodstream, which influences the absorption rate.

- pH Level: Weak acid medications (aspirin) are absorbed quickly across membranes of the GI tract. Weak base medications (antacid) cross the GI membrane slowly. Strong acid medication and strong base medication are not absorbed because they destroy cells.
- Medication Concentration: High concentration of medication absorbs rapidly. (Hint: Healthcare providers may prescribe a high dose of a medication as the first dose, called a loading dose, to quickly increase absorption and speed the therapeutic effect.)
- Medication Form: Pharmaceutical manufacturers add ingredients to a medication to increase or decrease the medication's absorption.

2.9 Bioavailability

Bioavailability is the percentage of a dose the reaches the bloodstream. One hundred percent bioavailability occurs when the medication is injected into a vein compared with between 20% and 40% for a medication administered orally. Medication particles that do not reach the bloodstream are either misdirected or destroyed during the absorption process. For example, some particles of a medication that is administered orally are destroyed by hydrochloric acid in the stomach. The dose of a medication reflects the bioavailability of the medication based on the route that it is administered to the patient. For example, a medication that is administered orally may have a dose four times higher than if the medication is administered intravenously. Factors that alter bioavailability are:

- Form: tablet, capsule, liquid, transdermal, suppository, and inhalation
- Route: oral, topical, parenteral, and rectal
- GI Tract: Dysfunction of the GI tract can alter the absorption of medication particles.
- Food: Some medications are better absorbed if taken with food, whereas for others, food slows down or blocks absorption of the medication.
- Medication: Interaction between two medications can increase or decrease absorption when both medications are taken together.
- Liver Metabolism: Liver dysfunction can prevent or delay the absorption of a medication.
- Concentration: Higher active ingredient in a medication form increases absorption.
- Cell Membrane: Layers of cell membrane affect absorption. Multilayer cell membrane slows absorption and single layer cell membrane increases absorption.
- Surface Area: A larger surface areas absorbs medication faster than a smaller surface area.

2.10 Medication Concentration

Medication concentration is the percentage of the active ingredient in a dose of medication. There are generally two levels of concentrations. These are:

- Primary Loading: A large concentration used to achieve a fast therapeutic effect
- Maintenance Dose: A typical concentration used to provide an ongoing therapeutic effect

2.11 Distribution

Medication particles in plasma are distributed throughout the body in blood plasma. Medication particles in blood plasma are referred to as free medication because particles are not bound to receptor sites. Only free medications can cause a pharmacological response.

Some medication particles bind to albumin or globulin protein in plasma, forming a medication–protein complex. Medication–protein complexes decrease the concentration of free medication in circulation because medication–protein complex molecules are too large to cross the blood vessel membrane, making these molecules unavailable for therapeutic purpose. Medication–protein complexes are reduced to protein and medication particles when the medication is excreted from the body. Protein is reabsorbed and the medication particle is excreted.

Medication affects the heart, liver, kidney, and brain first because these organs have good blood supply. Medication affects muscles and fat last. Four factors influence the effective distribution of medication. These are:

- Level of Plasma Protein: A low level of plasma protein can result in a build-up of medication, possibly reaching a toxic level. Plasma protein decreases in a condition called hypoalbuminemia, which is common in liver disease, kidney disease, and malnutrition.
- Blood Flow: Adequate blood flow is necessary to distribute medication particles. Low blood flow can cause medication pooling.
- Competing Medication: Two medications might compete for the same receptor site. Particles that do not bind to the receptor site can accumulate, reaching a toxic level. In addition, these medications may not have a therapeutic effect.
- Tumors, Abscesses, Exudates: These disorders impair the distribution of medication.

2.12 Medication Accumulation

Medication accumulates and forms a reservoir called *pooling*. There are two types of pooling. These are:

- Protein-binding: Protein-binding occurs when a medication binds to plasma proteins.
- Tissue-binding: Tissue-binding occurs when medication binds to tissues, such as fat-soluble medication binding to adipose tissues.

2.13 Elimination

Pooling medication is gradually absorbed and eliminated by biotransformation. Biotransformation occurs in the liver, where enzymes inactivate the medication by changing the medication into water-soluble compounds that can be excreted in urine, bile, feces, exhalation, sweat, and breast milk. Elimination of a medication is measured as the medication's half-life. A medication's half-life is the amount of time necessary for half of the medication's concentration to be eliminated from the body. Healthcare providers consider a medication's half-life when prescribing dosage to patients. A goal is to achieve a steady-state serum concentration of a medication to provide a therapeutic effect. It can take days for some medications to reach the steady-state serum concentration.

The pH of the urine influences the quantity of medication that can be excreted by the kidneys. Acidic urine eliminates weak base medication. Alkaline urine eliminates weak acid medication. The pH of the urine can be altered to increase elimination of specific medications. Kidney disease decreases the glomerular filtration rate (GFR), resulting in the reduction of medication that the kidneys can eliminate and can lead to medication toxicity. Decreased blood flow to the kidneys can have a similar effect.

A healthcare provider can purposely reduce the elimination of medication, thereby increasing the medication's therapeutic effect by administering medication that blocks the excretion of a medication. For example, probenecid blocks excretion of penicillin. In contrast, dialysis can be used to increase the excretion of medication, which is common in certain medication overdoses. Drugs can artificially be excreted through the use of hemodialysis, which is a common treatment in certain drug overdoses.

Medications metabolized by the liver are secreted into bile. Bile enters the intestine and is eliminated in feces. Fat-soluble medications are reabsorbed from bile into the bloodstream and returned to the liver to be metabolized and eliminated by the kidneys. This process is called the enterohepatic cycle. Medications that are not metabolized by the liver are eliminated by the lungs at a rate that corresponds to the patient's respiration rate. These are volatile medications, such as anesthetics and medications that are metabolized to CO_2 and H_2O. Side effects such as rashes and skin reaction are commonly seen at sweat and salivary glands. For example, a patient may report tasting the medication. Medication excreted into saliva is eventually swallowed, reabsorbed, and eliminated in urine. Medication can also be excreted by mammary glands and breast milk and can have a cumulative adverse effect on breastfeeding infants.

2.14   The First Pass Effect

The first pass effect occurs when medication is administered orally, is absorbed into the GI tract, and enters the bloodstream. Medication particles are transported through the portal vein into the liver, where the medication is metabolized. Medication can bypass the first pass effect by being administered sublingual (under the tongue) or buccal (between the gums and the cheek). These sites absorb medication directly into the bloodstream and avoid the stomach, where medication particles might be destroyed by hydrochloric acid.

2.15   Pharmacodynamics

Pharmacodynamics is the study of the medication's effect on the cell physiology and the mechanism of the pharmaceutical response. There are two types of effects. These are:

- Primary Effect: The reason the medication was administered to the patient
- Secondary Effect: The side effect or adverse effect of the medication on the patient.

For example, the primary effect of an antihistamine is to treat the symptoms of allergies. The secondary effect is drowsiness caused by depression of the central nervous system. The secondary effect is a desirable side effect if the patient requires bed rest. It is an adverse effect if the patient intends to drive a car.

2.16   Medication Time Response

Medication time response is the time period that passes between when the medication is administered to the patient and the pharmaceutical response. There are three types of medication time responses. These are:

- Onset Time Response: The minimum concentration of the medication to cause the initial pharmaceutical response
- Peak Time Response: The period when the medication has its highest blood or plasma concentration
- Duration: The length of time that the drug maintains the pharmaceutical response

All three response times must be considered when prescribing medication to determine when the medication becomes effective, most effective, and no longer effective, and when the medication will reach a toxic level.

2.17   Receptor Theory

The cell membrane has receptor sites referred to as reactive cellular sites. Receptor sites on cell membranes are proteins, glycoproteins, proteolipids, or enzymes.

A medication particle binds to receptor sites similar to how two pieces of a puzzle fit together. The pharmaceutical response results from this binding. The better the particle and receptor site fit together, the better is the pharmaceutical response. Binding either initiates a physiological response by the cell or blocks a cell's physiological response, depending on the medication. There are four families of receptors. These are:

- Rapid-Cell Membrane-Embedded Enzymes: A medication particle binds to the surface of the cell, causing an enzyme inside the cell to initiate a physiological response.

- Rapid-Ligand-Gated Ion Channels: The medication spans the cell membrane causing ion channels within the membrane to open resulting in the flow of primarily sodium and calcium ions into and out of the cell.
- Rapid-G Protein-Couple Receptor Systems: The medication binds with the receptor, causing the G protein to bind with guanosine triphosphate (GTP). An enzyme inside the cell then initiates a physiological response or results in the opening of the ion channel.
- Prolonged-Transcription Factors: The medication binds to the transcription factors on the DNA within the nucleus of the cell resulting in the transcription factor undergoing a physiological change.

2.18   Agonist and Antagonist

An agonist is a medication that causes a physiological response. An antagonist is a medication that blocks a physiological response. The effectiveness of an antagonist is described by the medication's inhibitory (I) action on the receptor site. For example, a medication with an inhibitory action of 50 (I_{50}) means the medication effectively inhibits the receptor response in 50% of the population.

Agonist and antagonist that lack specific and selective effects are referred to as nonspecific and have non-specificity properties. That is, each receptor can product a variety of physiological responses when the agonist or antagonist bind to the receptor site. For example, the cholinergic receptor is located in blood vessels, the heart, lungs, bladder, and eye. Different physiological responses occur when an agonist or antagonist binds to the site depending on the location of the site. It can change the heart rate, change blood pressure, change gastric acid secretion, change the size of bronchioles, change the size of pupils, and alter the bladder function.

2.19   Categories of Medication Action

Medications are categorized by the action it causes to the body. There are four types of actions. These are:

- Stimulation or Depression: These medications increase or depress cellular activity.
- Replacement: These medications replace an essential body compound, such as insulin and estrogen.
- Inhibition: These medications, such as penicillin, interfere with bacterial cell growth, resulting in limiting bacterial growth or eliminating bacteria.
- Irritation: These medications irritate cells to cause a natural response that has a therapeutic effect, such as irritating the colon wall to stimulate defecation.

2.20   Therapeutic Index and Therapeutic Range

The therapeutic index (TI) identifies the margin of safety of the medication. It is a ratio between the therapeutic dose in 50% of person/animals and the lethal dose in 50% of animals.

The therapeutic dose is written as ED_{50}, and the lethal dose in animals is written as LD_{50}. The closer that the ratio is to 1, the greater the danger of toxicity.

$$TI = LD_{50}/ED_{50}$$

Medications that have a low TI are said to have a narrow margin of safety and require that drug levels in the plasma be monitored and if necessary adjustments to the dosage be made to prevent a toxic effect from occurring.

The therapeutic range is a range of dosage that is safe to administer to a patient based on the therapeutic index. This range is also known as the therapeutic window. The therapeutic range is defined as between the minimum effective concentration (MEC) for achieving the pharmaceutical response and the minimum toxic concentration (MTC).

The therapeutic dose must be within the therapeutic range, which is also known as the therapeutic window. The therapeutic range is between the MEC for obtaining the desired pharmaceutical response and the MTC.

2.21   Peak and Trough Levels

The concentration of medications that have a low TI (a narrow margin of safety) must be routinely monitored by assessing peak and trough levels of the plasma concentration of the medication by drawing blood samples from the patient.

The peak level is the highest plasma concentration of the medication at a specific time. A peak level indicates the rate that a medication is absorbed by the body, which is influenced by the route the medication is administered to the patient.

The trough level is the lowest plasma concentration of the medication at a specific time. A trough level indicates the rate at which the medication is eliminated from the body.

Hint

The concentration of medication that has a narrow margin of safety should be monitored before administering each dose of the medication to assure that the plasma concentration of the medication in within therapeutic range.

2.22   Side Effects

A side effect of a medication is the physiological effect other than the desired effect. A side effect might be predictable or unpredictable. Likewise, a side effect might be desirable or undesirable such as an anaphylaxis reaction to a medication.

Side effects of a medication can be influenced by these factors:

- Gender: Women have a different proportion of fat and water, which affects absorption and distribution of the medication.
- Environment: Cold, heat, sensory deprivation, or overload and oxygen deprivation in high altitude can interact with medication.
- Time of Administration: The presence or absence of food in the gastrointestinal tract, corticosteroid secretion rhythm, circadian cycle, urinary excretion pattern, fluid intake, and drug-metabolizing enzyme rhythms all can influence the effect of the medication.
- Pathological State: A medication can react differently if the patient is experiencing pain, anxiety, circulatory distress, or hepatic, and/or renal dysfunction.
- Idiosyncrasy: This is an unpredictable and unexplainable effect that results from an over- or under response to the medication.
- Tolerance: This is a decreased physiological response after repeated administration of the medication.
- Drug Dependence: This is either a physical or psychological dependency on the medication. Physical dependency occurs when there is intense physical disturbance when the medication is withdrawn. Psychological dependency occurs when an emotional reliance on the medication develops.
- Medication Interaction: A medication increases or decreases the pharmaceutical response of a previously administered medication.
- Synergism: The interaction of two or more medication results in a more desirable pharmaceutical response.
- Potentiation: This occurs when concurrent administration of two medication increases the pharmaceutical response of one of those medications.
- Toxic Effect: The medication dosage exceeds the therapeutic range through either an overdose or accumulation of the medication.

- Tachyphylaxis: This is a tolerance to the medication caused by frequent dosages.
- Placebo Effect: The medication provides a psychological and possibly physical benefit, but no pharmaceutical response.
- Pharmacogenetic Effect: Genetic factors can alter the metabolism of the drug that results in an enhanced or diminished pharmaceutical response causes an unpredictable response.
- Body Mass: Body mass can caused an adverse reaction especially in children, elderly people, and patients whose body mass greatly differs from the average body mass.

2.23 Allergic Reactions

An allergic reaction occurs when the patient develops sensitivity to a medication. When a medication is first administered, the patient's immune system develops antibodies to the medication sensitizing the patient to the medication.

The next administration of the medication causes a reaction with the antibodies resulting in the production of histamine. Histamine causes allergic symptoms.

There are four types of allergic reactions. These are:

- Anaphylactic: This is an immediate allergic reaction that can result in anaphylactic shock, which can lead to sudden drop in blood pressure and edema of the bronchial mucosa causing bronchoconstriction.
- Cytotoxic Reaction: This is an autoimmune response the results in hemolytic anemia, thrombocytopenia, or lupus erythematosus (blood disorders). In some cases, it takes months for the reaction to dissipate.
- Immune Complex Reaction: This is referred to as serum sickness and results in angioedema, arthralgia (sore joints), fever, swollen lymph nodes, and splenomegaly (large spleen). The Immune complex reaction can appear up to 3 weeks after the drug is administered.
- Cell Mediated: This is an inflammatory skin reaction that is also known as delayed hypersensitivity.

Solved Problems

Medication Actions

2.1   What are the possible effects of a medication?

The possible effects of a medication are desired effect, side effect, and adverse effect.

2.2   How does a patient develop an allergic reaction to medication?

An allergic reaction occurs when the patient develops sensitivity to a medication. When a medication is first administered, the patient's immune system develops antibodies to the medication, sensitizing the patient to the medication. The next administration of the medication causes a reaction with the antibodies, resulting in the production of histamine. Histamine causes allergic symptoms.

2.3   What are the four types of allergic reactions?

The four types of allergic reactions are anaphylactic, cytotoxic, immune complex, and cell mediated.

Medication Activity

2.4   What is the pharmaceutical phase?

The pharmaceutical phase is the form of the medication such as a tablet, capsule, liquid, elixirs, or syrups.

2.5   What is the purpose of an inactive ingredient in a medication form?

The inactive ingredient is also called the excipient. This is a substance that does not cause the pharmaceutical response but helps delivers the medication. Inactive ingredients are used as fillers to give the medication shape, size, and assist in the delivery of medication, such as the coating around tiny particles of a time release capsule.

2.6   What is pharmacokinetics?

Pharmacokinetics is the study of how a medication is absorbed, distributed, metabolized, and excreted.

Medication Absorption

2.7   What is passive diffusion?

Medication particles move from a high concentration to a low concentration, similar to how water flows downstream. No energy is expended because particles are moving along the natural flow.

2.8   What is active diffusion?

Medication particles move against the natural flow. There is a higher concentration of plasma then there is of particles. Drug particles need enzyme or protein carriers to help particles move against the natural flow, such as to cross a membrane. Enzyme and protein carriers expend energy to move particles of the medication.

2.9   What absorption method are medication particles engulfed by a cell and pulled across a membrane?

The absorption method for medication particles engulfed by a cell and pulled across a membrane is pinocytosis.

2.10 What is an absorption rate?

Absorption rate is the time necessary for a medication to be absorbed by the body and begins when the medication is administered to the patient.

2.11 Name three factors that influence the absorption rate.

Circulation slows absorption when the medication is administered to a site that has poor circulation. The intravenous route of administration is nearly instantaneously absorbed. The intramuscular route of administration has slower absorption depending on the amount of blood vessels at the injection site. Subcutaneous tissue injection sites have a slower absorption rate than muscles. Exercise slows absorption because circulation is diverted from the stomach to other areas of the body

Medication Concentration

2.12 What is primary loading?

Primary Loading is a large concentration used to achieve a fast therapeutic effect.

2.13 What loading is used to provide ongoing therapeutic effect?

Maintenance dose is used to provide ongoing therapeutic effect.

Medication Distribution

2.14 What factors influence the effective distribution of medication?

The factors that influence the effective distribution of medication are level of plasma protein, blood flow, competing medication, tumors, abscesses, and exudates.

2.15   What adverse effect does low blood flow have on the distribution of medication?

Low blood flow can cause medication pooling.

2.16   What kinds of pooling can occur in the distribution of medication?

The kinds of pooling that can occur in the distribution of medication are protein binding and tissue binding.

2.17   What is protein-binding?

Protein-binding occurs when a medication binds to plasma proteins.

2.18   What is tissue-binding?

Tissue-binding occurs when medication binds to tissues, such as fat-soluble medication binding to adipose tissues.

Medication Elimination

2.19   How is the elimination of medication measured?

The elimination of a medication is measured as the medication's half-life. A medication's half-life is the amount of time necessary for half of the medication's concentration to be eliminated from the body.

2.20   What pH of urine is best to eliminate weak base medication?

Acidic urine eliminates weak base medication.

2.21   What effect would decreasing the GFR have on the elimination of medication?

Decreasing the GFR results in the reduction of medication that the kidneys can eliminate, which can lead to medication toxicity.

2.22   Why would it be beneficial to decrease the rate of elimination of a medication? How would a medical professional achieve this reduction?

Reducing the rate of elimination of a medication can be beneficial because it would increase the medication's therapeutic effect. A medical professional would obtain this decrease by administering a medication that blocks the excretion of the initial medication.

2.23   What is the first pass effect?

The first pass effect is when medication is administered orally, absorbed into the GI tract, and enters the bloodstream. Medication particles are transported through the portal vein into the liver where the medication is metabolized.

2.24   How is the first pass effect avoided?

Medication can bypass the first pass effect by being administered sublingual (under the tongue) or buccal (between the gums and the cheek). These sites absorb medication directly into the bloodstream and avoid the stomach, where medication particles might be destroyed by hydrochloric acid.

2.25   What is the medication time response?

Medication time response is the time period that passes between when the medication is administered to the patient and the pharmaceutical response.

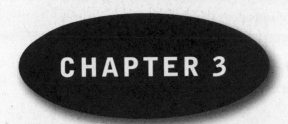

CHAPTER 3

Pharmacology and the Nursing Process

3.1 The Nursing Process

The nursing process is a method for making decisions on how to diagnose and treat a patient. There are five steps in the nursing process. These are:

- Assessment: Data collection. The nurse gathers subjective and objective patient data. Subjective data is information that the patient reports. Objective data is information that can be measured or observed.
- Diagnosis: The patient's problem(s) based on an analysis of assessment data. Diagnosis is a nursing diagnosis, which differs from a medical diagnosis.
- Planning: The proposed treatment as described in the patient's care plan. Each diagnosis has one or more specific expected outcomes called goals, an intervention for each, and a method to determine if the expected outcome is achieved.
- Implementation/Intervention: The execution of the plan.
- Evaluation: Determines if the intervention worked. If the intervention is not successful, the nursing process begins again with an assessment, diagnoses, and a revised care plan.

3.2 Assessment Related to Drugs

The nurse must make the following assessments before administering medication to the patient:

- The validity of the medication order: A valid medication must be written by a physician, dentist, physician assistant, or advance practice nurse and contain the date and time the order is written; name of the medication; dosage; route of administration; frequency of administration; how long the patient is to receive the medication; and signature.
- The brand or generic name for the medication: The brand name is the name chosen by the pharmaceutical manufacturer, and the generic name is the official medication name that is universally acceptable.
- When the medication is used: A comparison must be made to symptoms exhibited by the patient and the therapeutic effect of the medication and the dose prescribed by the healthcare provider.

- How the medication works: The nurse understands how the medication is absorbed, distributed, metabolized, and eliminated and is assured that all these mechanisms are functioning properly. In addition, the nurse must know the action, peak action, and duration of the action.
- Interactions with the medication: Food, herbal remedies, and other medications might alter the medication's action.
- The side effects and toxicity of the medication: The nurse can prepare to manage side effects and recognize the signs of toxicity.
- The signs and symptoms that must be monitored: Signs and symptoms of side effects, adverse reactions and toxicity can appear minutes, hours, or days after the medication is administered to the patient.
- The facts that the patient needs to know about the medication: Patient education enables the patient to self-administer the medication and report adverse reactions after he or she leaves the healthcare facility.
- The availability of the medication: Make sure that the healthcare facility stocks the medication.
- The medication's expiration date: This determines if the medication on hand has expired.
- The cost of the medication: Medication not covered by the patient's medical insurance must be paid for by the patient. The patient may not be able to afford the medication and therefore either refuse the medication or, if self-administering, take less than the prescribed dose. Medical insurance may cover the cost of a similar but less expensive medication, and the healthcare provider may be able to prescribe the less costly medication.

3.3   Patient Information

The nurse must review information about the patient to avoid adverse reactions to it. The nurse must determine if:

- The patient has any allergies to the drug or the food that might be given along with the medication
- The patient's condition has changed since the medication was ordered
- The patient's age may adversely affect the medication's metabolism
- The dose of a medication is appropriate, which may depend on the patient's weight
- Gender may adversely affect the medication's therapeutic response
- The patient is pregnant
- The patient's primary language is English or has a sufficient understanding of it
- The patient has any religious or cultural influence that would cause him or her to resist taking the medication
- The patient understands the purpose for taking the medication
- The patient has knowledge about the medication
- The patient has a medication history that includes vitamins, birth control, and herbal remedies
- The patient uses illegal drugs and/or alcohol
- The patient has developed a tolerance for the medication
- The patient has any genetic factors that might cause an adverse reaction from taking the medication
- The patient has any emotional factors that can affect his or her ability take the medication
- The patient has any contraindication for the medication based on vital signs and current laboratory and diagnostic tests
- The patient's mental status is sufficient to understand why medication is being administered
- The patient can afford the medication
- Family members or friends will be available at his or her side to monitor for side effects and toxicity
- The patient is scheduled for tests, procedures, or other activities at the same time as he or she is scheduled to receive the medication

- The patient is scheduled to receive medication during visiting hours
- The patient is required to have a procedure performed such as insertion of an IV or feeding tube before medication is administered

3.4   Nursing Diagnosis

A nursing diagnosis is a problem statement(s) describing the patient's actual or potential response to a health problem that the nurse is licensed and competent to treat based on guidelines developed by the North American Nursing Diagnosis Association (NANDA). A problem statement may include the cause of the problem and symptoms that manifested the problem.

Here are common nursing diagnoses related to medication therapy:

- "Knowledge deficit of disease and medication related to inability to understand English." This occurs when health care is provided in English, which is not understood by the patient.
- "Risk for injury related to side effects of medication." This occurs when narcotic analgesics administered for pain impair the patient's ability to drive a car.
- "Alteration in thought processes related to medication action." The patient's normal thought process is interrupted when the patient is administered barbiturates, sedatives, and mood-altering medication.
- "Constipation related to medication action or side effect." Intestinal movement is reduced when opioids such as morphine sulfate are administered to the patient.
- "Fluid volume deficit related to drug action." A diuretic such as furosemide (Lasix) increases urination, which can result in the patient retaining an inadequate fluid level.
- "Ineffective breathing pattern related to drug side effects." Respiratory rate can decrease as a side effect of administering opioids such as morphine sulfate to the patient.

3.5   Planning

After the nursing diagnosis is defined, a plan is developed describing how the healthcare team will treat the patient's problem(s). The plan must define:

- Goals: Each diagnosis has a goal statement that specifies an expected outcome of an intervention that addresses diagnosis. A goal statement can be a medical order focused on the patient that specifies a specific behavior that will occur at a specified time. For example, a goal for a patient in pain is to reduce pain from 8 to 4 on a scale of 0 to 10 in 4 hours. The patient should agree with and assist in achieving the goal, such as by taking medication.
- Deadlines: Realistic deadlines must be set for reaching each goal. For example, a realistic goal is that the frequency of coughing is decreased 48 hours after administering dextromethorphan (Robitussin DM). Avoid unrealistic goals such as decrease coughing will occur 2 hours after taking dextromethorphan (Robitussin DM), because this will frustrate the patient. Dextromethorphan (Robitussin DM) is not an instant cure for coughing.
- Measurement: Define a method for measuring whether or not the goal was achieved within the specified deadline. Some methods are objective, such as measuring the patient's temperature. Other methods are subjective, but just as valid, such as asking the patient to report pain on a scale of 0 to 10 or asking him or her if coughing has decreased.
- Implementation/Intervention: An intervention clearly states an action that must be taken to achieve the goal, such as administering medication to the patient. There are three types of interventions. These are:
  ○ Nurse-initiated Intervention: The nurse performs the intervention independently.
  ○ Healthcare Provider Intervention: The intervention is dependent on the healthcare provider, such as with prescribing medication.

- ○ Collaborative Intervention: An intervention is performed by multiple members of the healthcare team, such as the respiratory therapist, the healthcare provider, and the nurse.
- Evaluation: Assessment is made to determine if the goal is achieved. The plan is updated once all goals are achieved. If a goal is not achieved, then the patient is reassessed and a new goal is stated.

3.6 Teaching the Patient about Medication

The patient must be taught about all medication—both medication administered by the healthcare team and medication self-administered. When teaching:

- Teach in a comfortable environment.
- Use a common language.
- Use charts, graphs, audio, and video when appropriate.
- Provide time for questions and answers.
- Plan to teach over several sessions and avoid rushing.
- Provide instructional material that can be taken home.
- Write instructions using language that the patient understands.
- Demonstrate the proper administration of medication.
- Ask the patient to demonstrate the proper administration of medication. This assures that the patient has the visual acuity, manual dexterity, and mental capacity to administer the medication.

3.7 Prompt for Feedback

The best way to assure that your instructions are understood is to prompt the patient to give you feedback on your teachings. Ask the patient:

- What things help you take your medicine?
- What things prevent you from taking your medication?
- What would you do if you forget to take your medication?
- What would you feel if you are taking too much of the medication?
- What could you feel that are side effects of taking the medication?
- Is there anything you can do to reduce side effects of the medication?

Hint: Make sure that the patient and the patient's family can describe the signs and symptoms of an allergic response to the medication and signs and symptoms of toxicity.

3.8 Medication Plan

It is important that you can provide a way for a patient to manage a medication schedule that might involve self-administering several medications. Here are methods to use:

- A multi-compartment dispenser to hold a daily or weekly supply of medication
- A timer to remind the patient when to take medication
- Color-coded envelopes in which each color represents an hour or a day
- A written record of when medication should be administered and when it was administered

3.9   Impact of Cultural Influences in Medication Administration

Cultural influences are learned values, beliefs, customs, and behaviors that can affect administering medication to the patient. For example, a patient may avoid pain medication because of a fear of addiction to it. Likewise, a patient who is taking antihypertensive medication might also be eating garlic to help lower blood pressure. The combination could result in hypotension.

When cultural influences might have an adverse effect on medicating the patient, the healthcare provider should educate the patient about the benefits of taking the medication and the risks of substituting or combining cultural-based treatments. It is important that the healthcare provider remaining nonjudgmental about the patient's decision.

3.10   Culture-Based Communication

A patient's culture influences how to teach the patient about medication. Here are factors that influence communication in some cultures:

- Know that the woman is typically responsible for managing the family's health.
- Be mindful that the older man is often the authority figure who makes decisions about the family's health.
- Remember that eye contact might not be appropriate.
- Address the patient formally until given permission to address him or her in another way.
- Ask the patient how he or she wants to be addressed.
- Know how the patient perceives time such as day/night, sunrise/sunset to comply with the appropriate medication schedule.
- Maintain the patient's personal space.
- Ask permission to invade the personal space to perform a procedure.
- Remember that the patient may feel uncomfortable if you stand or sit too close or touch him or her.
- Consider food beliefs and rituals as related to illnesses.
- Evaluate the family's attitude toward the elderly. Elderly people are revered in some cultures and the family goes to great lengths to care for them. In other cultures, the family leaves elderly people to die peacefully without interference

3.11   Genetic Considerations

A patient's genetic makeup can influence his or her physiological response to medication. Therefore, it is critical for the healthcare provider to determine if the medication prescribed for a patient is likely to cause an adverse reaction based on genetic traits.

For example, a patient with Reye's syndrome has a genetic defect that prevents the liver from metabolizing aspirin. African Americans have a genetic factor that makes them less responsive to beta-blocking medication and antihypertensive medication.

A genetic factor in Asians causes an undesirable side effect when administered the standard dose of benzodiazepines (diazepam [Valium]) alprazolam [Xanax], tricyclic antidepressants, atropine, and propranolol [Inderal].

3.12   Maternity

Medications can cross the placenta and have an adverse effect on the fetus. The fetus has an immature metabolism and a slow excretion rate that can cause a pooling of the medication. Depending on the physiological effect of the medication, the fetus can be addicted to the medication and go through withdrawal after birth. This can occur with alcohol, barbiturates, and narcotics.

Some medication taken during the first trimester can have a teratogenic effect on the fetus. The teratogenic effect occurs when the medication is mutagenic (genetic mutation), causing fetal defects, or carcinogenic (causing cancer). Medications known to have the teratogenic effect are:

- Thalidomide: Causes abnormal limb development
- Cocaine: Causes miscarriages, fetal hypoxia (lack of oxygen), low birth weight, tremors, strokes, congenital heart disease, skull defects, and other malformations

Adverse effects of medication on the fetus can be avoided by reviewing the medication's Pregnancy Category (see 1.13 Pregnancy Categories) before administering the medication to the patient.

3.13   Pediatrics

Special care is given to prescribing and administering medication to children because of their immature bodies. Children typically lack the physiological maturity to absorb, metabolize, distribute, and excrete some medications. The dose of medication prescribed to children is based on weight or body surface area. For example, the prescription might read 2 ml per kilogram (kg). The nurse must weigh the child and then use the child's weight to calculate the dose.

Administering medication to the neonatal patient can be difficult because they are unable to metabolize the medication. The solution is to administer the medication through breast milk. That is, the medication is administered to the mother who is able to metabolize the medication. The medication is then passed into the breast milk, which is transferred to the neonatal patient during breastfeeding.

3.14   Elderly Patients

Elderly patients are susceptible to adverse side effects from medication because, as the body ages, the ability to absorb, metabolize, distribute, and excrete medication decreases and results in pooling of medication. Here are additional factors that influence the adverse side effects from medication in elderly people:

- Interactions between medications caused polypharmacy. (Polypharmacy occurs when new medications are prescribed without discontinuing current medication, resulting in an adverse interaction of medications.)
- Medication causing impaired mental and physical capacity, resulting in accidental injury
- Decreased sensitivity to medication caused by age, resulting in medication-induced disease
- Altered absorption of medication caused by increased gastric pH
- Decreased lean body mass, increased fat stores, decreased total body water, decreased serum albumin, and decreased cardiac output adversely affect the distribution of medication
- Enzyme activity decreases, causing changes in metabolism
- Decreased kidney function impairs excretion of the medication
- Decreased liver function impairs metabolism of the medication

3.15   Assessing Elderly People

It is important to gather a complete medication history to establish potential adverse side effects and barriers that prevent an elderly patient from being properly medicated. In assessing the medication history, the healthcare provider should:

- List all prescription and over-the-counter medication.
- List herbals, vitamins, and home remedies.

- Assess where prescribed medication is self-administered.
- Assess whether the patient can afford the medication.
- Determine if prescribed medication has unpleasant side effects.
- Determine the patient's medication schedule.
- Identify all healthcare providers who prescribe medication for the patient.
- Identify all pharmacies that provide medication to the patient.
- Determine if the patient has any barriers to taking medication safely.
- Ask if the patient skips medication and, if so, which medication is skipped.

Solved Problems

The Nursing Process

3.1   What is the assessment step in the nursing process?

Assessment is data collection. The nurse gathers subjective and objective patient data. Subjective data is information that the patient reports. Objective data is information that can be measured or observed.

3.2   What step of the nursing process executes the treatment plan?

The step of the nursing process that executes the treatment plan is intervention.

3.3   What are the steps in the nursing process?

The steps in the nursing process are assessment, diagnosis, planning, intervention, and evaluation.

Assessment Related to Drugs

3.4   Why is it important to know how the medication works before administering the medication to the patient?

The nurse understands how the medication is absorbed, distributed, metabolized, and eliminated, and is assured that all these mechanisms are functioning properly.

3.5   How long after a medication is administered will signs and symptoms of an adverse side effect appear?

An adverse side effect can appear minutes, hours, or days after the medication is administered to the patient.

3.6   Why should the nurse consider the cost of medication?

The patient may not be able to afford the medication and therefore either refuse the medication or, if self-medicated, take less than the prescribed dose. Medical insurance may cover the cost of a similar but less expensive medication and the healthcare provider may be able to prescribe the less costly medication.

Planning

3.7   What kinds of measurements are used to determine if a goal is achieved?

The kinds of measurements used to determine if a goal is achieved are objective measurements, such as measuring the patient's temperature, and subjective measurements, such as asking the patient to report pain on a scale of 0 to 10 or asking the patient if coughing has decreased.

3.8   What are the elements of a good patient plan?

The elements of a good patient plan are goals, deadlines, measurement, intervention, and evaluation.

3.9   Why is it important to set realistic goals for the patient when administering medication?

Setting a realistic goal manages the patient's expectations of the therapeutic effect of the medication. The goal should state how long after administering the medication the therapeutic effect will be realized.

3.10   What are the types of interventions used to treat a patient?

The types of interventions used to treat a patient are nurse-initiated intervention, healthcare provider intervention, and collaborative intervention.

Teaching about Medication

3.11   How can you be assured that the patient knows how to self-administer medication?

You can be assured that the patient knows how to self-administer medication by asking the patient to demonstrate how to self-administer the medication.

3.12   Name three aids that help teach patients about medication.

Three aids that help teach patients about medication are video, comfortable environment, and instructional material that can be taken home and read.

3.13   Name three capabilities a patient must have to self-administer medication.

Three capabilities a patient must have to self-administer medication are visual acuity, manual dexterity, and mental capacity.

3.14   What would you do if the patient lacks the capability to self-administer medication?

If the patient lacks the capability to self-administer medication, make sure that the patient's family learns and can demonstrate how to administer medication to the patient.

3.15   What adverse side effects should be explained to the patient and the patient's family?

The adverse side effects that should be explained to the patient and the patient's family are the signs and symptoms of an allergic response to the medication and the signs and symptoms of toxicity.

3.16   What methods can be used to assist the patient keep a schedule to self-administer medication?

The methods used to assist the patient with keeping a schedule of self-administered medication are a multi-compartment dispenser that is commonly used to hold a daily or weekly supply of medication, a timer that can remind the patient when to take medication, color-coded envelopes where each color represents an hour or a day, and a written record which tracks when medication should be administered and when it was administered.

Cultural Influence in Medication Administration

3.17   Give an example of how a patient's belief interferes with administering medication to the patient.

A patient may avoid pain medication, fearing addiction to the medication.

3.18   What should you do if your beliefs are contrary to the patient's beliefs?

If your beliefs are contrary to the patient's beliefs, remain nonjudgmental about the patient's decision.

3.19   How would you respond if the patient defers healthcare decisions to his elderly grandfather?

In certain cultures, the older man in the family is the authoritative figure who makes healthcare decisions for the family. Be sure to provide both the patient and the elderly grandfather with information about the patient if the patient grants you permission to do so.

Maternity, Pediatrics, Elderly

3.20   What is the teratogenic effect?

The teratogenic effect is when the medication is mutagenic (genetic mutation, causing fetal defects) or carcinogenic (causing cancer).

3.21   How can you prevent administering medication that might cause the teratogenic effect?

Review the medication's Pregnancy Category to determine if the medication causes the teratogenic effect.

3.22   How does a healthcare provider determine the correct dose for a child?

The dose of medication prescribed to children is based on weight or body surface area.

3.23   How can medication be administered to a neonate?

Administer the medication to the mother who will metabolize the medication and pass the medication to the neonate in breast milk during breastfeeding.

3.24   How come medication may be adversely distributed in elderly people?

Elderly people have decreased lean body mass, increased fat stores, decreased total body water, decreased serum albumin, and decreased cardiac output which adversely affect the distribution of medication.

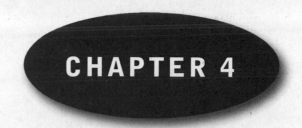

CHAPTER 4

Substance Abuse

4.1 Medication Misuse and Abuse

A medication is misused whenever a person indiscriminately uses the medication. A medication becomes abused when the person continually self-medicates, resulting in a physical and/or a psychological dependence on the medication. Any medication can be abused, not only medications with addictive properties.

A person is considered addicted to a medication if he or she experiences three or more of the following characteristics over 6 months.

- Tolerance: Tolerance occurs when an increasingly larger dose of the medication is required to achieve the same physiological reaction. Tolerance is not addiction. The healthcare provider increases the dose to achieve the same therapeutic effect and discontinues the medication once the treatment is completed.
- Withdrawal: Withdrawal is a physiological and/or psychological reaction a person experiences when a medication is no longer administered. Gradually decreasing the dose and/or frequency of medication reduces withdrawal symptoms.
- Increased Dosage: The patient increases the dosage, expecting to increase the physiological effect of the medication.
- Uncontrollable Use: A person addicted to medication has an uncontrollable urge to self-medicate.
- Taking Medication Is a Scheduled Event: Time is set aside daily to acquire and administer medication and time for the medication's effect to dissipate.
- Priority over Activities of Daily Life: Work, family, and other daily activities become secondary to the acquisition, administration, and recovery from the effects of medication.
- Addiction Continues Despite Negative Consequences: The patient continues self-medication regardless of the negative consequences.

4.2 Behavioral Patterns of Addiction

Medication abuse occurs gradually, so much so that the patient is unable to recognize the addiction and steadfastly denies that he or she is addicted. Addiction results in an altered mental state that leads to deviation from normal behavioral patterns. These deviations are:

- Being late for or missing appointments (i.e., work, school)
- Poor hygiene

- Disheveled appearance
- Strained family and social relationships
- Frequent medical attention
- Legal problems resulting from arrest
- Associations with unsavory characters
- Experiences with violent situations

4.3   Substance Abuse and Healthcare Professionals

Healthcare professionals are at risk for abusing medication for the following reasons:

- Performance Enhancement: Healthcare professionals at times are on duty for long stretches without sleep. Medication, some feel, boosts their performance to a level necessary to make split-second, lifesaving decisions.
- Self-Treatment: It is easy for a healthcare professional to diagnose his or her own condition and then administer medication to treat the disease. A high risk for abuse occurs when the treatment is for pain, depression, or anxiety because medications that treat these conditions are addictive.
- Easy Access: Medication in a healthcare facility can be diverted from patients with little chance of being detected.
- Recreational Use: Medication is a quick way to relax; however, as tolerance builds additional medication is necessary to achieve the desired effect.

4.4   Detecting Substance Abuse

Substance abusers go to great lengths to hide their addiction from family, friends, and colleagues. Therefore, they may not be disheveled and malnourished, which are stereotypical characteristics of a substance abuser.
   Regardless of their attempts to hide their abuse, substance abusers do have telltale signs. These are:

- Disorganization: Medication interferes with the ability to think logically and clearly, leading to becoming overwhelmed by the simple task of being organized.
- Frequent Absences: Medication can lead to unnatural periods of wakefulness and sleep, resulting in drowsiness and fatigue and the inability to continue a normal schedule of daily activities.
- Inability to Get Along: Interpersonal relationships diminish as a result of being disorganized, frequently absent, and focusing more on acquiring, administering, and experiencing the desired effects of the medication.
- Changes in Appearance: Appearance changes, although not necessarily appearing disheveled and malnourished. The same clothes might be worn two subsequent days or clothes are no longer pressed.
- Slow Responses During Off Hours: Response time slows and speech becomes slurred, showing signs of intoxication during off hours. Efforts are made to maintain normal response time while at work or school.

4.5   Delayed Detection with Healthcare Professionals

Detecting a healthcare professional who is a substance abuser is challenging because of a number of inherit conditions. These are:

- Healthcare professionals are less supervised than other workers and many times work totally independently.

- Healthcare professionals are not always assessed by other healthcare professionals because they self-diagnose. Therefore, signs of abuse go undetected.
- License suspension or revocation can occur if the healthcare professional acknowledges a substance abuse problem.
- The white wall of silence. No healthcare professional wants to report a colleague for substance abuse for fear the colleague will lose his or her license or expose the reporting person to litigation if the accusation is inadvertently false.
- The perception of being handicapped. The Rehabilitation Act (29USC, Section 706) requires employers to continue employment of a substance abuser as long as the employee can perform the job function and is not a threat to safety or property. The healthcare professional may be reassigned temporarily until recovery is completed.

Caution: Healthcare professionals have an ethical obligation to report colleagues who are suspected substance abusers for the safety of both patients and the colleague.

4.6 Testing for Substance Abuse

The most common method used to detect substance abuse is by testing bodily fluid. The presence or level of medication in the bodily fluid indicates that the medication might be being abused. Two bodily fluids commonly tested are:

1. Blood: This is typically used if the patient is suspected of overdosing or is poisoned.
2. Urine: This is the more commonly used testing method and can detect use of drugs used for up to a week before the test is performed.

Tests can produce a false positive or false negative. A false positive occurs when the findings detect medication when in fact no medication is present. For example, a test for methadone produces a false positive in the presence of antihistamine. When a test produces a positive result and the patient denies taking the medication, a second test is performed. A false negative occurs when the test does not detect medication when in fact medication is present.

Table 4.1 shows the length of time that traces of popular drugs remain in the body. The most commonly misused and abused drugs are listed in Table 4.2.

4.7 Why Substances Are Abused

Those who abuse medications generally do so because they:

- Feel frustrated
- Fear failure
- Feel bored
- Feel pressured by their peers
- Seek pleasurable behavior
- Are affluent and want to experiment
- Seek to escape from reality
- Feel inadequate; feel like a failure
- Feel ashamed and depressed
- Seek relief from conflicts

TABLE 4.1 Days That Substances Remain in the Body

DRUG	DAYS DETECTABLE IN URINE
Alcohol	Less than 1 day
Amphetamines	Up to 1 day
Barbiturates	Up to 1 day
Cocaine	Up to 2 days
Methadone	Up to 3 days
Marijuana	
Single use	Up to 6 days
Chronic use	Up to 29 days
Opioids: short-acting	Up to 1 days

TABLE 4.2 Commonly Misused/Abused Drugs as Reported by the National Surveillance Agency Drug Abuse Warning Network (DAWN)

DRUG	DESCRIPTION
Xanthines	A class of drugs that include caffeine and are used in coffee, tea, chocolate, and colas. These drugs affect the central nervous system (CNS) drugs. Most frequently abused drug.
Nicotine	Used in tobacco products. This drug affects the CNS drugs. One of the most frequently misused and abused.
Ethyl alcohol	Used in distilled spirits and beverage. This drug affects the CNS drugs. One of the most frequently misused and abused.
Anticholinergics	A class of drugs that includes Robinul, which is referred to as the "date rape" drug. This drug affects the CNS.
Steroids	A performance-enhancing drug that affects the CNS.
Amphetamines	A class of drugs that includes: Dextroamphetamine, dexies, and methamphetamine (crystal). Commonly referred to as "speed" and "crystal meth." This drug affects the CNS drugs.
Pentazocine	Creates a morphine-like effect. Also known as Talwin. This drug affects the CNS drugs.
L-dopa	Used to alleviate some of the symptoms of Parkinson's disease. This drug causes an alteration in feelings, thoughts, and perceptions.
Cocaine	A leading drug resulting in visits to the ER. This drug can cause tachycardia (fast heart rate), increase blood pressure, chills, fever, agitation, nervousness, confusion, inability to remain still, nausea, vomiting, abdominal pain, increased sweating, rapid breathing, large pupils and advance to CNS hemorrhage, congestive failure, convulsions, delirium, and death.
Heroin	A leading drug resulting in visits to the ER. Heroin is a pro-drug and is converted in the liver to morphine with the same side effects.
Morphine	A leading drug resulting in visits to the ER. Morphine is an opioid narcotic analgesic. Side effects include sedation, decreased blood pressure, increased sweating, flushed face, constipation, dizziness, drowsiness, nausea, and vomiting.
Acetaminophen	Commonly known as Tylenol. A leading drug resulting in visits to the ER. This medication is commonly used in overdoses and can cause serious kidney problems and death.
Aspirin	A leading drug resulting in visits to the ER. Aspirin abuse can cause gastric (stomach) irritation, which can lead to ulcers and subsequent gastric hemorrhage (bleeding).

DRUG	DESCRIPTION
Xanax	Alprazolam (Xanax) is an antianxiety and antipanic agent. Several of the side effects include episodes of violent and aggressive behavior, seizures, delirium, and other withdrawal reactions.
Marijuana/hashish	These are cannabis drugs that seem to act as a CNS depressant. The effects are mental relaxation, euphoria, and decreased inhibitions.
Diazepam	Commonly known as Valium and is used for short-term relief of anxiety symptoms. Side effects include drowsiness, fatigue, and ataxia (muscular incoordination). Overdose can result in somnolence (sleepiness), confusion, diminished reflexes, and coma.
Ibuprofen	This is a commonly used nonsteroidal antiinflammatory drug. Side effects and overdose can results in gastrointestinal bleeding or a metabolic acidosis.
PCP/PCP combinations	Phencyclidine (PCP) is a hallucinogenic drug that can cause violent and aggressive behavior.
Lorazepam	Commonly known as Ativan, which causes an alteration in thoughts, feelings, and perceptions.
Benzodiazepine	This medication can cause an alteration in thoughts, feelings, and perceptions.
Amitriptyline	Commonly known as Elavil. This medication is a mood elevator and can cause an alteration in thoughts, feelings, and perceptions.
Clonazepam	Commonly known as Klonopin. This medication is used to inhibit seizure activity. Side effects can be mild drowsiness, ataxia, and behavioral disturbances that are manifested as aggression, irritability, and agitation.
d-Propoxyphene	Commonly known as Darvon. This is an opioid analgesic that can cause an alteration in sensory perception, which includes euphoria, dizziness, drowsiness, hypotension, nausea, and vomiting.

4.8 Characteristics of Frequently Abused Medications

There are four characteristics that describe medications that are frequently abused:

1. The drug creates an altered state of consciousness.
2. Prolonged use of the drug creates a tolerance for the drug.
3. The desirable effect is quick.
4. Withdrawal symptoms develop if the drug is stopped after prolonged use. (Administering the drug is a fast way to treat withdrawal symptoms.)

4.9 Dependence versus Tolerance

Psychological and/or physical dependency occurs when withdrawal symptoms become unbearable. Relief comes only when a dose of the medication is administered. Tolerance occurs when the concentration of a medication no longer continues a desired effect because receptor sites adapt to the prescribed level of medication. Increasing the concentration of the medication is the only way to regain the desired effect. A patient can develop a pharmacological tolerance. A pharmacological tolerance occurs when prolong exposure to the medication increases the excretion of the medication, resulting in a lower concentration of medication in plasma.

4.10 Pathophysiological Changes

Substance abusers can exhibit pathophysiologic changes related to substance abuse. Pathophysiological changes are debilitating changes, including:

- Malnutrition
- Dehydration
- Hypovitaminosis
- Respiratory depression
- Sepsis
- Pulmonary emboli
- Pneumonia
- Endocarditis
- Human immunodeficiency virus
- Cellulites (infection in the tissues)
- Sclerosis (scaring of the veins)
- Phlebitis (irritation of veins)
- Skin abscesses

4.11 Commonly Abused Substances

There are three groups of drugs that are commonly abused. These are:

1. Cannabinoids
   a. Cannabis: Cannabis is an extraction from the leaves, stems, fruiting tops, and resin of the hemp plant (*Cannabis sativa*). Forms of cannabis are: hashish (most common), banji, ganga, charas, kif, and dagga.
   b. Hashish
      i. Classified as a controlled substance, a sedative-hypnotic, anesthetic, and psychedelic (capable of altering perception, thought, and feeling)
      ii. Depresses the central nervous system, resulting in mental relaxation, altered perception of time and space, loss of inhibitions, and euphoria within 15 minutes; lasts up to 4 hours
      iii. Progresses from relief to disinhibition, excitement, and respiratory and vasomotor depression with increased dosage
      iv. Ideas are disconnected and can experience gaps in memory
      v. It can be smoked as a cigarette, through a water pipe to reduce irritation of the acidic smoke, or ground into powder and mixed with food, delaying the absorption of the medication
      vi. Signs and symptoms: lightheadedness, loss of concentration, weakness, palpitations, tremors, postural hypotension, staggering gait (ataxia), and sense of floating
      vii. Metabolized in the liver
      viii. Eliminated in bile and feces
      ix. Trace amount of hashish is detectable in urine
      x. Affects the metabolism of amphetamines, opiates, barbiturates, atropine, and ethyl alcohol
      xi. Withdrawal symptoms: Minor discomfort for a few days; insomnia, anxiety, irritability for a few weeks; intermittent craving for a few months
      xii. Treatment: Exercise; no pharmacological intervention
2. Hallucinogens: Hallucinogens are natural or chemically synthesized medications that change perception of time, reality, and the environment by abnormal disruption and activation of serotonin. Some patients experience chronic mental disorders. Commonly used hallucinogens are:
   a. Lysergic acid diethylamide (LSD)
      i. Heightens perception, creates distortions of the body and visual hallucinations
      ii. Unpredictable mood swings from euphoria to depression and panic referred to as a "bad trip"
      iii. Causes hypertension, dilated pupils, hyperthermia, and tachycardia (rapid heart rate)
      iv. Takes effect within 20 minutes and last up to 2 hours

     v. Can lead to psychosis and trigger flashbacks called latent psychosis

    vi. Side effect: Acute panic attacks, paranoia, homicidal thoughts and actions

   vii. Toxic effect: Toxic delirium, exhaustion, feeling of emptiness, depression, and risk of suicide

  viii. Potential for long-term schizophrenic or psychotic reaction

    ix. LSD stimulates the uterus and could induce contractions in a pregnant woman

     x. Treatment: Talk the patient through the episode in a quiet, relaxed environment. If this fails, administer a benzodiazepine such as diazepam (Valium), with crisis intervention therapy.

    xi. Do not administer phenothiazines, such as chlorpromazine (Thorazine), because this can exacerbate a panic reaction and cause postural hypotension.

   xii. Do not administer large doses of tranquilizers or use restraints or isolation because these are more traumatic than therapeutic.

  b. Mescaline

     i. Extracted from the flowering heads of the peyote cactus

    ii. Mescaline crystalline power can be dissolved into tea or placed in capsules.

   iii. Causes hallucinogenic effects similar to LSD

   iv. Effects: Immediately and last 6 hours

    v. Excreted: Urine

   vi. Signs and Symptoms: Anxiety, hyperreflexia, static tremors, vivid visual hallucinations, abdominal pain, nausea, and diarrhea

  c. Psilocybin

     i. Extracted from Mexican mushrooms

    ii. Causes hallucinogenic effect similar to LSD except has a shorter duration

   iii. Effects: Half hour to an hour and lasts 6 hours

   iv. Signs and Symptoms: Pleasant mood; drowsiness and sleep; patient can be apprehensive, demonstrate poor performance and critical judgment; hyperkinetic compulsive movements, inappropriate laughter; pupils dilate, vertigo (dizziness), ataxia (stagger); paresthesias (numbness, tingling) and muscle weakness. The drug also induces drowsiness and sleep.

  d. Phencyclidine (PCP)

     i. Developed as a dissociative anesthetic (patient is awake but detached from surroundings and unresponsive to pain)

    ii. Not used for humans. Used in veterinary medicine.

   iii. Causes hallucinations that can result in assault, murder, and suicide.

   iv. Effect: Immediately, lasting 1 to 4 hours depending on concentration. Long-term results are unpredictable.

    v. Stages of Effect: First stage—change in body image and feeling depersonalized. Second stage—hearing and vision distortions. Third stage—feelings of estrangement, alienation, and apathy.

   vi. Metabolizes in the liver

   vii. Excreted: Urine

  viii. Signs and Symptoms: Flush, sweat profusely; rapid eye movement (nystagmus), double vision (diplopia), drooping eyelids (ptosis), sedated appearance, staggering gait (ataxia), and general numbness

   ix. Treatment: Keep in quiet dark room away from sensory stimuli. Protect from self-inflicted injuries. Do not talk down because patient can become violent and perceive the interaction as a personal attack. Administer Diazepam (Valium) or haloperidol (Haldol) for antianxiety and antipsychotic effects.

3. Inhalants: Inhalants are volatile hydrocarbons and aerosols used to dispense chemicals that create a euphoric effect when inhaled. Euphoria can last a few minutes or several hours. Repeated used can lead to loss of consciousness and heart failure. There are no specific antidotes; therefore, side effects are treated symptomatically. Long-term use damages the liver, kidney, central nervous system, brain, and bone marrow; and induces hearing loss and peripheral neuropathy (numbness, tingling). Commonly used inhalants are:

a. Airplane glue

b. Paint thinner

c. Paint

d. Hairspray

e. Deodorant

f. Typewriter correction fluid

g. Lighter fluid

h. Nitrous oxide

i. Xylene

j. Toluene

4.12 Assessment for Substance Abuse

Criteria for assessment for substance abuse are:

- Vital signs
- Pupil size
- Skin examination for needle marks and abscesses
- Nutrition
- Elimination patterns
- Sleep patterns
- History of HIV, cellulitis, endocarditis, and pneumonia

The following are commonly used nursing diagnoses for drug abuse patients:

- Knowledge deficit related to denial of problem
- Ineffective individual coping related to lack of support system
- Risk for violence to oneself or others related to drug use
- Altered health maintenance related to drug dependency
- Ineffective management of therapeutic regimen

Solved Problems

Medication Misuse

4.1   What is tolerance?

Tolerance occurs when an increasingly larger dose of the medication is required to achieve the same physiologic reaction. Tolerance is not addiction. The healthcare provider increases the dose to achieve the same therapeutic effect and discontinues the medication once the treatment is completed.

4.2   What is withdrawal?

Withdrawal is a physiological and/or psychological reaction a person experiences when a medication is no longer administered. Gradually decreasing the dose and/or frequency of medication reduces withdrawal symptoms.

4.3   Why would a patient increase dosage when self-medicating?

The patient increases the dosage, expecting to increase the physiological effect of the medication.

Patterns of Addiction

4.4 Name five behavioral patterns of addiction.
- Late for or missing appointments (i.e., work, school)
- Poor hygiene
- Disheveled appearance
- Strained family and social relationships
- Frequent medical attention

4.5 Name two reasons why healthcare professionals abuse medication.
- Performance Enhancement: Healthcare professionals at times are on duty for long stretches without sleep. Medication, some feel, boosts their performance to a level necessary to make split-second, lifesaving decisions.
- Self-Treatment: It is easy for a healthcare professional to diagnose his or her own condition and then administer medication to treat the disease. A high risk for abuse occurs when he or she treats for pain, depression, and anxiety because medications to treat these conditions are addictive.

4.6 Why is it difficult to detect substance abuse by healthcare professionals?

Healthcare professionals are less supervised and are not always assessed by other healthcare professionals. Healthcare professionals are reluctant to report suspicious coworkers for fear that the colleague will lose his or her license, and reporting someone could potentially mean exposing themselves to litigation if the accusation is inadvertently false.

Testing for Substance Abuse

4.7 What bodily fluid is most commonly tested for substances that are abused?

Urine is the bodily fluid most commonly tested for substance abuse because medication can be detected for up to 1 week.

4.8 What danger exists with testing for substance abuse?

Tests can produce a false positive or false negative.

4.9 What is a false positive?

A false positive occurs when the findings detect medication although in fact no medication is present.

4.10 What happens when the patient tests positive, but the patient states no medication was taken?

When a test produces a positive result and the patient denies taking the medication, then a second test is performed. The second test may be a different type of detection test than the first test.

4.11 Give an example of how a test can report a false positive for methadone.

A test for methadone produces a false positive in the presence of antihistamine.

4.12 For how long can you detect marijuana?

Single use can be detected for 6 days and chronic use for 29 days.

4.13 How long can you detect alcohol?

Alcohol can be detected for less than 1 day.

4.14 How long can you detect cocaine?

Cocaine can be detected for less than 2 days.

Medications That Are Abused

4.15 What is the effect of hashish?

Hashish depresses the CNS and results in mental relaxation, altered perception of time and space, loss of inhibitions, and euphoria within 15 minutes and lasts up to 4 hours.

4.16 What are the signs and symptoms of hashish intoxication?

The signs of symptoms of hashish intoxication are lightheadedness, loss of concentration, weakness, palpitations, tremors, postural hypotension, staggering gait (ataxia), and sense of floating.

4.17 Where is hashish eliminated?

Hashish is eliminated through bile, feces, and a trace amount in urine.

4.18 What are hallucinogens?

Hallucinogens are natural or chemically synthesized medications that change perception of time, reality, and the environment by abnormal disruption and activation of serotonin.

4.19 What is the commonly used name for lysergic acid diethylamide?

The commonly used name for lysergic acid diethylamide is LSD.

4.20 What are the effects of LSD?

The effects of LSD are heightened perception, imagined distortions of the body, and visual hallucinations.

4.21 What are the potential longer-term effects of LSD?

The potential longer-term effects of LSD are schizophrenic or psychotic reaction.

4.22 What medications should not be administered with LSD?

Phenothiazines such as chlorpromazine (Thorazine) are medications that should no be administered with LSD, because this can exacerbate panic reaction and cause postural hypotension.

4.23 Where is mescaline excreted?

Mescaline is excreted in urine.

4.24 What are the signs and symptoms of mescaline intoxication?

The signs and symptoms of mescaline intoxication are anxiety, hyperreflexia, static tremors, vivid visual hallucinations, abdominal pain, nausea, and diarrhea.

4.25 What is the commonly used name of phencyclidine?

The commonly used name of phencyclidine is PCP.

4.26 What was the therapeutic effect of phencyclidine before it was discontinued for human use?

The therapeutic effect of phencyclidine before it was discontinued for human use was dissociative anesthetic (patient is awake but detached from surroundings and is unresponsive to pain).

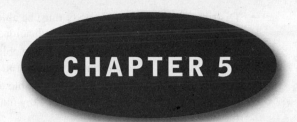

CHAPTER 5

Principles of Medication Administration

5.1 The Process of Medication Administration

Assess the patient before administering medication because the patient's condition can change since medication was prescribed. Assessing the patient also provides a baseline from which you can compare the patient's reaction to the medication. The assessment must consider:

Is the therapeutic action of the drug proper for the patient? Independently verify that the medication is proper for the patient. Compare the diagnosis with information about the medication from the medication manual. Answer the question, "Why was this medication prescribed?" Contact the healthcare provider who prescribed the medication if it is not obvious why the medication was prescribed.

Is the route best for the patient? Verify that the prescribed route is best for the patient. The patient's conditions might have changed since the medication was prescribed. For example, the healthcare provider might have prescribed that the medication be administered by mouth, but vomiting precludes administering medication using this route.

Is this the proper dose for the patient? Compare the prescribed dosage with the recommended dosage in the medication manual. The prescribed dosage should be within the range specified in the medication manual. Although the healthcare provider may vary the dosage because of the patient's condition, a dosage falling outside the specified range should be confirmed.

Assess for contraindications. Verify that the patient's current condition does not prevent the administration of the medication.

Assess for side effects and adverse reactions to the medication. Determine the medication's side effects and adverse reactions from the medication manual. Monitor the patient for signs and symptoms of side effects and adverse reactions to the medication and be prepared to deal with them. For example, an adverse effect of narcotic medication can be reversed by administering Narcan.

5.2 Assessment Required for Specific Medications

An assessment must be made to determine if the patient's body can handle the pharmacokinetics (see 2.6 Pharmacokinetics) of the medication. This assessment must consider:

- Absorption: The patient's body might be able to absorb the medication. Disturbances in the stomach and small intestine might disrupt absorption of the medication.

- Distribution: The patient's body must be able to distribute the medication. Distribution can be disrupted by low albumin (some medication binds to albumin) and impaired circulation.
- Metabolism: The patient's body must be able to break down (metabolize) the medication, which occurs in the liver. Inadequate liver function can prevent the metabolism of the medication.
- Excretion: The patient's body must be able to excrete the medication, which occurs in urine, bile, feces, respiration, saliva, and sweat. Any malfunction in these areas can reduce or prevent excretion of the medication.
- Age: The very young can have an immature ability to absorb, distribute, metabolize, and excrete medication. Elderly people have a reduced ability to handle medication because of aging systems. Both of these age groups are at higher risk of side effects and adverse effects of medication.
- Body Weight: Assessment of the patient's weight must be made before administering medication that is prescribed by weight. The patient's weight might have materially changed since it was entered into the patient's chart.
- Pharmacogenetics: Verify if parents, siblings, or other close relatives have had an adverse reaction to the medication.
- Time: Determine if the medication must be administered at a particular time. For example, stimulants are not administered at bedtime because the medication inhibits sleep.
- Food–medication interaction: Determine if food interacts with medication. A food–drug interaction may result in an adverse effect. At times, medication is taken with food to reduce an upsetting side effect of the medication. On the other hand, food can slow absorption for some medications.
- Medication–drug interaction: Determine if a combination medication might have an adverse or undesirable effect.
- Medication history: Assess the amount of medication that the patient has received to determine if she or he has received the maximum daily allowance according to the medication manual. Also determine if the patient has a tolerance for the medication and if she or he shows signs and symptoms of a toxic effect caused by the cumulative effect of the medication.

5.3   Administering Medication

After assessing the patient and determining that the medication can be safely administered to her or him, prepare to administer the medication by:

- *Checking the medication order*: Compare the medication order with the medication.
- *Checking the Medication Administration Record (MAR)*: Compare the medication order with the MAR. The MAR will indicate if the medication has already been administered to the patient or discontinued.
- *Checking all medications prescribed to the patient*: Review all medications, even medications that were administered previously to the patient, because the medication may have a long half-life and may have the potential to conflict with the medication being administered to the patient.
- *Checking the patient's allergies*: Review the patient's chart and ask the patient about allergies. The patient may not have recalled allergies when her or his history was taken for the chart.
- *Creating your own medication administration worksheet*: Include scheduled medications and patient's other medical activities, such as tests and procedures, on your worksheet to avoid scheduling conflicts.
- *Checking PRN medication*: These are unscheduled as-needed medications. Determine what and when PRN medications were given before administering medication to avoid potential conflict.

5.4   Preparing the Medication

Once assured that the medication can be administered properly, follow these steps for preparing it.

- Wash your hands to prevent infection.
- Prepare the medication in a quiet area where you are not interrupted. Do not prepare all medications for all patients at once.
- Double check the dosage calculation. Verify the dose with a colleague.
- Compare the contents of the patient's medication drawer against the MAR. The medication and dose must match. Sometimes the pharmacy substitutes a generic drug for a brand name. Look up the medication in the medication manual if you do not recognize the name of the medication.
- Check the name of the medication when you remove it from the drawer, prepare it, and before dispensing it.

5.5   Administering the Medication

After medication is prepared, administer it safely at the bedside by:

- Washing your hands.
- Introducing yourself to the patient.
- Asking the patient to state her or his complete name. The patient must say her or his name without your help if capable.
- Comparing the patient's name and number on her or his identification band against the patient's name and number on the MAR.
- Asking the patient if she or he has any allergies to food or medication. Be aware that patients who are allergic to shellfish might also be allergic to some medications.
- Examining the patient's identification band to see if she or he has allergies.
- Assisting the patient into a comfortable position to administer the medication.
- Asking the patient if she or he knows about the medication and why the medication is being administered.
- Making sure that the patient sees the medication (tablet or liquid). Stop immediately if the patient does not recognize the medication. Recheck the order.
- Making sure you have baseline vital signs, labs, and other patient data before administering the medication to be compared after the patient receives the medication to determine her or his reaction to the medication.
- Instructing the patient about side effects of the medication and taking precautions to assure the patient's safety, such as raising the side rails and instructing her or him to remain in bed until the side effects subside.
- Staying with the patient until all of the medication is ingested.
- Remembering that the patient has the right to refuse medication. Notify the healthcare provider if this occurs and document appropriately.
- Properly disposing of the medication and supplies used to administer the medication. Do not leave the medication at the patient's bedside unless required by the medication order.
- Washing hands before leaving the patient's room.
- Documenting in the MAR that you administered the medication to the patient and signing the MAR.
- Returning in the appropriate amount of time and evaluating the effectiveness of the medication.

5.6   Useful Tips When Administering Medication

- If the medication can taste bad, then give ice chips before administering it. Ice chips numb the taste buds.
- Always give bad-tasting medications first, followed by pleasant-tasting liquids to shorten the time when the patient experiences the bad taste.
- Use the liquid form of the medication when possible, because patients find it easier to ingest a liquid over a tablet.
- Administer medication to a patient who needs extra assistance taking it after you give medication to your other patients so you can devote time to assist this patient.

5.7   Avoiding Medication Errors

It is critical to avoid situations that frequently result in medication errors. Here are ways to avoid medication errors:

- Avoid distractions when preparing medication.
- Avoid conversations while preparing medication.
- Only administer medications that you prepare.
- Only pour or prepare medication from containers that have full labels that are easy to read.
- Do not transfer medication from one container to another.
- Do not pour medications directly into your hand.
- Do not give medications that have expired.
- Do not guess about medication and doses. Always ask the healthcare provider if you cannot read the order.
- Do not administer medications that are discolored, have sediment, or are cloudy unless this is a normal state for the medication.
- Do not leave medications by the bedside or with visitors.
- Keep medications in clear sight.
- Do not give medications if the patient says she or he has allergies to it or the medication group.
- Use both the patient's name and number on the identification band to identify the patient.
- Do not recap needles.
- Do not administer medication with food or beverages unless the medication can be given with food and beverages.

Hint: If an error occurs, assess the patient and then notify the nurse in charge and the physician. Follow the healthcare facility's policy for reporting error. Review the steps that caused the error to occur.

5.8   Proper Disposal of Medication

Strict policies exist that govern how unused medications and supplies are disposed of. Here are steps you should follow when disposing of medication:

- Discard needles and syringes in an appropriate container.
- Dispose of medication in the sink, toilet, or appropriate container, and not in the trash.
- Return controlled substances to the pharmacy.
- Dispose of a controlled substance in the presence of another licensed healthcare worker who is willing to provide a signed statement saying she or he witnessed the disposal.
- Discard unused solutions from ampules.

5.9 Administering Medication at Home

Provide the patient with information on how to administer medication at home. Explain:

- Store the medication properly. Medication should be kept at prescribed temperature controls.
- Always label the date and time when medication was opened.
- Keep the medication in a locked area or on her or his person.
- Self-assess when the medication has reached its onset and peak time; otherwise, the assessment might be misleading because the medication has not taken effect.
- Suspend further doses if the patient sees the signs and symptoms of an adverse reaction to the medication. Call the healthcare provider immediately.
- Note any side effect of the medication and how well the side effect is tolerated. Call the healthcare provider if there is a low tolerance. A different medication might be prescribed.

5.10 Controlling Narcotics

Special precautions are necessary for storing and handling narcotics. Here are the steps that must be taken to secure narcotics:

- Keep narcotics in a double-locked drawer or a closet that is protected with a computerized access system.
- One nurse per shift must keep the keys to the narcotic drawer on her or his person.
- A sign-out sheet must be used to control the inventory of narcotics.
- Document on the MAR when a patient is administered a narcotic.

Solved Problems

Patient Assessment

5.1   Why do you determine the reason that a medication is prescribed for a patient before administering the medication?

Independent verification assures that an error did not occur when the medication was prescribed by the healthcare provider.

5.2   What would you do if the medication is prescribed to be administered orally and the patient has stomach pains and is vomiting?

Hold the medication. Call the healthcare provider who prescribed the medication and ask for a new medication order, directing that the medication be administered using a different route.

5.3   Why is it important to assess the patient's condition for contraindications before administering medication?

Although the healthcare provider assessed the patient before prescribing the medication, the patient's condition might have changed since then. An updated assessment assures that the patient does not have any contraindications for the medication.

5.4   Why is it important to assess the patient's kidney function before administering medication?

Many medications are excreted in the urine. If the kidneys are not functioning properly, then the medication cannot be adequately excreted, resulting in the buildup of medication.

5.5 Why is age important to medication metabolism?

The very young can have an immature ability to absorb, distribute, metabolize, and excrete medication. Elderly people have a reduced ability to handle medication because of aging systems. Both of these age groups are at higher exposure to side effects and adverse effects of medication.

5.6 Why is it important to review the patient's medication history before administering medication?

Assess the amount of medication that the patient has received to determine if the patient has received the maximum daily allowance according to the medication manual. Also determine if the patient has a tolerance for the medication and if the patient shows signs and symptoms of a toxic effect caused by the cumulative effect of the medication.

5.7 Why is it important to review the time before administering medication?

Determine if the medication must be administered at a particular time. For example, stimulants are not administered at bedtime because the medication inhibits sleep.

5.8 Why is it important to know the patient's body weight before administering medication?

Assessment of the patient's weight must be made before administering medication that is prescribed by weight. The patient's weight might have materially changed since the patient's weight was entered into the patient's chart.

5.9 Why is it important to know the patient's albumin level before administering medication?

The patient's body must be able to distribute the medication. Distribution can be disrupted by low albumin (some medication binds to albumin) and impaired circulation.

5.10 What effect can food have on medication absorption?

Food slows absorption for some medications.

Medication Administration

5.11 How should you check the medication order?

Compare the medication order with the medication ordered for the patient.

5.12 Why should you make sure that the patient sees the medication before administering it?

Stop immediately if the patient does not recognize the medication. Recheck the order. Many patients who take scheduled medication are able to recognize the medication if in tablet or liquid form.

5.13 What do you do if the patient refuses the medication?

The patient has the right to refuse medication. Notify the healthcare provider if this occurs.

5.14 What do you do if the medication will leave a bad taste in the patient's mouth?

Give ice chips before administering the medication. Ice chips numb the taste buds. Always give bad-tasting medications first followed by pleasant-tasting liquids to shorten the time when the patient experiences the bad taste.

5.15 Name four ways to prevent common medication administration errors.

Avoid distractions when preparing medication. Only administer medications that you prepare. Do not guess about medication and doses. Always ask the healthcare provider if you cannot read the order.

5.16 What should you do if a medication error occurs?

If an error occurs, assess the patient and then notify the nurse in charge and the physician if the patient experiences adverse effects to the medication. Follow the healthcare facility's policy for reporting error. Review the steps that caused the error to occur.

5.17 How do you dispose of controlled substances?

Dispose of a controlled substance in the presence of another licensed healthcare worker who is willing to provide a sign statement saying that she or he witnessed the disposal. Return controlled substances to the pharmacy.

5.18 How do you dispose non-controlled substances?

Dispose of medication in the sink or toilet and not in the trash.

5.19 Where do you document the administration of medication?

Document the administration of medication in the MAR.

5.20 Why should you stay with the patient until all of the medication is ingested?

The patient may have difficulty swallowing the medication or may pretend to swallow the medication and later spit it out.

5.21 Why is it important to have baseline vital signs and labs before administering medication?

Make sure you have baseline vital signs, labs, and other patient data before administering the medication to be compared after the patient receives the medication to determine her or his reaction to the medication.

5.22 Why is it important compare the patient's identification band with the MAR and medication label?

The patient's identification band contains information that uniquely identifies her or him. This same information appears in the MAR and many times on the medication label.

5.23 Why is it important to ask the patient to state her or his name without your help before administering medication?

This helps to identify the patient; however, the patient's identification band is the best way to confirm her or his identity.

5.24 Why ask the patient if she or he has allergies before administering the medication?

The patient may have forgotten to make the allergies known when giving her or his medical history, therefore the allergies would not appear in the patient's medical record or identification band. Do not give medications if the patient says she or he has allergies to the medication or medication group.

5.25 What should you do if the patient exhibits adverse reaction to the medication?

Suspend further doses if the patient shows signs and symptoms of an adverse reaction to the medication. Call the healthcare provider immediately.

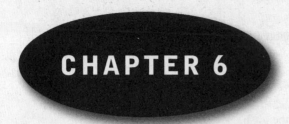

CHAPTER 6

Route of Administration

6.1 Medication and Routes

The route a medication is administered to the patient is the means in which the patient receives the medication. The routine influences the pharmacokinetics of the medication (see 2.6 Pharmacokinetics).

There are 11 routes for administering medication.

6.2 Oral Route

The oral route is medications administered by mouth in the form of tablets, capsules, and liquids. Oral medications are absorbed in the small intestines and have a peak time of 1 to 3 hours.

Precautions must be taken when administering medication using the oral route:

- No oral medication may be given to patients who are vomiting, lack a gag reflex, or are in an unresponsive state.
- Do not mix oral medication with large amounts of food or liquid. However, mixing food with applesauce and giving medication with water or juice is permissible, depending the medication. Food and liquid can alter the medication's effectiveness by interfering with absorption of the medication.

Tablets: These are administered using the oral route. The dosage of a tablet can be reduced by cutting the tablet into half or quarters. Some tablets can be crushed and mixed with food, such as applesauce, depending on the medication.

Capsules: These are administered using the oral route. Capsules must be taken whole and not crushed because medication in the capsule is enteric-coated for timed release. Capsules can be opened and the medication mixed with the food depending on the medication.

Liquid: Medication is also administered using the oral route. There are three forms of liquid medication:

- Elixir: A sweet, pleasant-smelling solution of alcohol and water used as a vehicle for medicine such as Robitussin
- Emulsion: A suspension of small globules of one liquid in a second liquid
- Suspension: A preparation of undissolved particles dispersed in a liquid such as bismuth subsalicylate (Pepto-Bismol)

To administer liquid medication:

- Dilute, shake, or stir the medication if required.
- Read the meniscus (curve in the surface of a liquid) at the lowest fluid level while pouring the liquid to determine the dose.
- Refrigerate open or reconstituted (mixed) liquid medication. Write the date and time on the label of when the medication was opened.

6.3 Sublingual and Buccal Medication Routes

Sublingual medications are administered under the tongue. Buccal medications are administered between the cheek and the gum. Both routes absorb medication quickly into the circulatory system because there is a vast network of capillaries beneath the thin layer of epithelium tissue in those areas.

To administer medication sublingually or buccally:

- No food or liquid should be ingested until the medication is completely absorbed.
- Medication can be administered sublingually to nonresponsive patients. There is minimal change of aspiration because sublingual medication is absorbed quickly.

6.4 Transdermal Route

The transdermal route (patch) delivers medication through the skin providing a consistent blood level of medication.

To administer medication transdermally:

- Do not alter the patch in any way.
- Remove the patch before applying another patch.
- Apply the patch onto the specified area of the body.
- Alternate the sites of the patch on the body.
- Wear gloves when administering the patch; otherwise, you may absorb the medication.
- Place the patch on a clean, dry, hairless area where the skin is intact.

Hint: Transdermal medication may need to be prepared before fixing the transdermal applicator to the skin. Medication is provided in a tube and a pad of paper patches. Each paper patch has measurement lines. The medication is applied by squeezing it onto the paper patch and is measured by using the measurement lines.

6.5 Topical Route

The topical route administers medication to the skin to provide therapeutic effect directly to the affected skin site. Topical medication is administered in three ways:

- By glove
- With a tongue blade
- With a cotton-tipped applicator or cotton ball

To administer topical medication:

- Use medically clean or sterile techniques if skin is not intact.
- Stroke or pat the medication onto the skin.
- Provide patient comfort if medication is applied in a painful area of the skin.
- Use a firm touch when administering medication in an itchy (pruritic) site. A light touch increases itching.
- Always use a gloved hand when applying topical medication; otherwise, the medication will be absorbed by your fingers.

6.6   Instillation Route

The instillation route consists of administering medication by drops, ointments, or sprays. Special care must be taken to prevent the spread of the disease when instilling the medication. When administering medication to the eye using the instillation route:

- Wash hands.
- Apply clean gloves.
- Ask the patient to look toward the ceiling.
- Pull down the lower eye lid, exposing the conjunctival sac.
- Administer the medication.
- Avoid placing medication on the cornea. The cornea might be damaged and cause the patient discomfort.
- Ask the patient to close his or her eyes for 1 to 2 minutes after the medication is administered.

When instilling eye drops:

- Administer the prescribed number of drops into the center of the conjunctival sac.
- Avoid touching the eyelid and eye lashes with the dropper.
- Release the lower eye lid.
- Press the lacrimal duct (inner corner of the eye) with sterile cotton balls or tissues for 1 to 2 minutes to prevent the medication from being absorbed through the lacrimal canal.

When instilling eye ointment:

- Squeeze a half inch of ointment into the conjunctival sac.
- Explain that vision might be temporarily blurred.

When administering medication to the ear using the instillation route:

- Wash your hands.
- Apply clean gloves.
- Keep the medication at room temperature.
- Ask the patient to tilt his or her head toward the unaffected side.
- Straighten the external ear canal.
- For patients 3 years old or older: Pull the auricle up and back.
- For patients less than 3 years old: Pull the auricle down and back.
- Administer the prescribed number of drops into the ear.
- Avoid touching the ear with the dropper. The dropper will become contaminated.
- Ask the patient to continue to tilt his or her head for 2 to 3 minutes.

When administering medication to the nose using the instillation route, first ask the patient to blow his or her nose. When instilling nose drops:

- If the infection is in the frontal sinus, ask the patient to put his or her head back.
- If the infection is in the ethmoid sinus, ask the patient to move his or her head to the affected side.
- Administer the prescribed number of drops.
- Ask the patient to tilt his or her head backward for 5 minutes.

When instilling nose sprays:

- Ask the patient to close the unaffected nostril.
- Ask the patient to tilt his or her head to the side of the closed nostril.
- Spray the medication in to the open nostril.
- Ask the patient to hold his or her breath or open the closed nostril and breathe through the nostril, depending on the medication.

6.7 Inhalation Route

The inhalation route administers medication using an inhaler. Medication is absorbed in the bronchioles. There are two types of inhalers:

- Hand-held nebulizer: Changes liquid medication into a fine spray
- Metered Dose Inhaler (MDI): Sprays a fixed dose of medication each time the device's button is pressed

Nine percent of the medication sprayed reaches the bronchioles. Using a spacer increases the delivery of medication to the bronchioles to 21%. The spacer is a funnel-like device that attaches to the mouthpiece of the meter dose inhaler. When administering medication using an inhaler:

- Sit the patient up (in a semi-Fowler or high Fowler position).
- Remove the cap.
- Hold the inhaler upright.
- Shake the inhaler.
- Ask the patient to tilt his or her head back slightly.
- Ask the patient to breathe out.
- Insert the inhaler.
- Press down on the inhaler button.
- Ask the patient to breathe in slowly for 3 to 5 seconds.
- Ask the patient to hold his or her breath for 10 seconds. This enables the medication to enter the bronchioles.
- Wait 1 minute before administering a second inhalation.
- Repeat this process according the healthcare provider's orders.

6.8 Nasogastric and Gastrostomy Tubes Route

The nasogastric tube and gastrostomy tube routines are used to administer medication when the patient is unable to swallow or ingest.

- *Nasogastric Tube (NG)*: This is a tube passed through the nose and into the stomach providing direct access to the stomach. It is used to administer medication, for temporary feeding, and to remove stomach contents.

- *Gastrostomy Tube (GT)*: This is a tube inserted through the skin into the stomach. It is used to administer medication and for permanent feeding.

When administering medication through the nasogastric or gastrostomy tube:

- Check the position of the nasogastric tube (the gastrostomy is surgically positioned), using one of the following methods:
  - Check the stomach content.
    - Using a syringe, inject 20 ml of air into the tube.
    - Aspirate the gastric contents.
    - Check the pH of the gastric contents—a pH less than 5 indicates that the tube is positioned properly.
    - Using a syringe, inject 10 ml of air into the tube.
  - Listen for air.
    - Using a stethoscope, listen over the stomach for the rush of air. If you hear the rush of air, then the tube is positioned properly.
- Remove the plunger from a syringe.
- Close the clamp on the tube.
- Attach the syringe to the tube.
- Open the clamp on the tube.
- Pour medication into the syringe.
- Allow the medication to flow from the syringe down the tube.
- Flush the tube with 50 ml of water.
- Close the clamp on the tube.
- Remove the syringe.

6.9 Suppositories Route

The suppositories route is used to administer medication through the rectum or vagina. The rectum contains many capillaries that increase the absorption of the medication. Rectal suppositories are used when:

- The upper GI tract is not functioning.
- The medication has an offensive taste or foul odor.
- Digestive enzymes change the chemical integrity of the medication.

When administering a rectal suppository:

- Provide privacy.
- Lay the patient on the left side (Sims position).
- Wash your hands.
- Apply clean gloves.
- Lubricate the suppository with a water-soluble lubricant.
- Ask the patient to breathe through his or her mouth to relax the anal sphincter.
- Insert the suppository.
- Ask the patient to remain in position for 20 minutes.

When administering a vaginal suppository:

- Wash your hands.
- Apply clean gloves.

- Place the patient on her back with legs flexed at the knees (lithotomy position).
- Insert the suppository using an applicator.
- Clean the vaginal area after insertion.

6.10 Parenteral Route

A parenteral route is used to inject medication into the patient. There are four parenteral routes: intradermal (ID), subcutaneous (SC), intramuscular (IM), and intravenous (IV). The healthcare provider determines the choice of route based on the medication, desired onset, and the patient's needs.

6.11 Intradermal Parenteral Route

The intradermal parenteral route is an injection that is given slightly below the surface of the skin where the medication is not absorbed into the bloodstream. The area of the skin is hairless, lightly pigmented, and thinly keratinized, providing a clear view of the site. The intradermal parenteral route is used to determine if there is a reaction to the medication, which is signified by a blister (wheal) on the injection site.

Injections are made using a 26- to 27-gauge needle and a 1 ml syringe calibrated in 0.01 ml increments. The typical injection is 0.01 to 0.1 ml. Sites for intradermal injections are:

- Inner aspect of forearm
- Scapular area of back
- Upper chest
- Medial thigh sites

When administering medication using the intradermal parenteral route:

- Wash your hands.
- Apply clean gloves.
- Cleanse the area of the site in a circular motion using alcohol or Betadine.
- Hold the skin taut.
- Position the bevel of the needle up.
- Insert the needle at a 10- to 15-degree angle. (Visualize the outline of the needle through the skin.)
- Inject slowly to form a wheal.
- Slowly remove the needle.
- Do not massage the area.
- Mark the site with a pen.
- Ask the patient not to wash the site until the healthcare provider assesses it.
- Assess the site in 24 to 72 hours. The diameter of the wheal increases if there is an allergic response.
- Assess the hardness of the wheal—not its redness—if used for a tuberculosis test.

6.12 Subcutaneous Parenteral Route

The subcutaneous parenteral route is an injection into the skin (subcutaneous) where the medication is slowly absorbed into the capillaries, resulting in a slower onset than intramuscular and intravenous parenteral routes. The subcutaneous parenteral injection site should have an adequate fat pad and injections must be rotated to prevent lipodystrophy. Lipodystrophy is the loss of fat under the skin, resulting in effective absorption of the medication. Subcutaneous parenteral injection sites are:

- Abdomen
- Upper hips

- Upper back
- Lateral upper arms
- Lateral thighs

Injections are made using a 25- to 27-gauge needle that is 1/2 or 5/8 inches in length and with a 1- to 3-ml syringe calibrated 0.5 to 1.5 ml. (Syringes for insulin are measured in units, not ml.) When administering medication using the subcutaneous parenteral route:

- Wash your hands.
- Apply clean gloves.
- Cleanse the area of the site in a circular motion using alcohol or Betadine in to out.
- Pinch the skin.
- Insert the needle at 45- to 90-degree angle. (A 45-degree angle is preferred when there is a small amount of subcutaneous tissue.)
- Release the skin.
- Inject slowly.
- Quickly remove the needle.
- Gently massage the site (not if heparin or insulin is injected).
- Apply a band-aid as necessary.

6.13 Intramuscular Parenteral Route

The intramuscular parenteral route is an injection given into the muscle. Doses greater than 3 ml for an adult and 1 ml for a child should be divided into two injections using different syringes. Table 6.1 shows injection sites.

Injections are made using a 20- to 23-gauge needle that is 1 to 1.5 inches in length and a 1- to 3-ml syringe. When administering medication using the intramuscular parenteral route:

- Wash your hands.
- Apply clean gloves.
- Cleanse the area of the site in a circular motion using alcohol or Betadine in to out.
- Flatten the skin at the injection site.
- Insert the needle at a 90-degree angle into the muscle between your thumb and index finger.
- Release the skin.
- Aspirate to check for blood. If blood is returned, then prepare another injection for a different site.
- Slowly inject the medication.
- Quickly remove the needle.
- Gently massage the area unless contraindicated by the medication.

6.14 Z-Track Injection Technique

The Z-track injection technique prevents medication from leaking back in the subcutaneous tissue after the injection and is used for administering medication that might cause visible permanent skin discoloration. When using the Z-track injection technique:

- Wash your hands.
- Apply clean gloves.
- Cleanse the area of the site in a circular motion using alcohol or Betadine in to out.
- Pull the skin to one side and hold it.

TABLE 6.1 Injection Sites

INJECTION SITE	DESCRIPTION
Ventrogluteal (hip)	• Relatively free of major nerves and vascular branches • Well-defined bony anatomic landmarks • For IM or Z-track injections • Locate the site by placing the heel of your hand on the greater trochanter of the femur with the thumb pointed toward the umbilicus. • The index finger marks the anterosuperior iliac spine. The middle finger traces the iliac crest curvature. The space between the index and middle fingers is the injection site.
Dorsogluteal (buttocks)	• Good site for IM and Z-track injections • Danger to major nerves and vascular structures near site • Easy to give subcutaneously when trying to give an IM because the fat is often very thick
Deltoid (upper arm)	• Preferred site for vaccines • Easily accessible • Muscle mass is small compared to other sites • Use a 5/8- to 1.5-inch long needle • Locate the acromion process of the scapula and the deltoid. Measure two to three fingers below the acromion process on the lateral midline of the arm to identify the proper site. Inject at a 90-degree angle.
Vastus lateralis (front of thigh)	• Preferred site for infants younger than 7 months • It has a relatively large muscle mass • Free from major nerves and vascular branches • Site is a hand's breadth below the greater trochanter and above the knee • Inject at a 45-degree angle toward the knee

- Insert the needle at a 90-degree angle.
- Aspirate to check for blood. If blood is returned, then prepare another injection for a different site.
- Inject the medication as you hold the skin to one side.
- Withdraw the needle.
- Release the skin.

6.15 Minimize Pain Parenteral Route

Minimize painful discomfort of an injection by using these techniques:

- Ask the patient to relax his or her muscle. There is less pain when medication is injected into a relaxed muscle.
- Replace the needle with a new needle after drawing up the medication.
- Ask the patient to lay on his or her side and flex the knees.
- Position the patient on his or her side with knees flexed if you are using the ventrogluteal site.
- Position the patient flat on the abdomen with toes turned inward if using the dorsogluteal site.
- Do not inject into sensitive or hardened tissues.
- Compress the tissue at the injection site.
- Wait for the antiseptic to dry before injecting the medication.
- Dart the needle to reduce puncture pain.

- Ask the patient to cough and inject slowly while coughing.
- Withdraw the needle quickly and straight.

6.16   Intravenous Parenteral Route

The intravenous (IV) parenteral route directly injects medication into the circulatory system, providing rapid onset. The IV should be inserted in the dorsal vein but can also be inserted into the:

- Cephalic vein (arm)
- Cubital vein (arm)—only in an emergency. The cubital vein is used for withdrawing blood.
- Dorsal vein (hand)

An IV uses a 21- or 22-gauge needle (larger bore for thicker medication) that is 1 to 1.5 inches in length. IV lines are inserted with a butterfly needle or an angiocatheter that ranges from 14 gauge for whole blood or fractions of blood to 18 gauge for rapid infusion. Medication is frequently delivered to the patient through the IV using controllers and pumps that control the infusion of medication.

When administering medication using the intravenous parenteral route:

- Wash your hands.
- Apply clean gloves.
- Cleanse the area of the site in a circular motion using alcohol or Betadine.
- Apply a tourniquet above the site.
- Insert the butterfly or catheter into the vein until blood returns.
- Remove the tourniquet.
- Stabilize the needle or catheter.
- Dress the site.
- Add IV fluid/medication and set flow rate.
- Monitor flow rate, skin color and temperature, distal pulses, insertion side for infiltration, and side effects of the medication.

Solved Problems

Oral Route

6.1   What is a medication route?

A medication route is the way the medication is administered to a patient.

6.2   When should the oral route not be used to administer medication?

Do not use the oral route if the patient is vomiting, lacks the gag reflex, or is unresponsive.

6.3   How can the dose of a tablet be reduced?

The dose of a table can be reduced by dividing the tablet in half or into quarters.

6.4   Can capsules be crushed?

Capsules must be taken whole because a capsule contains medication that is enteric coated for timed release.

6.5   What is an elixir liquid?

An elixir liquid is a sweet, pleasant-smelling solution of alcohol and water that is used as a vehicle for medicine such as Robitussin.

6.6   How do you measure the level of a liquid when pouring the liquid in a cup?

Measure the level of a liquid in a cup by reading the meniscus (curve in the surface of a liquid) at the lowest fluid level while pouring the liquid to determine the dose.

Transdermal Route

6.7   What is the benefit of using the transdermal route?

The benefit of the transdermal route is that the medication is delivered at a consistent level over time.

6.8   Why should you remove the existing transdermal patch before applying a new transdermal patch?

Two transdermal patches applied at the same time increase the dose of the medication.

6.9   Why should you use gloves when applying a transdermal patch?

Medication in the transdermal patch can be absorbed by your fingers if they are exposed to the medication side of the transdermal patch.

Topical Route

6.10   Name three ways of applying medication using the topical route.

The three ways of applying medication using the topical route are by glove, with a tongue blade, or with a cotton-tipped applicator.

6.11   How would you apply medication using the topical route to an itchy patch of skin?

Use a firm touch when administering medication in an itchy (pruritic) site. A light touch increases itchiness.

Instillation Route

6.12   Why do you press the lacrimal duct with sterile cotton balls or tissues after administering eye medication?

Press the lacrimal duct (inner corner of the eye) with sterile cotton balls or tissues for 1 to 2 minutes to prevent the medication from being absorbed through the lacrimal canal.

6.13   How much ointment should be squeezed onto the conjunctival sac?

Squeeze a half-inch of ointment onto the conjunctival sac.

6.14   When instilling medication into the ear of a 5-year-old child, in which direction do you pull the auricle?

For a child who is 3 years old or older, pull the auricle up and back.

6.15   In what position should the patient move his or her head when instilling drops for an ethmoid sinus infection?

If the infection is in the ethmoid sinus, ask the patient to move his or her head to the affected side.

Inhalation Route

6.16 How do you increase the efficiency of a metered dose inhaler?

Nine percent of the medication sprayed reaches the bronchioles. Using a spacer increases the delivery medication to the bronchioles to 21%. The spacer is a funnel-like device that attaches to the mouthpiece of the metered dose inhaler.

6.17 What position should the patient be in when using the metered dose inhaler?

When using the metered dose inhaler, the patient should be in semi-Fowler or high Fowler position.

6.18 What should you ask the patient to do after inhaling medication?

Ask the patient to hold his or her breath for 10 seconds. This enables the medication to enter the bronchioles.

6.19 What is a metered dose inhaler?

A metered dose inhaler (MDI) is a device that sprays a fixed dose of medication each time its button is pressed.

Nasogastric and Gastrostomy Tubes Route

6.20 What is a nasogastric tube?

A nasogastric tube (NG) is a tube passed through the nose and into the stomach, providing direct access to the stomach. It is used to administer medication, temporary feeding, and to remove stomach contents.

6.21 What is the first thing to do before administering medication in a nasogastric tube?

Before administering medication in a nasogastric tube, check the position of the nasogastric tube.

6.22 When checking the gastric contents to determine the position of a nasogastric tube, what should be the pH of the gastric contents?

The gastric contents should have a pH of less than 5.

Parenteral Route

6.23 What is the onset of medication administered using the intravenous parenteral route?

The onset of medication administered using the intravenous parenteral route is immediate.

6.24 Name three ways to reduce pain and discomfort when giving an injection.

Three ways to reduce pain and discomfort when giving an injection are to dart the needle, compress the tissue at the injection site, and ask the patient to relax the muscle. There is less pain when medication is injected into a relaxed muscle.

6.25 Where is the first place to start an IV?

The IV should be inserted in the dorsal vein, but can also be inserted into the cephalic or cubital vein.

6.26 When would you use the cubital vein?

The cubital vein is used for withdrawing blood.

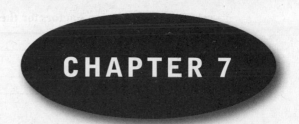

CHAPTER 7

Dose Calculations

7.1   Medication Measurements

Medication is measured using the metric system and the apothecaries' system. The metric system is used to measure medication in a healthcare facility and used when prescribing and recording the medication in the patient's chart. The apothecaries' (household) system is used by patients who self-administer medication.

The metric system uses grams to measure weight and liters to measure volume, as shown in Table 7.1. Prefixes are used to indicate the value (Table 7.2). The apothecaries' system uses ounces and pounds for weight and teaspoon, and tablespoon to measure volume. Table 7.3 contains conversion factors for the apothecaries' system and metric system.

TABLE 7.1 Units and Their Equivalents

UNIT	PURPOSE	EQUIVALENTS
Gram	Weight	1 kilogram (kg) = 1000 grams (g)
		1 gram (g) = 1000 milligrams (mg)
		1 milligram = 1000 micrograms (mcg)
Liter	Volume	1 liter (L) = 1000 milliliters (ml) = 1000 cubic centimeters (cc)
		1 milliliter (ml) = 1 cubic centimeter (cc)

TABLE 7.2 Prefixes Used in Medication

PREFIX	VALUE	DESCRIPTION
Kilo	1000	One thousand times
Centi	0.01	One hundredth part of
Milli	0.001	One thousandth part of
Micro	0.000001	One millionth part of

TABLE 7.3 **Conversion Factors for the Apothecaries' System and Metric System**

WEIGHT	
2.2 pounds (lb)	1 kilogram (kg)
VOLUME	
1 ounce	30 ml
16 ounces	480 ml
33.3 ounces	1000 ml
1 liter	1000 ml
60 drops (gh)	1 teaspoon (tsp)
1 teaspoon (tsp)	5 ml
1 tablespoon (tbsp)	15 ml
2 tablespoons (tbsp)	1 ounce = 30 ml

7.2 Converting Metric Units

The medication order may prescribe medication in a metric unit that is different from the metric unit of the medication delivered by the pharmacy. Before calculating the proper dose for the patient, you need to use like metric units; therefore, you might need to convert metric units.

For example, the medication order may be prescribed in grams and the pharmacy delivers medication in milligrams. You must convert grams to milligrams before calculating the dose that will be administered to the patient.

Converting from one metric unit to another metric unit is performed by following these steps:

- Determine if the prescribed metric unit is larger or smaller than the metric unit of the medication delivered by the pharmacy.
- Convert from a smaller unit to a larger unit by dividing the value by 1000 by moving the decimal three places to the left.
- Convert from a larger until to a smaller unit by multiplying the value by 1000 by moving the decimal three places to the right.
- Remember that 1 milliliter (ml) = 1 cubic centimeter (cc).

Example: Small Unit to Large Unit

The healthcare provider prescribed 300 milligrams (mg) of medication. The pharmacy delivers medication in grams (g). You must convert milligrams to grams.

Convert a smaller unit to a larger unit by dividing the value by 1000

$$300 \text{ mg}/1000 = 0.3 \text{ g}$$

Example: Large Unit to Small Unit

The healthcare provider prescribed 0.9 g of a medication. The pharmacy delivers medication in milligrams. You must convert grams to milligrams.

Convert a large unit to a small unit by multiplying the value by 1000:

$$0.9 \text{ g} \times 1000 = 900 \text{ mg}$$

Hint: Always place a zero to the left of the decimal when the quantity is not a whole number. This is a legal requirement and avoids errors when reading the value. Do not use trailing zeros following the decimal.

Incorrect: .9
Correct: 0.9

7.3 Converting Metric Units to Apothecaries' System Units

Patients use the apothecaries' system to measure medication when they self-medicate; however, the medication may be delivered in metric units. Therefore, the healthcare provider must convert the prescribed dose from metric units to units of the apothecaries' system. Use factors in Table 7.3 to convert values. The most common conversions are milliliters to teaspoons, tablespoons, or cups. A cup is measured in ounces. Another common conversion is pounds to kilograms.

Example: Milliliters to Ounces

The healthcare provider prescribed 240 ml of a medication. The patient has an 8-oz cup. You must convert milliliters to ounces and then ounces to cups.

Table 7.3 states that there are 30 milliliters per ounce.

$$240 \text{ ml} / 30 \text{ ml} = 8 \text{ oz}$$
$$8 \text{ oz} / 8 \text{ oz per cup} = 1 \text{ cup}$$

Example: Pounds to Kilograms

The healthcare provider prescribed 3 mg of a medication per kilogram of the patient's weight. The patient weighs 150 pounds. You must convert pounds to kilograms and then multiply the patient's weight in kilograms by the prescribed dose of medication.

Table 7.3 states there are 2.2 pounds per kilogram.

$$150 \text{ lb} / 2.2 \text{ lb} = 68.181 \text{ kg}$$
$$68.181 \text{ kg} \times 3 \text{ mg} = 205.5 \text{ mg}$$

7.4 Calculating the Desired Dose

The dose prescribed by the healthcare provider may not be available in the healthcare facility. For example, the healthcare provider may order 15 mg tablets of Inderal and the healthcare facility has 10 mg tablets of Inderal.

You must calculate the dose to administer to the patient. In this example, you must determine how many 10 mg tablets of Inderal to give the patient so that the patient receives the full 15 mg dose that is prescribed by the healthcare provider.

There are two methods used to calculate the dose to administer to the patient. These are the formula method and the ratio-proportion method. Both methods produce the same results.

7.5 The Formula Method

The formula method contains four elements:

- D = Desired dose, which is the dose specified in the medication order
- H = Have dose, which is the dose on hand
- Q = Quantity, which is the number of tablets on hand or whatever form of the medication
- X = Dose to administer to patient

The formula is:

$$D / H \times Q = X$$

For example, the medication order is 15 mg tablets of Inderal. This is the Desired dose. The pharmacy has 10 mg tablets of Inderal. This is the Have and Quantity. Insert these values into the formula:

$$15 \text{ mg} / 10 \text{ mg} \times 1 \text{ tablet} = X$$
$$1.5 \times 1 \text{ tablet} = X$$
$$1.5 \text{ tablets} = X$$

The patient must receive 1.5 tablets of Inderal to receive the 15 mg that the healthcare provider prescribed.

Hint: Be sure that all values are in the same unit before calculating the formula.

The formula method is used for any form of medication. For example, a healthcare provider prescribed 500 mg of Ampicillin Sodium. The pharmacy has 250 mg capsules of Ampicillin Sodium. Here is how you calculate the number of capsules to administer to the patient:

$$500 \text{ mg} / 250 \text{ mg} (1 \text{ capsule} = X$$
$$2 \times 1 \text{ capsule} = X$$
$$2 \text{ capsules} = X$$

The patient must receive two capsules of Ampicillin Sodium to receive the 500 mg that the healthcare provider prescribed.

Parenteral route injections are also calculated using the formula method. Suppose the healthcare provider ordered 375 mg of Ampicillin. The pharmacy delivers a solution of 250 mg in 5 milliliters. How many milliliters should be administered to the patient? Here is how this is calculated:

$$375 \text{ mg} / 250 \text{ mg} \times 5 \text{ ml} = X$$
$$1.5 \times 5 \text{ ml} = X$$
$$7.5 \text{ ml} = X$$

The patient must receive an injection of 7.5 ml of Ampicillin to receive the 375 mg prescribed by the healthcare provider.

Hint: Make sure to label all terms in the formula with the appropriate unit to avoid errors.

7.6　Ratio-Proportion

The ratio-proportion method applies the ratio of the on-hand medication to the medication order to calculate the correct dose. Here are the components of the ratio-proportion formula. The ratio of the left side of the equation equals the ratio on the right side of the equation. The left side of the equation is the ratio of the medication on hand. The right side of the equation is the medication ordered by the healthcare provider. X is the quantity of the medication that will be administered to the patient.

Have : Quantity = Desired : X quantity

The healthcare provider ordered 40 mg of a medication. The pharmacy has 80 mg of the medication in 1 milliliter of solution.

80 mg: 1 ml = 40 mg : X ml

Here is how to perform the calculation:

1. Multiply the two values that are closest to the equal signs. These are referred to as the means.

$$1 \text{ ml} \times 40 \text{ mg} = 40 \text{ mg/ml}$$

2. Multiply the two values that are farthest from the equal signs. These are referred to as the extremes.

$$80 \text{ mg / ml} \cdot X = 80 \text{ mg / ml } X$$

3. Restate the equation

$$80 \text{ mg / ml } X = 40 \text{ mg / ml}$$

4. Divide both sides of the equation by 80 mg/ml.

$$\frac{80 \text{ mg/ml}}{80 \text{ mg/ml}} X = X \qquad \frac{40 \text{ mg/ml}}{80 \text{ mg/ml}} = 0.5 \text{ mg/ml}$$
$$80 \text{ mg/ml } X = 0.5 \text{ ml}$$

7.7   Calculating the IV Flow Rate

Medication using the intravenous route is measured by flow rate. Flow rate, also known as the drip rate, is the number of drops of medication the patient receives in a minute. In order to calculate the flow rate you need to know:

- The volume of fluid that is to be infused
- The amount of time of the infusion
- The drip factor, which is specified on the IV tubing used for the infusion

The Flow Rate formula is:

- Total Fluid × Drip Factor / Infusion Time in minutes = Flow Rate in drops (gtt) per minute

Hint: The drip factor for microdrip tubing is 60, but is not specified on the tubing. The drip factor is not calculated if an infusion pump is used. The infusion pump is set at number of milliliters per hour.

Example: The healthcare provider ordered 250 ml of 5% D/W to infuse over 10 hours. The pharmacy delivers an IV bag of 250 ml of 5% D/W. You use Microdrip tubing, which has a drip factor of 60. Calculate the flow rate.

1. Change 10 hours to minutes
   10 hours × 60 minutes = 600 minutes
2. 250 ml × 60 drip factor / 600 minutes = Flow Rate
3. 250 ml × 60 drip factor = 15,000
4. 15,000 / 600 minutes = 25 gtt/minutes

Hint: Carry out the calculation to the tenth. Express the flow rate in a whole number.

7.8   Pediatric Dose Calculation Formula

Some pediatric medications are prescribed by weight in kilograms. There are 2.2 lb per kilogram (see Table 7.3). To calculate the pediatric dose you need to know:

- D = Desired dose per kilogram ordered
- W = Patient's weight in kilogram
- H = Have on hand

- Q = Quantity on hand
- X = Dose to administer to patient

The pediatric medication formula is:

$$((D \cdot W) / H) \times Q = X$$

Example: The healthcare provider prescribed Elixir of Digoxin 15 mcg per kilogram. The patient weighs 66 lb. The pharmacy delivers 50 mcg per milliliter.

1. Convert 66 lb to kilograms

$$66 \text{ lb} / 2.2 \text{ lb} = 30 \text{ kg}$$

2. Enter values into the formula

$$((15 \text{ mcg} \times 30 \text{ kg}) / 50 \text{ mcg}) \times 1 \text{ milliliter} = X$$

3. Calculate the formula

$$(450 \text{ mcg} / 50 \text{ mcg}) \times 1 \text{ milliliter} = X$$
$$9 \text{ mcg} \times 1 \text{ milliliter} = X$$
$$9 \text{ mcg} = X = \text{dose to administer to the patient}$$

Hint: Truncate kilogram weight to three decimal values. Do not round the kilogram weight.

7.9 Heparin Dose Calculation Formula

The heparin calculation is a two-step process.

1. Calculate number of heparin units in a milliliter of the IV fluids.
2. Calculate the number of milliliters to administer per hour to the patient.

To calculate the pediatric dose you need to know:

- HU = Have heparin units
- QH = Quantity of heparin
- HUml = Heparin units per milliliter
- D = Desired heparin units
- X = Dose of heparin per hour to administer to the patient

The heparin formula is:

- HU / QH = HUmL
- D / HUmL = X

Example: The healthcare provider ordered heparin to be infused at 800 U per hour. The pharmacy delivers 25,000 U in 250 ml of D5W.

1. First, calculate the heparin units per milliliter

$$25,000 \text{ U} \div 250 \text{ ml} = 100 \text{ U/ml}$$

2. Second, calculate the dose of heparin per hour to administer to the patient.

- 800 U (100 U/ml = 8 ml/hr
- 8 ml/hr = X

Hint: Heparin is always infused using an infusion pump.

7.10 Dopamine Dose Calculation Formula

There are three steps necessary to calculate the proper dose of dopamine to administer to the patient. These are:

1. Calculate the concentration of dopamine in the IV fluid.
2. Calculate the patient's weight in kilograms.
3. Calculate the dose to administer to the patient.

To calculate the pediatric dose you need to know:

- C = Concentration of dopamine in the IV fluid
- W = Patient's weight in kilograms
- T = Time of the infusion in minutes
- D = Desired dose
- H = Have dopamine
- Q = Quantity of fluid
- X = Dose to administer to patient

The dopamine formula is:

- H ÷ Q = C
- W lb ÷ 2.2 lb = W
- D × W × T ÷ C = X

Example: The healthcare provider ordered dopamine 3 mcg/kg/min. The patient weighs 165 pounds. The pharmacy delivers dopamine 400 mg in 250 D5W.

1. First, calculate the concentration of dopamine in the IV fluid.

   Since the medication order is in micrograms and the dopamine is in milligrams, you need to convert milligrams to micrograms.

$$400 \text{ mg} \times 1000 = 400,000 \text{ mcg}$$
$$400,000 \text{ mcg} / 250 \text{ ml} = 1600 \text{ mcg}$$
$$1600 \text{ mcg} = C$$

2. Second, convert the patient's weight to kilograms.

$$165 \text{ lb} / 2.2 \text{ lb} = 75 \text{ kg}$$

3. Third, calculate the dose to administer to the patient.

$$(3 \text{ mcg} \times 75 \text{ kg} \times 60 \text{ min}) / 1600 \text{ mcg} = X$$
$$(255 \text{ mcg} \times 60 \text{ min}) / 1600 \text{ mcg} = X$$

$$13,500 \text{ mcg} / 1600 \text{ mcg} = 8.437 \text{ ml/hr} = 8 \text{ ml/hr}$$
$$8 \text{ ml/hr} = X$$

Solved Problems

Calculating the Desired Dose

7.1 The healthcare provider ordered Gentamicin 1.50 mg PO qd. The pharmacy delivers Gentamicin 0.75 mg/2 tablet. How many tablets should be administered to the patient?

$$(1.5 \text{ mg} / 0.75 \text{ mg}) \times 1 \text{ tablet} = 2 \text{ tablets}$$

7.2 The medication order is for Motrin 0.8 g and the pharmacy delivered Motrin 400 mg per tablet. How many tablets will you administer to the patient?

$$0.8 \text{ g} \times 1000 = 800 \text{ mg}$$
$$400 \text{ mg} / 800 \text{ mg} = 0.5 \text{ tablet}$$

7.3 The healthcare provider ordered Capoten 3 mg PO q8h. The pharmacy delivers Capoten 6 mg/1 tablet. How many tablets would you administer to the patient?

$$3 \text{ mg} / 6 \text{ mg} = 0.5 \text{ tablet}$$

7.4 The medication order is for Decadron 2 mg and the pharmacy delivered Decadron 0.5 mg per tablet. What dose would you administer to the patient?

$$2 \text{ mg} / 0.5 \text{ mg} = 4 \text{ tablets}$$

7.5 The healthcare provider ordered GoLYTELY 1 gallon PO qd. The patient has a 12 ounce cup available at home. How many cups of GoLYTELY should the patient take?

$$1 \text{ gallon} = 128 \text{ ounces}$$
$$128 \text{ ounces} / 12 \text{ ounces} = 11 \text{ cups}$$

Calculating the IV Flow Rate

7.6 The healthcare provider ordered Gentamicin 4 gm diluted in 200 ml of Normal Saline IV over 2 hours. Use tubing with a 10 gtt/ml drip factor. What is the drip rate?

$$2 \text{ hrs} \times 60 \text{ minutes} = 120 \text{ minutes}$$
$$200 \text{ ml} \times 10 \text{ gtt} / 120 \text{ minutes} = 16.6 \text{ gtt/minute} = 17 \text{ gtt/minute}$$

7.7 The healthcare provider ordered 50 ml Normal Saline IV over 30 minutes. Use tubing with a 10 gtt/ml drip factor. What is the drip rate?

$$50 \text{ ml} \times 10 \text{ gtt} / 30 \text{ minutes} = 16.6 \text{ gtt/minute} = 17 \text{ gtt/minute}$$

Calculating the Weight Based Dose

7.8 The healthcare provider ordered Ampicillin 20 mg per kilogram. The patient weighs 157 lb. The medication label reads 50 mg per 1 milliliter. What dose will you administer to your patient?

$$157 \text{ lb} / 2.2 \text{ lb} = 71.363 \text{ kg}$$
$$((20 \text{ mg} \times 71.363 \text{ kg}) / 50 \text{ mg}) \times 1 \text{ ml} = 28.5 \text{ ml}$$

7.9   The healthcare provider ordered Zofran 140 mg/kg/day q8h. The patient weighs 77 lb. The pharmacy delivers Zofran 250 mg/1 ml. How many milliliters per dose will you administer to the patient?

$$77 \text{ lb} / 2.2 \text{ lb} = 35 \text{ kg}$$
$$24 \text{ hr} / 8 \text{ hr} = 3 \text{ doses per day}$$
$$((140 \text{ mg} \times 35 \text{ kg}) / 250 \text{ mg}) \times 1 \text{ ml} = 19.6 \text{ ml per day}$$
$$19.6 \text{ ml} / 3 \text{ doses} = 6.5 \text{ ml per dose}$$

7.10   The healthcare provider ordered Zovirax 2 mg/kg/day q12h. The patient weighs 160 lb. The pharmacy delivers Zovirax 50 mg/1 tablet. How many tablets per dose will you administer to the patient?

$$160 \text{ lb} / 2.2 \text{ lb} = 72.73 \text{ kg}$$
$$24 \text{ hr} / 12 \text{ hr} = 2 \text{ doses per day}$$
$$((2 \text{ mg} \times 60 \text{ kg}) / 50 \text{ mg}) \times 1 \text{ tablet} = 3 \text{ tablets per day}$$
$$3 \text{ tablets} / 2 \text{ doses} = 1\tfrac{1}{2} \text{ tablets per dose}$$

7.11   The healthcare provider ordered Benadryl 35 mg/kg/day q12h. The patient weighs 82 lb. The pharmacy delivers Benadryl 250 mg/10 ml. How many milliliters per dose will you administer to the patient?

$$82 \text{ lb} / 2.2 \text{ lb} = 37.272 \text{ kg}$$
$$24 \text{ hr} / 12 \text{ hr} = 2 \text{ doses per day}$$
$$((35 \text{ mg} \times 37.272 \text{ kg}) / 250 \text{ mg}) \times 10 \text{ ml} = 52.18 \text{ ml per day}$$
$$52.18 \text{ ml} / 2 \text{ doses} = 26 \text{ ml per dose}$$

7.12   The healthcare provider ordered Dilantin 60 mg/kg/day q4h. Your patient weighs 130 lb. The pharmacy delivers Dilantin 125 mg/1 ml. How many milliliters per dose will you administer to your patient?

$$130 \text{ lb} / 2.2 \text{ lb} = 59.1 \text{ kg}$$
$$24 \text{ hr} / 4 \text{ hr} = 6 \text{ doses per day}$$
$$((60 \text{ mg} \times 59.1 \text{ kg}) / 125 \text{ mg}) \times 1 \text{ ml} = 28.368 \text{ ml per day}$$
$$28.368 \text{ ml} / 6 \text{ doses} = 4.7 \text{ ml per dose}$$

7.13   The healthcare provider ordered Cleocin 20 mg per kilogram per day q6h. The patient weighs 125 lb. The medication label reads 175 mg per 5 milliliters. What dose will you administer to the patient?

$$125 \text{ lb} / 2.2 \text{ lb} = 56.818 \text{ kg}$$
$$24 \text{ hr} / 6 \text{ hr} = 4 \text{ doses per day}$$
$$((20 \text{ mg} \times 56.818 \text{ kg}) / 175 \text{ mg}) \times 5 \text{ ml} = 32.467 \text{ ml per day}$$
$$32.467 \text{ ml} / 4 \text{ doses} = 8.1 \text{ ml per dose}$$

7.14   The healthcare provider ordered Lithostat 5 mg/kg. The patient weighs 150 lb. The pharmacy delivers Lithostat 150 mg/1 tablet. How many tablets will you administer to the patient?

$$150 \text{ lb} / 2.2 \text{ lb} = 68.181 \text{ kg}$$
$$((5 \text{ mg} \times 68.181 \text{ kg}) / 150 \text{ mg}) \times 1 \text{ tablet} = 2 \text{ tablets}$$

7.15   The healthcare provider ordered Ampicillin 25 mg/kg/day q8/h. The patient weighs 65 lb. The pharmacy delivers Ampicillin 125 mg/1 ml. How many milliliters per dose will you administer to the patient?

$$65 \text{ lb} / 2.2 \text{ lb} = 29.545 \text{ kg}$$
$$24 \text{ hr} / 8 \text{ hr} = 3 \text{ doses per day}$$
$$((25 \text{ mg} \times 29.545 \text{ kg}) / 125 \text{ mg}) \times 1 \text{ ml} = 5.909 \text{ ml per day}$$
$$5.909 \text{ ml} / 3 \text{ doses} = 1.97 \text{ ml per dose} = 2 \text{ ml per dose}$$

7.16 The healthcare provider ordered Benylin 15 mg/kg. The patient weighs 30 lb. The pharmacy delivers Benylin 50 mg/1 tablet. How many tablets will you administer to the patient?

$$30 \text{ lb} / 2.2 \text{ lb} = 13.636 \text{ kg}$$
$$((15 \text{ mg} \times 13.636 \text{ kg}) / 50 \text{ mg}) (1 \text{ tablet} = 4 \text{ tablets})$$

Calculating the Heparin Dose

7.17 The healthcare provider ordered heparin 4000 U SC. The pharmacy delivers 20,000 U heparin per 150 ml. How many milliliters will you administer to the patient?

$$20,000 \text{ U} / 150 \text{ ml} = 133.33 \text{ concentration}$$
$$4000 \text{ U} / 133.33 = 30 \text{ ml}$$

7.18 The healthcare provider ordered heparin 6000 U SC. The medication label reads 20,000 U heparin per 100 ml. How many milliliters will you administer to the patient per hour?

$$20,000 \text{ U} / 100 \text{ ml} = 200 \text{ concentration}$$
$$6000 \text{ U} / 200 = 30 \text{ ml}$$

7.19 The healthcare provider ordered heparin 3500 U SC. The pharmacy delivers 25,000 U heparin per 200 ml. How many milliliters will you administer to the patient?

$$25,000 \text{ U} / 200 \text{ ml} = 125 \text{ concentration}$$
$$3500 \text{ U} / 125 = 28 \text{ ml}$$

7.20 The healthcare provider ordered heparin 800 U per hour. The pharmacy delivers 20,000 U heparin in 2000 ml normal saline. How many milliliters will you administer to the patient per hour?

$$20,000 \text{ U} / 2000 \text{ ml} = 10 \text{ concentration}$$
$$800 \text{ U} / 10 = 80 \text{ ml}$$

7.21 The healthcare provider ordered heparin 800 U SC. The pharmacy delivers 25,000 U heparin per 500 ml. How many milliliters will you administer to the patient?

$$20,000 \text{ U} / 500 \text{ ml} = 40 \text{ concentration}$$
$$800 \text{ U} / 40 = 20 \text{ ml}$$

Calculating the Dopamine Dose

7.22 The healthcare provider ordered dopamine 6 mcg per kg per min for a patient that weighs 150 lb. The pharmacy delivers dopamine 800 mg in 500 D5W. How many milliliters will you administer to the patient per hour?

$$150 \text{ lb} / 2.2 \text{ lb} = 68.181 \text{ kg}$$
$$800 \text{ mg} \times 1000 = 800,000 \text{ mcg}$$

$$800,000 / 500 = 1600 \text{ concentration}$$
$$(6 \text{ mcg} \times 68.181 \times 60 \text{ min}) / 1600 \text{ mcg} = 15.3 \text{ ml}$$

7.23 The healthcare provider ordered dopamine 12 mcg per kg per min for a patient that weighs 170 lb. The pharmacy delivers dopamine 800 mg in 500 D5W. How many milliliters per hour will set the infusion pump?

$$170 \text{ lb} / 2.2 \text{ lb} = 77.272 \text{ kg}$$
$$800 \text{ mg} \times 1000 = 800,000 \text{ mcg}$$
$$800,000 / 500 = 1600 \text{ concentration}$$
$$(12 \text{ mcg} (77.272 \times 60 \text{ min}) / 1600 \text{ mcg} = 34.8 \text{ ml}$$

7.24 The healthcare provider ordered dopamine 10 mcg per kg per min for a patient that weighs 85 lb. The pharmacy delivers dopamine 400 mg in 250 ml D5W. How many milliliters will you administer to the patient per hour?

$$85 \text{ lb} / 2.2 \text{ lb} = 38.636 \text{ kg}$$
$$400 \text{ mg} \times 1000 = 400,000 \text{ mcg}$$
$$400,000 / 250 = 1600 \text{ concentration}$$
$$(10 \text{ mcg} \times 38.636 \times 60 \text{ min}) / 1600 \text{ mcg} = 14.5 \text{ ml}$$

7.25 The healthcare provider ordered dopamine 10 mcg per kg per min for a patient that weighs 170 lb. The pharmacy delivers dopamine 800 mg in 500 D5W. How many milliliters will you administer to your patient per hour?

$$170 \text{ lb} / 2.2 \text{ lb} = 77.272 \text{ kg}$$
$$800 \text{ mg} \times 1000 = 800,000 \text{ mcg}$$
$$800,000 / 500 = 1600 \text{ concentration}$$
$$(10 \text{ mcg} \times 77.272 \times 60 \text{ min}) / 1600 \text{ mcg} = 29 \text{ ml}$$

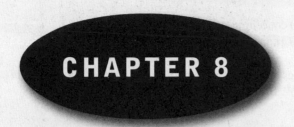

CHAPTER 8

Herbal Therapy

8.1   Understanding Herbal Therapy

Herbs are plants or parts of plants that have a proven therapeutic effect but are unregulated by the Food and Drug Administration. Herbs may be raw materials for pharmaceutical medication such as digitalis (from the foxglove herb), aspirin (from the salicin herb), and taxol (from the pacific yew tree).

Pharmaceutical medication is medication that is approved by the Food and Drug Administration and has proven guidelines for compounding and standards of purity. Herbal therapies lack these. Some healthcare providers, especially outside the United States, prescribe herbs as the first treatment of certain diseases.

Herbs are not typically prescribed in the United States. These reasons are:

- Healthcare insurance does not pay for herbal therapy.
- Herbal therapies are not patented, making them less attractive to the pharmaceutical industry.
- Few pharmacy schools offer courses in botanical remedies.
- Pharmaceutical courses focus more on misuse of herbal therapies than their therapeutic use.
- Herbal therapies lack quality standards.
- The Food and Drug Administration is not required to approve herbal therapies.

8.2   Lack of Uniform Information

There is a lack of uniformity of the information about the use, dosage, side effect, and contraindications of herbal therapies. Likewise there are not any qualitative monographs that provide guidelines for compounding and standards of purity, which are well defined for pharmaceutical medications.

The National Institute of Health, Office of Alternative Medicine is setting out to research herbal therapies and other alternative therapies. The United States Pharmacopeia (USP), the World Health Organization (WHO), and the American Herbal Pharmacopeia (AHP) are developing herbal therapeutic monographs.

8.3   Herbal Therapies and Patients

Increasingly, patients are using herbal therapies to treat their diseases. Many of these patients self-prescribe and self-medicate without advice from a healthcare provider. Although patients may receive the desired therapeutic effect of herbal therapies, patients are exposed to the following risks:

- Lack of standards for compounding, purity, and manufacturing cause a lack of uniformity of herbal products in the market.

- Herbal products may not be carefully measured.

- Doses may vary.

- Herbal therapy may be contraindicated when used with pharmaceutical medication taken by the patient.

- Herbal therapy may interact with other herbal therapies and pharmaceutical medication, causing an undesired side effect for the patient.

- Self-prescribed herbal therapies do not usually appear in the patient's medical records, risking the possibility that the healthcare provider will prescribe pharmaceutical medications that are contraindicated with the herbal therapy.

- Anyone can sell herbal therapies without approval from the government or medical community.

- There is a lack of oversight by regulatory authorities.

- There is a lack of backstop mechanism. Patients typically use the same pharmacy. The pharmacy's computerized records flag any potentially hazardous interaction with a prescription. A backstop mechanism usually is not in place for herbal therapies.

8.4   Forms of Herbal Therapies

After an herb is removed from the source of nutrition, enzyme activities begin to decay the herb immediately. The enzyme action is slowed by drying the herb to remove moisture. Therapeutic material is extracted from the herb to produce a reliable dose by:

- Isolating the part that contains the therapeutic material
- Soaking the part in alcohol, water, olive oil, or vegetable oil

Herbal therapeutic materials can take a number of forms:

- Herbal Oils: Oils are made by soaking the therapeutic material in olive oil or vegetable oil and then heating the herb for an extended time. The oil concentrates the therapeutic material and extends its life if stored properly.

- Herbal Salves: Salves are semisolid fatty preparations such as balms, creams, and ointments. Salves are prepared similarly to herbal oils, except after the herb soaks in oil, melted wax is mixed with the oil. The balm, cream, and ointment are then formed, as when wax cools and hardens.

- Herbal Teas: Teas are made by soaking fresh or dried herbs in boiling water. Tea is formed when the herb blends with the water. Herbal tea is refrigerated and used as a drink or bath water, or used on the skin.

- Herbal Tinctures: Tinctures are liquid extracts of the herb. Tinctures contain ingredients that do not dissolve in water. Tinctures are made by soaking fresh or dried herbs in alcohol, causing their water- and fat-soluble components to concentrate. Alcohol is used to preserve the herbal concentrate for 1 year. Water is used for people who do not consume alcohol.

- Herbal Capsules: Capsules contain dried, pulverized powder of the therapeutic material. Some herbal capsules contain oil, soaked herbals, or herbal juices.

- Herbal Tablets: Tablets are dried, pulverized therapeutic material that is combined with stabilizers and binders and compressed into a tablet. A stabilizer assures that the herb retains its therapeutic effect. A binder acts like glue to hold together the powdery mixture and stabilizer.

- Herbal Syrups: Syrups are made by drying the herb and soaking it in water or oil and then adding a sweetener to the mix. The sweetener is usually honey or sugar mixture heated until syrup forms.

8.5   Hazards of Herbal Therapeutics

Herbal therapies expose patients to potential hazards. Common hazards are:

- Toxicity occurs when the herbal therapies cascara and senna (laxatives) are taken with digoxin (which treats irregular heart rhythm).
- Toxicity occurs when the herbal therapies juniper and dandelion (diuretics causing increased urination) are taken with lithium (a psychiatric medication).
- Liver damage occurs when herbal therapy comfrey (which relieves swelling from abrasions and sprains) is used internally as an expectorant
- Palpitations might occur with ephedra herbal therapy (which offers an energy boost and weight loss). Ephedra, known as ma huang, contains ephedrine and pseudoephedrine, a stimulant that causes bronchodilation

8.6   Herbal Therapy and the Nursing Process

An assessment must be made to determine if the patient is undergoing herbal therapy. Ask the patient about herbs. If the patient seems knowledgeable about it, then assume that the patient might have undertaken herbal therapy with or without direction from a healthcare professional.

Determine which herbal therapies the patient is employing, the reason for taking them, and the brand of herbs being used. (Some packages employ their own standards.)

- Dosage
- Frequency
- Side effects

Ask the patient what over-the-counter medication she or he has been taking. (Over-the-counter medications are typically not found in the patient's medication records.)

Assess whether the patient's current condition is a side effect of herbal therapy:

- Altered nutritional balance
- Nausea, diarrhea, headache, and fatigue
- Toxic effect from interactions with prescribed medications
- Rash

Ways to intervene:

- Monitor the patient's response to conventional and herbal therapy, looking for adverse side effects.
- Consult with dietitians and other healthcare specialists to assure that the patient's nutrition remains balanced.
- Tell the patient to notify the healthcare provider if she or he changes herbal brand.
- Explain the rationale for herbal therapy.
- Tell the patient to notify the healthcare provider if the patient plans to substitute herbals for conventional therapies.
- Tell the patient to read the labels of herbal containers, over-the-counter medications, and prescribed medications to assure that there are no contraindications.
- Explain the optimal storage for the herbal remedy.
- Explain about foods that increase or decrease the action of herbs.
- Explain foods to avoid.
- Explain the potential side effects of herbs.

- Explain symptoms to report immediately to the healthcare provider.
- Explain the correct preparation for use of herbals.
- Explain that herbs are a medicine that is less potent than conventional medication.
- Explain that some medications act faster when combined with herbal therapy.
- Explain that it is important to note the scientific name of the herb, the manufacturer's contact information, and the batch and lot number of the package.

8.7 Avoiding Common Herbal Therapy Errors

- Do not take if you are pregnant or trying to become pregnant.
- Do not take if you are breast feeding.
- Do not give to babies or young children.
- Do not take large quantities.
- Do not stop prescribed medication before contacting your healthcare provider.
- Do not delay seeking healthcare if you experience adverse symptoms.
- Keep herbs away from children.
- Buy herbs where the plant and quantities are listed on the package.
- Use fresh herbs.
- Remember that herbals are not miracle cures.
- Do not use expired herbs. (Herbs have a short half-life.)

8.8 Common Herbal Therapies

- Aloe Vera (Aloe barbadensis): Aloe vera juice treats minor burns, insect bites, and sunburn, and is a powerful laxative when taken internally. In small doses, it increases menstrual flow.
- Chamomile (Matricaria recutita): Chamomile is dried flower heads used in herbal tea for relief of digestive and gastrointestinal (GI) disruptions and infant colic. Chamomile has a sedative effect. Chamomile can cause hives and bronchoconstriction in patients who are allergic to daisy or ragweed.
- Cinnamon: Cinnamon reduces blood sugar levels and increases the natural production of insulin. Cinnamon lowers blood cholesterol.
- Dong Quai (Angelica sinensis): Dong quai is used for menstrual cramps and to regulate the menstrual cycle. Dong quai can cause fever and excessive menstrual bleeding. Experts suggest avoiding using dong quai.
- Echinacea (Echinacea angustifolia): Echinacea enhances immunity by increasing white blood cells, activating granulocytes, and increasing cells in the spleen. The Echinacea leaf combats respiratory and urinary infections and is used to treat snakebite. The Echinacea root is used to treat flu symptoms. Patients with autoimmune disease and abnormal T-cell functions should avoid Echinacea. Patients who take Echinacea should do so for 8 weeks. Do not stop taking Echinacea after 1 week.
- Garlic (Allium sativum): Garlic lowers cholesterol and triglyceride levels, decreases blood pressure, and reduces the clotting capability of blood. Garlic is an antibiotic for internal and external treatment of infections and wounds. Warm garlic oil is used to treat earaches.
- Ginger (Zingiber): Ginger increases the effectiveness of the immune system and is used to treat stomach and digestive disorders, including motion sickness. Ginger relieves nausea and pain, swelling, and stiffness from osteoarthritis and rheumatoid arthritis.
- Ginkgo (Ginkgo biloba): Ginkgo dilates cerebral arteries and increases the uptake of oxygen and glucose. Ginkgo is used to treat dementia syndromes, intermittent claudication (decreased circulation in the legs), vertigo (dizziness), and tinnitus (ringing in the ears). Ginkgo improves cognition

(thinking) and may be helpful treating Alzheimer's disease, early stroke, and Raynaud's phenomenon (circulatory disorder). Patients who take Ginkgo may experience headache and GI disturbance.

- Ginseng (Panax ginseng): Ginseng is taken for short-term relief of stress and as an energy boost. Ginseng improves digestion. Ginseng may overstimulate chronic inflammatory conditions such as arthritis.
- Kava kava (Piper methysticum): Kava kava root promotes sleep and relaxes muscles. Kava kava tea combats urinary tract infections. Kava kava can be used with herbs such as valerian and St. John's Wort for anxiety.
- Licorice (Glycyrrhiza glabra): Licorice has physiological effects similar to aldosterone (antihypertensive) and corticosteroids (antiinflammatory).
- Peppermint (menthe piperita): Peppermint stimulates appetite, aids in digestion, and treats bowel disorders when taken internally. Hot peppermint tea stimulates circulation, reduces fever, clears congestion, and helps restore energy. Peppermint is used to treat tension headache when rubbed on the forehead and is as effective as extra-strength Tylenol in relieving headache.
- Psyllium (Plantago): The psyllium seed is a laxative and treats hemorrhoids, colitis, Crohn's disease, and irritable bowel syndrome.
- Sage (Salvia officinalis): Sage dry leaves heal wounds. Sage tea (from leaves) soothes a sore throat when gargled. Sage dries breast milk and reduces hot flashes.
- St. John's Wort (Hypericum perforatum): St. John's wort, known as herbal Prozac, treats depression, anxiety, and psychogenic disturbance similar to monoamine oxidase (MAO). Patients who use St. John's Wort do not have to avoid tyramine-rich foods, which is the case with patients who take MAO. St. John's Wort is a dietary supplement.
- Saw palmetto (Serenoa repens): Saw palmetto relieves symptoms of benign prostatic hypertrophy (enlarged prostate) and other urinary conditions. Saw palmetto is an expectorant and treats for colds, asthma, bronchitis, and thyroid deficiency.
- Valerian (Valeriana officinalis): Valerian is a mild sedative and induces sleep similar to benzodiazepines (Benadryl). Valerian has an odor of "dirty socks," reducing the risk for an overdose. Valerian may lead to habituation and addiction.
- Yarrow (Achillea millefolium): Yarrow stops bleeding wounds and is used for healing. Yarrow reduces pain and heavy bleeding resulting from menstrual irregularities and helps to regulate the menstrual cycle. Yarrow enhances circulation, lowers blood pressure, and has an antispasmodic, antimicrobial effect and antiinflammatory effect on skin and on mucous membranes. Dermatitis (skin rash) is a common side effect of using yarrow. Yarrow should not be used for patients who have epilepsy or during pregnancy.

Solved Problems

Nature of Herbal Therapies

8.1   Name three reasons why herbal therapies are not prescribed in the United States.

Healthcare insurance does not pay for herbal therapy, herbal therapies lack quality standards, and pharmaceutical courses focus more on misuse of herbal therapies than on their therapeutic use.

8.2   What information is lacking about herbal therapies?

There is a lack of uniform information about the use, dosage, side effect, and contraindications of herbal therapies, and there are not any qualitative monographs.

8.3   What is the purpose of a qualitative monograph?

A qualitative monograph provides guidelines for compounding and standards of purity of a medication.

8.4   What government agency or medical association is responsible for approving herbal therapies?

No approval by a government agency or medical association is necessary for herbal therapies.

Risk of Herbal Therapies

8.5   Name three risks of herbal therapies.

The dose may vary; herbal therapy may be contraindicated for combination with pharmaceutical medication taken by the patient; and the lack of standards for compounding, purity, and manufacturing causes a deficiency of uniformity of herbal products on the market.

8.6   What is a backstop mechanism for herbal therapy?

Patients typically use the same pharmacy. A backstop mechanism is the pharmacy's computerized records, which flag any potentially hazardous interaction with a prescription. A backstop mechanism is not in place for herbal therapies.

8.7   Why is it risky that herbal therapies do not usually appear in a patient's medical record?

Self-prescribed herbal therapies do not usually appear in the patient's medical records, creating a risk that the healthcare provider will prescribe pharmaceutical medication that is contraindicated with the herbal therapy.

Forms of Herbal Therapies

8.8   What is the advantage of herbal oil?

The advantage of herbal oil is that the oil concentrates the therapeutic material and extends its life if stored properly.

8.9   How are herbal salves made?

Salves are semisolid fatty preparations such as balms, creams, and ointments. Salves are prepared similar to herbal oils except after the herb soaks in oil, melted wax is mixed with the oil. The balm, cream, and ointment are formed when the wax cools and hardens.

8.10   How is herbal tea used?

Tea is made by soaking fresh or dried herbs in boiling water. Tea is formed when the herb blends with the water. Herbal tea is refrigerated and used as a drink, bath water, or used on the skin.

8.11   What is inside an herbal capsule?

Capsules contain dried, pulverized powder of the therapeutic material. Some herbal capsules contain oil, soaked herbals, or herbal juices.

8.12   What components are used to make an herbal tablet?

Tablets are dried, pulverized therapeutic material that is combined with stabilizers and binders and compressed into a tablet.

8.13   What is a stabilizer?

A stabilizer is a substance that assures that the herb retains its therapeutic effect.

8.14   What is a binder?

A binder acts like glue to hold together the powdery mixture and stabilizer.

8.15   What is used to sweeten herbal syrup?

The sweetener is usually honey or sugar mixture heated until a syrup forms.

Types of Herbal Therapies

8.16   What is the therapeutic effect of don quai?

Dong Quai is used for menstrual cramps and to regulate the menstrual cycle.

8.17   What is the adverse effect of don quai?

Dong quai can cause fever and excessive menstrual bleeding. Experts suggest avoiding using don quai.

8.18   What is the therapeutic effect of chamomile?

Chamomile is dried flower heads used in herbal tea for relief of digestive and GI disruptions and infant colic. Chamomile has a sedative effect.

8.19   What is the therapeutic effect of garlic?

Garlic lowers cholesterol and triglyceride levels, decreases blood pressure, and reduces clotting capability of blood. Garlic is an antibiotic for internal and external treatment of infections and wounds. Warm garlic oil is used to treat earaches.

8.20   What is the therapeutic effect of ginger?

Ginger increases the effectiveness of the immune system and is used to treat stomach and digestive disorders, including motion sickness. Ginger relieves nausea and relieves pain, swelling, and stiffness from osteoarthritis and rheumatoid arthritis.

8.21   What is the adverse effect of ginseng?

Ginseng may overstimulate chronic inflammatory conditions such as arthritis.

Assessing Herbal Therapies

8.22   What makes you suspicious that a patient is undergoing herbal therapy?

The patient seems knowledgeable about herbal therapies.

8.23   Why should a patient use one brand of herbs?

The manufacturer of the brand might employ their own standards for preparing and packing herbs.

8.24   What should you ask once the patient reports undergoing herbal therapy?

Ask the patient what over-the-counter medication she or he has been taking. (Over-the-counter medications are typically not found in the patient's medication records.)

8.25   Name three side effects of herbal therapy that might appear in a patient who is undergoing herbal therapy.

Three side effects of herbal therapy that might appear in a patient who is undergoing herbal therapy are altered nutritional balance, nausea, and fatigue.

8.26   Name one thing should you do to reduce the herbal therapy risk for a patient.

Tell the patient to read labels of herbal containers, over-the-counter medications, and prescribed medications to assure that there are no contraindications.

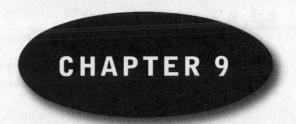

CHAPTER 9

Vitamins and Minerals

9.1 Vitamins

Vitamins are organic chemicals found in food required for metabolic activities for tissue growth and healing. A small quantity of vitamins is provided by a well-balanced diet and is adequate for normal health. A larger quantity of vitamins, more than what can be supplied by a well-balanced diet, is necessary if the patient is undergoing rapid growth, is pregnant, or has a debilitating illness. These patients require vitamin supplements.

A vitamin deficiency occurs when there is an insufficient quantity of vitamins for metabolism, such as when the patient's intake of vitamins is less than that required for his or her metabolism. Patients such as alcoholics and elderly people may not have a well-balanced diet or have difficulty absorbing food. Patients who have conditions that increase metabolism may use up their vitamin supply quicker than they can absorb food.

Conditions that increase metabolism are:

- Infection
- Fever
- Diarrhea
- Inflammatory diseases
- Cancer
- Inability to use vitamins
- Hemodialysis
- Hyperthyroidism
- Surgery
- Fad diets
- Pregnant women
- Growing children
- Athletics

9.2 A Well-Balanced Diet

A well-balanced diet contains the proper quantity of vitamins and minerals for a healthy life. The United States Department of Agriculture (USDA) defines a well-balanced diet with a guideline presented as a food pyramid. The food pyramid is organized into five color-coded groups, each with a general recommendation. These are:

- Grains: Three ounces of whole grain bread, rice, cereal, crackers, or pasta every day (orange)
- Vegetables: Eat more dark green vegetables, orange vegetables, beans, and peas (green)
- Fruits: Fresh, frozen, dry, or canned fruit. Drink fruit juices sparingly. (red)
- Milk: Calcium rich foods. Choose lactose-free products. (blue)
- Meat and beans: Low-fat and lean meat and poultry. Bake, broil, or grill. Eat more fish, beans, peas, nuts, and seeds. (purple)

The USDA's web site (http://www.mypyramid.gov/pyramid/index.html) calculates portions for each group based on a person's age, gender, and the amount of exercise he or she performs daily.

9.3 Recommended Dietary Allowance

The recommended dietary allowance (RDA) specifies the daily dose for each vitamin along with food sources that contain the vitamin. Table 9.1 contains the recommended dietary allowance as published by the USDA and the National Academy of Sciences Food and Nutrition Board (http://www.iom.edu).

9.4 Fat-Soluble Vitamins

Fat-soluble vitamins are absorbed by the intestinal tract using the same mechanism that absorbs fat. Conditions that interfere with fat absorption interfere with fat-soluble vitamin absorption. Fat-soluble vitamins are stored in the liver, fatty tissues, and muscle, and are excreted in urine. They remain in the body longer than water-soluble vitamins.

Vitamin A (Acon, Aquasol)

Vitamin A is used for treatment of acne and other skin disorders. It helps to maintain epithelial tissue, eyes, hair, and bone growth. Excess vitamin A causes a toxic effect. Vitamin A is stored in the liver for up to 2 years and can result in inadvertent toxicity. Vitamin A–caused birth defects can occur if greater than 6000 international units (IU) are taken during the pregnancy.

VITAMIN A	
Dose for deficiency	100,000–500,000 IU daily × 3 d; then 50,000 IU × 14 d
Maintenance	10,000–20,000 IU q.d. × 60 d
Pregnancy category	A; PB: UK; $t_{1/2}$: weeks–months
Deficiency conditions	Treats vitamin A deficiency, prevents night blindness, treats skin disorders, promotes bone development
Side effects	Headache, fatigue, drowsiness, irritability, anorexia, vomiting, diarrhea, dry skin, visual changes
Adverse reactions	Evident only with toxicity; leucopenia, aplastic anemia, papilledema, increased intracranial pressure, hypervitaminosis A (loss of hair and peeling skin)
Contraindications	Mineral oil, cholestyramine, alcohol, and antilipemic drugs decrease the absorption of A. It is excreted through urine and feces.

TABLE 9.1 RDA Recommended Dietary Allowances

VITAMIN	FOOD SOURCES	RDA
Fat-soluble		
A	Whole milk, butter, eggs, leafy green and yellow vegetables and fruits, liver	Male: 1000 mcg or 5000 IU Female: 800 mcg or 4000 IU Preg: 1000 mcg; 5000 IU Lactating: 1200 mcg; 6000 IU
D	Fortified milk, egg, yolk, tuna, salmon	Male and female: 40–80 mcg; mcg 200–400 IU
E	Whole grain cereals, wheat germ, vegetable oils, lettuce, sunflower seeds	Male: 10 mg/d; 15 IU Female: 8 mg/d; 12 IU Preg: 10–12 mg/d
K	Leafy green vegetables, liver, cheese, egg yolk	Male: 70–80 mcg/d Female: 60–65 mcg/d Taking broad-spectrum antibiotics: 140 mcg/d Preg: 65 mcg/d
Water-Soluble		
C Ascorbic acid	Citrus fruits, tomatoes, leafy green vegetables, potatoes	Male and female: 60 mg/d Preg: 70 mg/dl Lact: 95 mg/dl
B_1 Thiamine	Enriched breads and cereals, yeast, liver, pork, fish, milk	Male: 1.5 mg Female: 1.1 mg Preg: 1.5 mg Lact: 1.6 mg
B_2 Riboflavin	Milk, enriched breads and cereals, liver, lean meat, eggs, leafy green vegetables	Male: 1.4–1.7 mg Female: 1.2–1.3 mg Preg: 1.6 mg Lact 1.8 mg
B_3 Niacin	Eggs, meat, liver, beans, peas, enriched bread and cereals	Male and female: 15–20 mg
B_6 Pyridoxine	Lean meat, leafy green vegetables, whole grain cereals, yeast, bananas	Male: 15–19 mg/d Female: 13–15 mg/d Preg: 18 mg/d Lact: 20 mg/d
B_{12}	Liver, kidney, fish, milk	Male and female: 3 mcg/d Preg: 4 mcg/d
Folic acid	Leafy green vegetables, yellow fruits and vegetables, yeast, meat	Male and female: 400 mcg/d Preg: 600–800 mcg/d Lact: 600–800 3 mcg/d

Vitamin D

Vitamin D, with aid from bile salts, is absorbed in the small intestine and excreted in bile, feces, and minimally in urine. Vitamin D is needed to absorb and metabolize calcium and phosphorus. The liver converts vitamin D into the inactive form of calcifediol. The kidneys convert the inactive form of calcifediol to the active form of calcifediol. The active form of calcifediol combines with the parathyroid hormone (PTH) and calcitonin to regulate calcium and phosphorus metabolism by causing the reabsorption of calcium and phosphorus by bone. A low serum calcium level causes increased usage of vitamin D.

There are two forms of vitamin D:

- D$_2$ (ergocalciferol): This is a synthetically fortified form of vitamin D.
- D$_3$ (cholecalciferol): This is the natural form of vitamin D produced in the skin by ultraviolet sunlight.

VITAMIN D	
Dose for deficiency	Mild deficiency: 50–125 mcg/dL
	Moderate to severe: 2.5–7.5 mg/d; 2500–7500 mcg
Maintenance	Male and female: 40–80 mcg; 200–400 IU
Pregnancy category	A
Deficiency conditions	Rickets, deficit of phosphorus and calcium in blood
Side effects	None significant
Adverse reactions	Excess of 40,000 IU results in hypervitaminosis D and may cause hypercalcemia (an elevated serum calcium level). Early symptoms of toxicity are anorexia, nausea, and vomiting.
Contraindications	Hypercalcemia, hypervitaminosis D, or renal osteodystrophy with hyperphosphatemia. Use with caution in patients with arteriosclerosis, hyperphosphatemia, hypersensitivity to vitamin D, and renal or cardiac impairment.

Vitamin E

Vitamin E protects oxidation of the heart, arteries, and cellular components. It prevents hemolysis (rupture) of red blood cells. Vitamin E is absorbed in the GI tract and stored in all tissues, especially in the liver, muscle, and fatty tissues. Most excess vitamin E is excreted in bile and feces, and the rest in urine.

VITAMIN E	
Dose for deficiency	Malabsorption: 30–100 mg/d
	Severe deficit: 1–2 mg/kg/d or 50–200 IU/kg/d
Maintenance	Male: 10 mg/d; 15 IU
	Female: 8 mg/d; 12 IU
	Preg: 10–12 mg/d
Pregnancy category	A (C if used in doses greater than RDA)
Deficiency conditions	Breakdown of red blood cells
Side effects	None significant
Adverse reactions	Large doses may cause fatigue, weakness, nausea, GI upset, headache, and breast tenderness, and may prolong the prothrombin time (PT; clotting time)
Contraindications	Patients taking warfarin (anticoagulant) should have their PT monitored closely. Iron and E should not be taken together because iron can interfere with the body's absorption and use of vitamin E.

Vitamin K

Vitamin K is used to synthesize prothrombin and clotting factors VII, IX, and X, and is an antidote for oral overdose of anticoagulant. Vitamin K is in leafy green vegetables, liver, cheese, and egg yolk, and is synthesized by intestinal flora.

There are four forms of vitamin K:

- K_1 (phytonadione): The active form of vitamin K. Requires bile salts to be absorbed. Prevents hemorrhage. Available as Mephyton, AquaMEPHYTON, and Konakion.
- K_2 (menaquinone): Synthesized by intestinal flora. Requires bile salts to be absorbed.
- K_3 (menadione): Commercially synthesized. Does not require bile salts to be absorbed.
- K_4 (menadiol): Commercially synthesized. Does not require bile salts to be absorbed. Available as Synkayvite.

VITAMIN K

Dose for deficiency	5–15 mg/d (based on PT laboratory results)
Maintenance	Male: 70–80 mcg/d
	Female: 60–65 mcg/d
	If taking a broad-spectrum antibiotic: 140 mcg/d
	Pregnancy: 65 mcg/d
Pregnancy category	C
Deficiency conditions	Increased clotting time leading to increased bleeding and hemorrhage
Side effects	Occasional pain, soreness and swelling at IM injection site; pruritic erythema (itchy redness) with repeated injections; flushed face, unusual taste
Adverse reactions	Rare: Severe reaction immediately following IV administration (cramplike pain; chest pain, dyspnea, facial flushing, dizziness, rapid/weak pulse, rash, profuse sweating, hypotension; may progress to shock, cardiac arrest)
Contraindications	Last few weeks of pregnancy and in neonates; Use with caution: asthma and impaired hepatic function

Hint: Remember fat-soluble vitamins as: addict spelled ADEK.

9.5   Water-Soluble Vitamins

Water-soluble vitamins are absorbed in water in the small intestine and excreted in urine, except for folic acid. They are not stored in the body; therefore, the body requires a continuous supply of water-soluble vitamins.

Vitamin C

Vitamin C is used to metabolize carbohydrates, for tissue repair and capillary endothelium, and for synthesis of protein, lipids, and collagen. Vitamin C is also needed for absorption of iron and folic acid metabolism. Vitamin C is found in citrus fruits, tomatoes, leafy green vegetables, and potatoes. Excess serum levels of vitamin C are excreted without any negative effects. Vitamin C is commercially available as Ascorbicap, Cecon, Cevalin, and SoluCap C.

VITAMIN C

Dose for deficiency	Adult per day is 50 to 100 mg. Severe deficit (scurvy) PO: IM: IV: 150–500 mg/d in one to two divided doses. 500–6000 mg/day for treatment of upper respiratory infections, cancer, or hypercholesterolemia
Maintenance	45–60 mg/d
Pregnancy category	C
Deficiency conditions	Prevents and treats C deficiency (scurvy); increases wound healing; for burns; sickle cell crisis; deep vein thrombosis. Megavitamin therapy (massive doses) of vitamins is not recommended; it can cause toxicity.

Side effects	Headaches, fatigue, drowsiness, nausea, heartburn, vomiting, diarrhea. Vitamin C with aspirin or sulfonamides may cause crystal formation in the urine (crystalluria); and can also cause a false negative occult (blood) stool result and false positive sugar result in the urine when tested by the Clinitest method.
Adverse reactions	Kidney stones, crystalluria, hyperuricemia. Massive doses can cause diarrhea and GI upset.
Contraindications	Large doses can decrease the effect of oral anticoagulants; oral contraceptives can decrease C concentration in the body; smoking decreases serum levels of C. Use with caution in renal calculi (kidney stones); gout, anemia, sickle cell, sideroblastic, and thalassemia.
Drug–lab–food interactions	Decreased ascorbic acid uptake when taken with salicylates; may decrease effect of oral anticoagulants; may decrease elimination of aspirins.

Vitamin B Complex

Vitamin B complex consists of four vitamins:

- B_1 (thiamine): Treats peripheral neuritis from alcoholism or beriberi
- B_2 (riboflavin): Treats scaly dermatitis, cracked corners of the mouth, inflammation of the skin and tongue, and dermatologic problems
- B_3 (niacin): Treats pellagra (dietary deficiency of niacin) and hyperlipidemia. Can cause GI irritation and vasodilatation results in a flushing sensation
- B_6 (pyridoxine): Treats symptoms of neuritis causes by isoniazid (INH) therapy for tuberculosis

VITAMIN B COMPLEX

Dose for deficiency	Thiamine: 30–60 mg/d
	Riboflavin: 5–25 mg/d
	Prophylactic: 3 mg/d
	Nicotinic acid or niacin: Prevention: 5–20 mg/d
	Deficit: 50–100 mg/d
	Pellagra: 300–500 mg in three divided doses
	Hyperlipidemia: 1–2 g/d in three divided doses
	Pyridoxine: 25–100 mg/d
	Isoniazid therapy prophylaxis: 25–20 mg/d *Peripheral neuritis*: 50–200 mg/d
Maintenance	Thiamine:
	Male 1.5 mg
	Female 1.1 mg
	Pregnancy 1.5 mg
	Lactation 1.6 mg
	Riboflavin:
	Male 1.4–1.7 mg
	Female 1.2–1.3 mg
	Pregnancy 1.6 mg
	Lactation 1.8 mg
	Nicotinic acid or niacin:
	Male 15–19 mg/d
	Female 13–15 mg/d
	Pregnancy 18 mg/d

	Lactation 20 mg/d
	Pyridoxine:
	Male 2.0 mg/d
	Female 1.6 mg/d
	Pregnancy 2.1 mg/d
	Lactation 2.2 mg/d
Pregnancy category	A (C if dose is more than RDA)
Deficiency conditions	Thiamine-sensory disturbances, retarded growth, fatigue, anorexia
	Riboflavin-visual defects, such as blurred vision and photophobia, cheilosis, rash on nose; numbness of extremities
	Niacin or nicotinic acid–retarded growth, pellagra, headache, memory loss, anorexia, insomnia
	Pyridoxine-neuritis, convulsions, dermatitis, anemia, lymphopenia
Side effects	Thiamine: Rate skin rash, pruritus, or wheezing after a large IV dose
	Riboflavin: Orange-yellow discoloration in urine
	Niacin or nicotinic acid-flushing, pruritus, feelings of warmth; high doses: dizziness, arrhythmias, dry skin, hyperglycemia, myalgia, nausea, vomiting, diarrhea
	Pyridoxine: Occasional: Stinging at IM injection site; Rare: headache, nausea, somnolence; high doses cause sensory neuropathy (paresthesia, unstable gait, clumsiness of hands)
Adverse reactions	Thiamine: Rare anaphylaxis after a large IV dose
	Riboflavin: None known
	Niacin or nicotinic acid: Cardiac arrhythmias may occur rarely
	Pyridoxine: Long-term megadoses may produce sensory neuropathy
Contraindications	Thiamine: Patients with renal dysfunction
	Riboflavin: Patients with renal dysfunction
	Niacin or nicotinic acid: Hypersensitivity to niacin or tartrazine; active peptic ulcer, severe hypotension, hepatic dysfunction, arterial hemorrhaging. *Caution:* Diabetes mellitus, gallbladder disease, gout, history of jaundice or liver disease.
	Pyridoxine: IV therapy in cardiac patients; *Caution:* Mega dosage in pregnancy

Folic Acid (Folate, Vitamin B$_9$)

Folic acid is needed for cell growth and DNA synthesis. Folate is the active form of folic acid. One third is stored in the liver; the rest is stored in other tissues. Folic acid is excreted in bile and a small amount in urine. Folic acid deficiency occurs when there is disruption of the small intestine's absorption ability, resulting in disruption of cell growth. Poor nutrition, chronic alcoholism, and pregnancy can also lead to folic acid deficiency. After 2 to 4 months of folic acid deficiency the patient will exhibit nausea, diarrhea, anorexia, fatigue, stomatitis, alopecia, and blood dyscrasias (megaloblastic anemia, leucopenia, and thrombocytopenia). Folic acid is found in yeast, meat, leafy green vegetables, and yellow fruits and vegetables.

FOLIC ACID	
Dose	1–2 mg/d
Maintenance	Male and female 400 mcg/d
	Pregnancy 600–800 mcg/d
	Lactating 600–800 mcg/d

Pregnancy category	A (C if > RDA)
Deficiency conditions	Decreased white blood cell (WBC) count and clotting factors, anemias, intestinal disturbances, depression; may decrease the risk of colon cancer
Side effects	None significant
Adverse reactions	High doses of folic acid can mask signs of B_{12} deficiency, which is a risk in elderly people. Patients taking phenytoin (Dilantin) for seizures should be cautious about taking folic acid because it can increase the risk of seizures.
	During the first trimester of pregnancy, folic acid deficiency can affect the development of the central nervous system (CNS) of the fetus; this can lead to neural tube defects (NTDs) such as spina bifida, a defective closure of the bony structure of the spinal cord, or anencephaly, lack of brain mass formation
Contraindications	Pernicious, aplastic, normocytic, refractory anemias

Vitamin B_{12}

Vitamin B_{12} is needed for cell growth, DNA synthesis, hematopoiesis (developing red blood cells in bone marrow), maintenance of the nervous system's integrity, and to help convert folic acid into folate. Vitamin B_{12} requires the intrinsic factor produced by gastric parietal cells to be absorbed in the body. Vitamin B_{12} binds to the transcobalamin II protein and is then transferred to tissues. Vitamin B_{12} is stored for up to 3 years in the liver and is excreted in urine. Vitamin B_{12} deficiency occurs in malabsorption syndromes (cancer, celiac disease, and certain drugs), gastrectomy, Crohn's disease, liver diseases, and kidney diseases. Vitamin B_{12} deficiency can also occur with patients who are on a strict vegetarian diet. Vitamin B_{12} is found in liver, kidney, fish, and fortified milk.

VITAMIN B_{12}	
Dose	100 mg/dl 14 d
	Pernicious anemia: 40–100 mcg/d or 1000 mcg/wk × 3 wk
Maintenance	Male and female: 3 mcg/d
	Pregnancy: 4 mcg/d
Pregnancy category	A (C if use doses > RDA)
Deficiency conditions	Pernicious anemia, deficiency caused by inadequate diet or intestinal malabsorption, hemolytic anemia, hyperthyroidism, bowel and pancreatic malignancies, gastrectomy, GI lesions, neurologic damage, malabsorption syndrome, metabolic disorders, renal disease
Side effects	Occasional: diarrhea, itching
Adverse reactions	Rare allergic reaction; may produce peripheral vascular thrombosis, pulmonary edema, hypokalemia, congestive heart failure
Contraindications	History of allergy to cobalamin; folate-deficient anemia, hereditary optic nerve atrophy

9.6   Vitamins and Assessment

Before administering vitamin therapy, the patient must be assessed for:

- Vitamin deficiency: Vitamin therapy can result in toxicity if the patient does not have a vitamin deficiency.
- Debilitating disease and GI disorders: The patient must be able to absorb, metabolize, and excrete vitamins used in vitamin therapy.

- Cause of the vitamin deficiency: Inadequate nutrient intake is a common cause for vitamin deficiency. Educate the patient on the importance of maintaining a balanced diet.

9.7   Vitamins and Vitamin Supplements

Develop a plan that provides the patient with an adequate supply of vitamins. In addition to a well-balanced diet, the patient might be prescribed vitamin supplements. Remember that:

- Vitamin supplements are administered with food to promote absorption.
- Vitamin supplements should be stored in light-resistant containers.
- Liquid vitamin supplements are administered using a calibrated dropper.
- Vitamin supplements are administered via intramuscular injection if the patient is unable to take by mouth.

9.8   Vitamins and Teaching

Teaching the patient the importance of vitamins lowers the risk that he or she will develop a vitamin deficiency. The patient can go to the USDA web site (http://www.mypyramid.gov/pyramid/index.html) to calculate a well-balanced diet for his or her age, gender, and the amount of exercise performed daily.

The patient should be taught to:

- Take the prescribed amount of the vitamin.
- Read the label on containers before purchasing or ingesting vitamins, and especially note the expiration date.
- Missing vitamins for a few days is not a cause for concern.
- Do not take megavitamins over a prolonged time.
- Do not take vitamin A with mineral oil because it interferes with the absorption of vitamin A.
- Vitamin C does not cure a cold.
- Do not take megadoses of vitamin C with aspirin or sulfonamides.
- Excessive alcohol can cause vitamin B–complex deficiencies.
- Call the healthcare provider if you experience nausea, vomiting, headache, loss of hair, and cracked lips. These might be signs and symptoms of hypervitaminosis A—too much vitamin A.
- Call the healthcare provider if you experience anorexia, nausea, and vomiting. These might be signs and symptoms of hypervitaminosis D—too much vitamin D.

9.9   Minerals

Minerals are inorganic compounds extracted from meats, eggs, vegetables, and fruits that form bones, teeth, and are used for metabolism.

Iron (Ferrous Sulfate, Gluconate, or Fumarate)

Iron is used to regenerate hemoglobin. Iron is absorbed in the intestine and enters plasma as heme. Iron is stored as ferritin in the liver, spleen, and bone marrow. Five to twenty milligrams of iron are required daily. Iron deficiency causes anemia. Iron is found in liver, lean meats, egg yolks, dried beans, green vegetables (i.e., spinach), and fruit. Women who are pregnant should increase their iron intake as specified by the healthcare provider. Large doses of iron are prescribed in the second and third trimesters. The patient must adhere to the prescribed dose in the first trimester to avoid birth defects. Iron supplements are recommended for patients who are unable to intake iron sufficiently through diet. Iron supplements should be taken with food to avoid GI discomfort. Iron absorption is substantially decreased if taken with antacids, tetracycline (antibiotic), and food. Vitamin C increases iron absorption. Iron toxicity can occur in children if 10 or more ferrous sulfate (3-g) tablets are taken at one time. Death can occur in 12 hours.

IRON

Dose	Adult 50 mg/day
	Infant and child dose of iron, ages 6 months to 2 years old is 1.5/mg/kg.
	Ferrous sulfate for therapeutic use 600–1200 mg/day in divided doses
Maintenance	Ferrous sulfate for prophylactic use is 300–325 mg/day
Pregnancy category	A; PB = UKt$_{1/2}$: UK
Treatment	Given to correct or control iron-deficiency anemia
Side effects	GI discomfort, nausea, vomiting, diarrhea, constipation, epigastric pain. Elixir may stain teeth.
Adverse reactions	Pallor, drowsiness. Life-threatening: cardiovascular collapse, metabolic acidosis
Contraindications	Avoid a megadose in the first trimester because it might cause birth defects.

Copper

Copper helps form red blood cells and connective tissues. Copper is a cofactor enzyme that initiates metabolic reactions in the body. Copper is necessary to produce norepinephrine and dopamine (neurotransmitters). Copper is absorbed in the intestine. Foods rich in copper are shellfish (crabs and oysters), liver, nuts, seeds (sunflower, sesame), legumes, and cocoa. Copper deficiency results in anemia, causes decreased hair and skin pigmentation, decreased white blood count, intolerance to glucose, and mental retardation in young patients. Excess serum levels of copper indicate Wilson's disease, which results in the accumulation of copper in the liver, brain, cornea, and kidney.

COPPER

Dose	1.5–3 mg/day
Maintenance	1.5–3 mg/day
Pregnancy category	A (C if > RDA dose)
Deficiency conditions	Anemia, decreased WBCs, glucose intolerance, decreased skin and hair pigmentation, and mental retardation in the young
Side effects	None significant
Adverse reactions	Vomiting and diarrhea
Contraindications	None known

Zinc

Zinc helps in wound healing and maintaining taste and smell. Zinc stimulates enzymes involved in the production of insulin, sperm, DNA synthesis, and the immune system. Zinc supplements larger than 150 mg can result in decreased high-density lipoprotein (HDL) cholesterol *and* copper deficiency, and can weaken the immune response. Zinc supplements should not be taken with antibiotics because it inhibits tetracycline (antibiotic) absorption. Wait 2 hours after taking any antibiotic before taking zinc.

ZINC

Dose	12–19 mg/day
Maintenance	12–19 mg/day
Pregnancy category	A (C if taken in doses > RDA)
Deficiency conditions	Growth retardation, diarrhea, vomiting, delay in puberty, weakness, dry skin,

	delay in wound healing
Side effects	None known
Adverse reactions	Anemia, increased LDL cholesterol, muscle pain, fever, nausea, vomiting
Contraindications	Do not take with tetracycline.

Chromium

Chromium is involved in controlling non–insulin-dependent diabetes by increasing the effects of insulin on cells. Chromium is in meat, whole grain cereals, and brewer's yeast.

CHROMIUM	
Dose	50–200 mcg/d considered within the normal range for anyone >6 years of age. (There is no RDA.)
Maintenance	50–200 mcg/d is considered within the normal range for anyone >6 years of age. (There is no RDA.)
Pregnancy category	A
Deficiency conditions	Inability to properly use glucose
Side effects	None known
Adverse reactions	May cause hypoglycemic reaction in patients who are taking insulin or an oral hypoglycemic agent
Contraindications	Monitor blood glucose levels in diabetic patients

Selenium

Selenium is a cofactor for antioxidant enzymes that protects protein and nucleic acids from damage caused by oxidation. Selenium might have an anticarcinogenic (anticancer) effect and may reduce the risk of lung, prostate, and colorectal cancer in a dose greater than 200 mcg. However, this dose can cause weakness, loss of hair, dermatitis, nausea, diarrhea, and abdominal pain. Selenium is found in meats (especially liver), seafood, eggs, and dairy products.

SELENIUM	
Dose	40–75 mcg (high doses for males and lower doses for females)
Maintenance	40–75 mcg (high doses for males and lower dose for females)
Pregnancy category	A
Deficiency conditions	Heart disease
Side effects	Causes a garliclike odor from the skin and breath in large doses
Adverse reactions	Disorders of nervous system and digestive system and loss of hair with doses >200 mcg
Contraindications	None known

Solved Problems

Vitamins

9.1　What are vitamins?

Vitamins are organic chemicals found in food that are required for metabolic activities for tissue growth and healing.

9.2 What is a vitamin deficiency?

A vitamin deficiency occurs when there is an insufficient quantity of vitamins for metabolism and the patient's intake of vitamins is less than that required for metabolism.

9.3 Name three causes of vitamin deficiency.

Three causes of vitamin deficiency are malnutrition, increased metabolism, and decreased absorption.

9.4 What is a well-balanced diet?

The USDA defines a well-balanced diet with a guideline that is presented as a food pyramid.

9.5 Is a well-balanced diet the same for everyone?

A well-balanced diet is based on a person's age, gender, and amount of exercise performed daily.

9.6 What is a recommended dietary allowance (RDA)?

The RDA specifies the daily dose for each vitamin along with food sources that contain that vitamin.

9.7 What are sources of vitamin D?

The sources of vitamin D are fortified milk, egg, yolk, tuna, and salmon.

9.8 What form of vitamin K is synthesized by intestinal flora?

The form of vitamin K that is synthesized by intestinal flora is K_2 (menaquinone).

9.9 What are sources for ascorbic acid?

The sources for ascorbic acid are citrus fruits, tomatoes, leafy green vegetables, and potatoes.

9.10 What are fat-soluble vitamins?

Fat-soluble vitamins are vitamins that are absorbed by the intestinal tract using the same mechanism that absorbs fat.

9.11 Name the fat-soluble vitamins.

The fat-soluble vitamins are vitamin A, vitamin D, vitamin E, and vitamin K.

9.12 What is does vitamin E do?

Vitamin E protects the oxidation of the heart, arteries, and cellular components. It prevents hemolysis (rupture) of red blood cells.

9.13 What vitamin helps metabolize calcium and phosphorus?

Vitamin D helps metabolize calcium and phosphorus.

9.14 What is the natural form of vitamin D?

D_3 (cholecalciferol) is the natural form of vitamin D and is produced in the skin by ultraviolet sunlight.

9.15 What does vitamin K do?

Vitamin K is used to synthesize prothrombin and clotting factors VII, IX, and X and is an antidote for oral overdose of anticoagulant.

9.16 What are sources of vitamin K?

Vitamin K is in leafy green vegetables, liver, cheese, and egg yolk and is synthesized by intestinal flora.

9.17 Name the water-soluble vitamins.

The water-soluble vitamins are vitamin C, vitamin B complex, folic acid, and vitamin B_{12}.

9.18 What does folic acid do?

Folic acid is needed for cell growth and DNA synthesis.

9.19 How are vitamin supplements handled?

Vitamin supplements are administered with food to promote absorption, are stored in light-resistant containers, and are administered (liquid) using a calibrated dropper.

9.20 What can excessive alcohol cause?

Excessive alcohol can cause vitamin B–complex deficiencies.

Minerals

9.21 What is a mineral?

Minerals are inorganic compounds that form bones and teeth, and are used for metabolism.

9.22 What are sources of minerals?

The sources of minerals are meats, eggs, vegetables, and fruits.

9.23 How should pregnant women adjust their iron intake?

Pregnant women should increase their iron intake as specified by the healthcare provider. Large doses of iron are prescribed in the second and third trimesters. The patient must adhere to the prescribed dose in the first trimester to avoid birth defects.

9.24 What is the effect of vitamin C on iron?

Vitamin C increases iron absorption.

9.25 What does zinc do?

Zinc helps in wound healing and maintaining taste and smell.

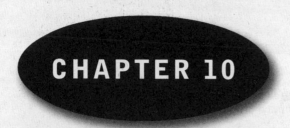

CHAPTER 10

Fluid and Electrolyte Therapy

10.1   Body Fluids

The majority of body fluid is water. Water is a solvent that transports solutes (salts, nutrients, and wastes) throughout the body. Body fluids are stored in compartments:

- Intracellular (ICF): Intracellular is inside cells and consists of 40% of body weight
- Extracellular (ECF): Extracellular is outside cells and consists of 20% of body weight. Extracellular has subcompartments:
  - Interstitial space: Space between cells, including lymph fluid
  - Transcellular fluid: Fluid in the gastrointestinal (GI) tract, cerebrospinal space, aqueous humor, pleural space, synovial space, and the peritoneal space
  - Plasma fluid
  - Bone and connective tissues fluid

10.2   Electrolytes

An electrolyte is a salt that splits into ions when placed into water. An ion is an electrically charged particle that is either positively or negatively charged. A positively charged ion is called a cation and a negatively charged ion is called an anion.

- Cations: Sodium (Na^+), potassium (K^+), calcium (Ca^{2+}), and magnesium (Mg^{2+}) are electrolytes that are cations
- Anion: Chloride (Cl^-), bicarbonate (HCO_3^-), phosphate (PO_4^-), and sulfate (SO_4^-)

An electrolyte is stored intracellularly (inside the cell) or extracellularly (outside the cell).

- Intracellular electrolytes are potassium, magnesium, and some calcium.
- Extracellular electrolytes are sodium and some calcium.

An electrolyte is measured as a millimole per liter (mmol/L). A millimole is the atomic weight of the electrolyte in milligrams. For example, the atomic weight of sodium is 23 milligrams. Therefore, 23 milligrams of sodium is measured as 1 mmol of sodium.

10.3   Fluid Movement

Fluid moves into and out of cells by osmotic pressure. Osmotic pressure is pressure exerted by the flow of water through a semipermeable membrane, separating two solutions with different concentrations of solute.

Osmotic pressure is determined by the concentration of the electrolytes and other solutes in water. A higher concentration outside the cell causes electrolytes to move inside the cell. A lower concentration outside the cell causes electrolytes to move outside the cell.

Osmotic pressure is expressed as osmolarity or osmolality. Osmolality is the concentration of body fluids. Tonicity is the effect bodily fluid has on cellular volume and is used to measure the concentration of intravenous solutions. Serum osmolality instead of tonicity is used to indicate the concentration of solutes in body fluids.

10.4   Fluid Concentration

Concentration determines the replacement fluid for a patient whose fluids and electrolytes are imbalanced. Replacement fluids are replaced orally (by mouth or nasogastric tube) or parenterally with IV fluids (intravenously or subcutaneously).

There are three types of fluid concentration:

- Iso-osmolar: A fluid is the same concentration of particles of solute as water: Osmolality of 275 to 295 mOsm/dg.
- Hypo-osmolar: A fluid is a lower concentration of particles of solute than water. Osmolality less than 275 mOsm/dg.
- Hyper-osmolar: A fluid is a higher concentration of particles of solute than water. Osmolality greater than 295 mOsm/dg.

10.5   Intravenous Fluids

IV fluids are defined by osmolality:

- Isotonic: The concentration is the same as concentration of intracellular fluid (iso-osmolar range 240 to 340 mOsm/L).
- Hypotonic: The concentration is less than the concentration of intracellular fluid (hypo-osmolar range less than 240 mOsm/L). Moves fluid from extracellular space into inside cells.
- Hypertonic: The concentration is more than the concentration of intracellular fluid (hyper-osmolar range greater than 340 mOsm/L). Moves fluid from inside cells into extracellular space.

10.6   Classification of Intravenous Solutions

- Crystalloids: Crystalloids are replacement and maintenance fluid therapy. These include dextrose, saline, and lactated Ringer's solutions.
- Colloids: Colloids are volume expanders that increase the patient's fluid volume. These are:
  - Dextran: Increases fluid volume, but does not carry oxygen and interferes with platelet function, which results in prolonged bleeding times.
  - Amino acids: Provide protein, calories, and fluid and are administered to patients who have hypoproteinemia.
  - Hetastarch: Treats or prevents shock and is administered when blood is not available. This too is not a substitute for whole blood. Decreases platelet and hematocrit counts when in an isotonic solution. Not used for patients who have bleeding disorders, congestive heart failure (CHF), and renal dysfunction.

- ○ Plasmanate: Contains protein and fluid. Treats shock where there is a loss of plasma, but not a loss of red blood cells. Not administered to patients who have anemia, increased blood volume, or CHF.
- Lipids: Lipids are a fat emulsion used to provide essential fatty acids for prolonged parenteral nutrition. Also used for IV therapy that extends longer than 5 days.

10.7   Blood and Blood Products

Blood and blood products are:

- Whole blood: Contains all blood products and is used to treat severe anemia
- Packed Red Blood Cells: Contain all blood products except plasma and are used to decrease circulatory overload and reduce the risk of reactions to antigens contained in plasma
- Plasma: Is the liquid component of blood and contains mostly water, proteins, glucose, minerals, hormones, and carbon dioxide
- Albumin: Is protein in blood

10.8   Fluid Replacement

Water is 30 ml/kg of body weight. A patient weighing 150 lb weighs 68 kg (150 lb/2.2 lb/kg) and has 2240 ml of water.

Each day the patient loses:

- 400 to 500 ml of water through evaporation from the skin
- 400 to 500 ml of water through breathing
- 100 to 200 ml of water in feces
- 1000 to 1200 ml of water in urine

A patient must take in 1900 to 2400 ml of fluid per day maintain fluid-electrolyte balance. Age and medical conditions influence the daily amount of water. Disease and its treatment increase water output, requiring an increased water intake. A fever causes the loss of 2185 to 2760 ml of water each day.

10.9   Replacing Fluid

When replacing fluid:

- Establish baseline vital signs.
- Establish baseline weight.
- Review hematocrit and BUN and report elevations.
  - ○ Elevated hematocrit and BUN indicates dehydration.
  - ○ Elevated BUN greater than 60 mg/kl indicates renal impairment.
- Measure urine output.
  - ○ Normal urine output is greater than 35 ml/h.
- Review urine specific gravity (SG).
  - ○ The normal range is 1.005 to 1.030.
  - ○ Greater than 1.030 indicates dehydration.
- Verify proper osmolality when IV fluids are ordered.
- Monitor fluid intake and output.

- Weigh the patient daily.
- Monitor for signs and symptoms of excess fluid volume.
  - Cough
  - Dyspnea (difficulty breathing)
  - Jugular vein distention (JVD) (neck vein engorgement = edema)
  - Moist rales (abnormal breath sounds)
- Monitor for signs and symptoms of fluid volume deficit (dehydration).
  - Thirst
  - Dry mucous membranes
  - Poor skin turgor
  - Decreased urine output
  - Tachycardia
  - Slight decrease in systolic blood pressure
- Monitor IV site for infiltration or phlebitis.
  - Not red
  - Not swollen
  - Not hot
  - Not hard

10.10 Risk of Replacing Fluid

The potential risks of replacing fluids are:

- Risk for fluid volume excess. Too much replacement fluid or fluid is infused too rapidly.
- Risk for fluid volume deficit. Not enough fluid is replaced.
- Altered tissue perfusion. Decreased blood circulation or inadequate fluid replacement reduces circulation to tissues.

10.11 Potassium

Potassium is an electrolyte (cation) inside cells and is used to transmit and conduct neuro-impulses and maintain cardiac rhythms. Potassium regulates intracellular osmolality. Potassium also promotes cell growth by moving into cells of new tissues and leaves cells during the breakdown of dead tissues. Potassium is used to contract skeletal and smooth muscles.

Muscles contract when potassium moves out the cell and is replaced by sodium (see 10.16 Sodium). Sodium is outside the cell. Potassium and sodium reverse positions to repolarize the muscle. The sodium-potassium pump located in cell membranes maintains the potassium and sodium balance. The sodium-potassium pump uses adenosine triphosphate (ATP) to pump potassium into the cell and sodium out of the cell.

Intake of potassium occurs from the diet. Potassium is excreted mostly in urine and some in feces. The normal serum potassium is 3.5 to 5.3 milliequivalents per liter (mEq/L). Serum potassium less than 2.5 mEq/L or greater than 7.0 mEq/L can cause cardiac arrest. Kidney disease causes serum potassium to be outside the normal range.

10.12 Hyperkalemia

Hyperkalemia is a serum potassium level greater than 5.3 mEq/L that can be caused by:

- Impaired renal excretion (most common)
- Massive intake of potassium

- Medication:
  - Potassium-sparing diuretics (Aldactone and Dyrenium)
  - Angiotensin-converting enzyme (ACE) inhibitors (Vasotec and Prinivil) reduce secretion of potassium by the kidneys.

Signs and symptoms of hyperkalemia are:

- Nausea
- Cold skin
- Grayish pallor skin
- Hypotension
- Confusion
- Irritability
- Abdominal cramps
- Oliguria (decreased urine output)
- Tachycardia, then bradycardia
- Muscle weakness leading to flaccid paralysis
- Numbness or tingling in the extremities
- ECG: Peaked T waves

10.13   Responding to Hyperkalemia

It is critical to reduce the potassium level quickly to avoid seizures and cardiac arrhythmias that can lead to death. You must:

- Restrict intake of potassium-rich foods.
- Administer diuretics and ion-exchange resins (Kayexalate [retention enema]) to increase the excretion of potassium.
- Remember that dialysis therapy excretes potassium.
- Remember that administering insulin and glucose parenterally forces potassium back inside cells.
- Remember that administering sodium bicarbonate intravenously corrects the acidosis (elevate pH).
- Remember that administering calcium gluconate intravenously decreases the irritability of the heart.

10.14   Hypokalemia

Hypokalemia is a serum potassium level less than 3.5 mEq/L caused by:

- Diarrhea
- Vomiting
- Fistulas
- Nasogastric suctioning
- Diuretics
- Hyperaldosteronism
- Magnesium depletion
- Diaphoresis
- Dialysis
- Increased insulin

- Alkalosis
- Stress (increases epinephrine)
- Starvation
- Low potassium in diet

Signs and symptoms of hypokalemia are:

- Leg cramps
- Muscle weakness
- Vomiting
- Fatigue
- Decreased reflexes
- Polyuria
- Irregular pulse
- Bradycardia

Abnormal ECG:

- Depressed ST segment
- Flattened T wave
- Presence of U wave
- Premature ventricular contractions

10.15   Responding to Hypokalemia

It is critical to increase the potassium level quickly to avoid cardiac arrhythmias that can lead to death. You must:

- Increase dietary intake of potassium—bananas, dried fruits, fruit juices, vegetables, or potassium supplements.
- Administer potassium chloride supplements (Table 10.1) orally with juice or water to reduce gastric irritation (onset takes 30 minutes).
- Remember that the central IV line is used for rapid infusion in critical conditions. Infuse less than 10 to 20 mEq per hour of 40 mEq/L added to 1000 ml of intravenous solution. It should not contain more than 60 mEq/L of potassium chloride (KCL). Monitor for pain at IV site. Call the healthcare provider if urine output is less than 30 ml/hour.
- Never administer potassium as an intravenous push or intravenous bolus. This causes immediate cardiac arrest that cannot be reversed with CPR.
- Do not give potassium to patients who have renal insufficiency, renal failure, or Addison's disease.
- Do not give potassium if the patient has hyperkalemia, severe dehydration, acidosis, or takes potassium-sparing diuretics.
- Administer potassium cautiously for cardiac or burn patients.

10.16   Sodium

Sodium is an electrolyte (cation) in extracellular fluid (tissue spaces and vessels) and regenerates and transmits nerve impulses. Sodium affects water distribution inside and outside cells. Sodium also combines readily in the body with chloride (CL) or bicarbonate (HCO_3) to promote acid-base balance (Ph).

TABLE 10.1 **Potassium Supplements**

POTASSIUM SUPPLEMENTS	DESCRIPTION
10% Potassium chloride	20 mEq/15 ml oral
20% Potassium chloride	40 mEq/16 ml oral
10% Kaochlor	Oral
Potassium triplex (potassium acetate, bicarbonate, citrate)	Oral rarely used
Kaon (potassium gluconate)	Enteric-coated tablet. Maintenance 20 mEq in one to two divided doses
Kaon-Cl (potassium chloride)	Enteric-coated tablet. Maintenance 20 mEq in one to two divided doses
Slow-K (potassium chloride)	Enteric-coated tablet. Maintenance 8 mEq
Kaochlor (potassium chloride)	Correction 40–80 mEq in three to four divided doses
K-Lyte (potassium bicarbonate)	Effervescent tablet. Correction 40–80 mEq in three to four divided doses
K-Lyte/Cl (potassium chloride)	Effervescent tablet. Correction 40–80 mEq in three to four divided doses
K-Dur (potassium chloride)	Effervescent tablet. Correction 40–80 mEq in three to four divided doses
Micro-K (potassium chloride)	Effervescent tablet. Correction 40–80 mEq in three to four divided doses
Potassium chloride	Clear liquid in multi-dose vial or ampule 2 mEq/ml
Potassium chloride	IV 20–40 mEq diluted in 1 L of IV solution

Muscles contract when sodium moves inside the cell, replacing potassium (see 10.11 Potassium). Sodium and potassium reverse positions to repolarize the muscle. The sodium-potassium pump located in cell membranes maintains the potassium and sodium balance.

Dietary sodium is absorbed in the GI tract. The sodium balance is regulated by the kidneys. When sodium concentration is low, urine is retained. When sodium concentration is high, then there is increased urine. Sodium is also excreted in perspiration and feces.

Sodium is measured in milliequivalents per liter (mEq/L). The normal range of serum sodium is 135 to 145 mEq/L. Sodium moves outside the normal range when there is too much or too little water or if there is a high or low concentration of sodium.

10.17 Hypernatremia

Hypernatremia occurs when serum sodium is greater than 145 mEq/L as a result of:

- Sodium concentration is increased and water volume is unchanged.
- Water volume is decreased and sodium concentration is unchanged.

The patient experiences hyperosmolality—a higher than normal concentration of sodium—causing water to shift out of cells and into extracellular space, resulting in cellular dehydration.

Hypernatremia is caused by:

- Inadequate water intake or dehydration
- Inability of the hypothalamus gland to synthesize antidiuretic hormone (ADH), which is required by the kidneys to regulate sodium.
- Inability of the pituitary gland to release ADH

- Nonresponse of the kidneys to ADH
- Diabetes insipidus
- Excess sodium intake

Signs and symptoms of hypernatremia are:

- Agitation
- Restlessness
- Weakness
- Seizures
- Twitching
- Confusion
- Coma
- Intense thirst
- Dry swollen tongue
- Edematous (swollen) extremities

10.18   Responding to Hypernatremia

It is critical to decrease the sodium level slowly to move water back into cells. Decreasing sodium quickly can result in cerebral edema (brain swelling). You must:

- Administer an IV of 5% dextrose in water or a hypotonic saline solution to replace water.
- Restrict sodium intake.
- Monitor weight.
- Assess extremities for edema (swelling).
- Monitor breath sounds and respiration for signs of heart failure.
- Avoid canned foods, lunch meats, ham, pork, pickles, potato chips, and pretzels.
- Avoid adding salt to foods.

10.19   Hyponatremia

Hyponatremia occurs when serum sodium is less than 135 mEq/L as a result of:

- Increased water volume, but sodium concentration is normal
- Loss of sodium, but water volume is normal

Hyponatremia is caused by:

- Profuse sweating
- Major trauma
- Surgery
- Excessive volume of water ingested
- Syndrome of inappropriate anti-diuretic hormone (SIADH), which causes water retention and sodium loss
- Addison's disease
- Diarrhea
- Vomiting

- Diuretics (loses water and salt)
- Burns
- Wound drainage

Signs and symptoms of hyponatremia are:

- Fatigue
- Headache
- Muscle cramps
- Nausea
- Seizures
- Coma

10.20   Responding to Hyponatremia

Increase the sodium level slowly. You must:

- Treat the underlying cause.
- Administer hypertonic saline solution IV such as 3% NaCl to restore the serum sodium level.
- Replace lost fluid.
- Monitor vital signs.
- Track fluid intake and output.
- Observe serum sodium levels.
- Monitor dietary sodium intake.
- Listen to breath sounds and take note of signs of respiratory distress.
- Advise against drinking excessive amounts of pure water on a hot day or after extreme exercise.
- Replace fluids orally with an electrolyte solution.

10.21   Calcium

Calcium is an electrolyte in extracellular fluid and intracellular fluid and assists in nerve impulse transmission, blood clotting, muscle contraction, and formation of teeth and bone. Calcium combines with phosphate in bone and albumin in serum.

Dietary sources of calcium are dairy products, eggs, green leafy vegetables, broccoli, legumes, nuts, and whole grains. (Less than 30% of calcium in food is absorbed.) Calcium is absorbed in the small intestine. The amount of absorption depends on the serum calcium level and availability of vitamin D. There is reduced absorption of calcium if there is a high serum calcium level or a low vitamin D level.

There are three forms of calcium in serum:

- Free ionized: This is the active form of calcium and is half the total calcium in the body.
- Protein bound: This is calcium that is bound to albumin.
- Complex: This is calcium combined with phosphate, citrate, or carbonate.

Serum calcium (all forms) ranges between 8.5 and 10.5 mg/dl. Serum ionized calcium is normally (4–5 mg/dl). Table 10.2 contains medication that increases and decreases serum calcium.

There is a balance between calcium and phosphorus. An increase in serum calcium decreases serum phosphorus. An increase in serum phosphorus decreases serum calcium.

The parathyroid hormone (PTH), calcitonin, and vitamin D regulate calcium.

TABLE 10.2 **Medications That Increase and Decrease Serum Calcium**

DECREASES SERUM CALCIUM	INCREASES SERUM CALCIUM
Magnesium sulfate	Calcium salts
Propylthiouracil (propacil)	Vitamin D
Colchicines	IV lipids
Pliamythin (Mithramycin)	Kayexalate androgens
Neomycin	Diuretics (thiazides, chlorthalidone [Hygroton]
Acetazolamide	
Aspirin	
Anticonvulsants	
Glutethimide (Doriden)	
Estrogens	
Aminoglycosides (gentamicin, amikacin, tobramycin)	
Phosphate preparations: oral, enema, and IV (sodium phosphate, potassium phosphate)	
Corticosteroids (cortisone, prednisone)	
Loop diuretics (furosemide [Lasix])	

Low serum calcium: PTH moves calcium from bone into serum and increases reabsorption of calcium by the kidneys. Absorption of calcium also occurs in the GI tract.

High serum calcium: Calcitonin (produced by the thyroid gland) causes bone to absorb serum calcium and increases urine to excrete calcium. The GI tract decreases the absorption of calcium.

10.22   Hypercalcemia

Hypercalcemia occurs when the serum calcium level is higher than 10.3 mg/dl and there is a low serum phosphorus level.

Hypercalcemia can be caused by:

- Renal failure
- Immobility
- Cancer
- Hyperparathyroidism
- Excess intake of calcium supplements (Tums)
- Excess use of antacids
- Prolonged diarrhea
- Excess use of diuretics

Signs and symptoms (may be asymptomatic) of hypercalcemia are:

- Nausea
- Vomiting
- Constipation
- Anorexia
- Abdominal pain
- Polyuria (frequent urination)

- Polydipsia (extreme thirst)
- Decreased memory
- Mood swings
- Confusion
- Depressed reflexes
- Muscular weakness
- Bone pain
- Fractures
- Kidney stones
- Hypertension
- Cardiac arrhythmias
- Coma

10.23   Responding to Hypercalcemia

High serum calcium level needs to be lowered quickly. You must:

- Treat the underlying causes.
- Verify normal kidney function.
- Administer isotonic saline IV for hydration (only if kidneys are functioning).
- Have the patient drink 3000 to 4000 ml of fluid to excrete the calcium in urine (only if kidneys are functioning).
- Administer furosemide (Lasix) or ethacrynic acid (Edecrin) loop diuretics after hydration (only if kidneys are functioning).
- Remember that hemodialysis lowers calcium levels (only if kidneys are not functioning).
- Remember that administering synthetic calcitonin lowers serum calcium.
- Remember that administering plicamycin (Mithracin) increases absorption of calcium in bone.
- Emphasize a low-calcium diet.
- Tell patient to perform weight-bearing activities.
- Protect the patient who experiences neuromuscular effects.

10.24   Hypocalcemia

Hypocalcemia occurs when the serum calcium level is lower than 8.5 mg/dl and there is a high serum phosphorus level. Fractures may occur because of demineralization (calcium loss from the bones).
    Hypocalcemia is caused by:

- Hypoparathyroidism
- Removal or injury to parathyroid gland
- Hypomagnesium associated with alcoholism
- Ingestion of phosphates
- Inadequate intake of dietary calcium or vitamin D

Signs and symptoms of hypocalcemia are:

- Depression
- Memory loss

- Confusion
- Hallucinations
- Numbness and tingling (face, mouth, hands, and feet)
- Muscle spasms (face, mouth, hands, and feet)
- Hyperreflexia
- Ventricular tachycardia

10.25   Responding to Hypocalcemia

Serum calcium level needs to be increased. You must:

- Use caution when replacing calcium. Calcium increases the action of digoxin, leading to cardiac arrest. There is also a risk for tetany and seizures.
- Administer dietary calcium (green leafy vegetables, fresh oysters, and milk products) up to 1500 mg/day.
- Administer vitamin D.
- Administer calcium PO in tablet, capsule, or powder form.
  - Calcium carbonate (Os-cal, Tums, Caltrate, Megacal): 650- to 1500-mg tablets
  - Calcium gluconate (Kalcinate): 500- to 1000-mg tablets
  - Calcium lactate: 325- to 650-mg tablets
  - Calcium citrate: 950-mg tablets
- Administer calcium IV
  - Calcium chloride IV: 10 ml
  - Calcium gluceptate: 5 ml
  - Calcium gluconate: 10 ml
  - Mix with 5% dextrose in water.
  - Do not mix with a saline solution. Sodium encourages the loss of calcium.
  - Monitor for tissue infiltration, which can cause tissue necrosis and sloughing.
  - Do not add calcium to bicarbonate or phosphorus because it precipitates form.
- Remember: no alcohol and caffeine. These inhibit calcium absorption.
- Advise the patient to exercise to decrease bone loss.
- Remember: Do not overuse antacids.
- Remember: Do not overuse laxatives.
- Advise an increase of fruits and fiber for bowel elimination.

10.26   Magnesium

Magnesium is an electrolyte (cation) in intracellular fluid and is considered a sister cation to potassium. A decrease in potassium means a decrease in magnesium. Magnesium is involved in metabolizing carbohydrates, protein, and nucleic acids and is associated with neuromuscular excitability. Nuts, whole grains, cornmeal, spinach, bananas, and oranges provide dietary magnesium.

Normal serum magnesium level is 1.5 to 2.5 mEq/L. Magnesium is absorbed in the GI tract and then excreted in urine. PTH (see 10.21 Calcium) influences the balance of magnesium.

10.27   Hypermagnesemia

Hypermagnesemia occurs when serum magnesium level is greater than 2.5 mEq/L because of excessive intake of magnesium salts contained in laxatives (magnesium sulfate, milk of magnesia, magnesium citrate) and antacids (Maalox, Mylanta, DiGel). Patients who take lithium are at risk for hypermagnesemia.

Signs and symptoms of hypermagnesemia are:

- Lethargy
- Drowsiness
- Weakness
- Paralysis
- Cardiac arrhythmias
- Heart block
- Loss of deep tendon reflexes
- Hypotension

Hint: Calcium gluconate is given in an emergency to reversal hypermagnesemia. This can cause hypomagnesemia.

10.28   Responding to Hypermagnesemia

The serum magnesium level needs to be decreased. You must:

- Withdraw magnesium supplements.
- Administer calcium gluconate IV. Calcium antagonizes the effect of magnesium.
- Administer diuretics IV (only if kidneys are functioning).
- Administer dialysis (only if kidneys are not functioning).

10.29   Hypomagnesemia

Hypomagnesemia occurs when the serum magnesium level is less than 1.5 mEq/L caused by long-term administration of saline infusions, diuretics, antibiotics, laxatives, and steroids. Hypomagnesemia increases the action of digitalis, resulting in digitalis toxicity.

Signs and symptoms of hypomagnesemia are:

- The patient may be asymptomatic until serum magnesium levels reach 1.0 mEq/L.
- Tremors
- Twitching of the face
- Ventricular tachycardia
- Ventricular fibrillation
- Hypertension
- Pregnancy-induced hypertension (toxemia)

10.30   Responding to Hypomagnesemia

Serum calcium level needs to be increased slowly; otherwise, there is a risk for cardiac arrest. You must:

- Administer intravenous magnesium sulfate on an infusion pump.
- Monitor signs of magnesium toxicity.
- Watch for hot flushed skin.
- Monitor anxiety.
- Watch for lethargy.
- Monitor hypotension.

- Watch for laryngeal stridor.
- Monitor ECG.
- Take seizure precautions.

10.31 Phosphorus

Phosphorus is an electrolyte (anion) in intracellular fluid that is converted by the body into phosphate. Phosphorus is involved in the function of red blood cells, muscles, the nervous system, acid-base buffering, and metabolizing carbohydrates, proteins, and fats. Phosphorus is mostly stored in bones, absorbed in the GI tract, and excreted in urine and a small amount in feces.

The normal range of serum phosphorus is 2.5 to 4.5 mg/dl. Phosphorus is regulated by PTH (see 10.21 Calcium) and the kidneys. As serum calcium level increases, serum phosphorus level decreases.

10.32 Hyperphosphatemia

Hyperphosphatemia occurs when the serum phosphorus level is greater than 4.5 mg/dl. This is caused by:

- Kidney disease
- Underactive parathyroid glands
- Acromegaly
- Rhabdomyolysis
- Healing fractures
- Untreated diabetic ketoacidosis
- Bone diseases
- Excess phosphate-containing laxatives
- Excess milk
- Chemotherapy for neoplastic disease
- Excess vitamin D
- Decrease in magnesium levels
- Increased phosphorus levels during the last trimester of pregnancy

Signs and symptoms of hyperphosphatemia are:

- Hyperreflexia
- Soft tissue calcification
- Nausea
- Vomiting
- Hypocalcemia
- Tachycardia
- Anorexia
- Tetany

10.33 Responding to Hyperphosphatemia

Serum phosphorus level needs to be decreased. You must:

- Treat the underlying cause.
- Take seizure precautions.
- Administer sevelamer (Renagel).

- Administer calcium supplements.
- Administer phosphorus-binding salts.
- Restrict foods high in phosphorus.

10.34   Hypophosphatemia

Hypophosphatemia occurs when serum phosphorus level is less than 2.5 mg/dl. This is caused by:

- Decreased serum magnesium
- Alcohol withdrawal
- Diabetic ketoacidosis
- Excess intake of carbohydrates
- Hyperventilation
- Severe dehydration

Signs and symptoms of hypophosphatemia are:

- Muscle weakness
- Rhabdomyolysis
- Confusion
- Osteomalacia
- Coma

10.35   Responding to Hypophosphatemia

The serum phosphorus level needs to be increased. You must:

- Administer phosphorus supplements (Neutra-Phos PO).
- Administer sodium phosphate IV.
- Administer potassium phosphate IV.
- Assess vital signs.
- Assess changes in mental status.
- Take seizure precautions.

Solved Problems

Body Fluids

10.1   What are the two general compartments where bodily fluids are stored?

Adminisfy The two general compartments where bodily fluids are stored are intracellular and extracellular.

10.2   What is the function of water in the body?

Water is a solvent that transports solutes (salts, nutrients, and wastes) throughout the body.

Electrolytes

10.3   What is an electrolyte?

An electrolyte is a salt that splits into ions when placed in water. An ion is an electrically charged particle that is either positively or negatively charged.

10.4   What electrolytes are stored inside the cell?

Intracellular electrolytes are potassium, magnesium, and some calcium.

10.5   How are electrolytes measured?

An electrolyte is measured as a millimole per liter (mmol/L). A millimole is the atomic weight of the electrolyte in milligrams. For example, the atomic weight of sodium is 23 milligrams. Therefore, 23 milligrams of sodium is measured as 1 mmol of sodium.

10.6   How does fluid move in and out of cells?

Fluid moves into and out of cells by osmotic pressure. Osmotic pressure is pressure exerted by the flow of water through a semipermeable membrane separating two solutions with different concentrations of solute.

10.7   How is osmotic pressure expressed?

Osmotic pressure is expressed as osmolarity or osmolality. Osmolality is the concentration of body fluids.

10.8   What is tonicity?

Tonicity is the effect bodily fluid has on cellular volume and is used to measure the concentration of intravenous solutions.

10.9   What is iso-osmolar?

Iso-osmolar is a fluid in the same concentration of particles of solute as water. Osmolality is 275 to 295 mOsm/dg.

10.10   What is hyper-osmolar?

Hyper-osmolar is a fluid in a higher concentration of particles of solute than water. Osmolality is greater than 295 mOsm/dg.

10.11   What is hypotonic IV fluid?

Hypotonic IV fluid occurs when the concentration is less than the concentration of intracellular fluid (hypo-osmolar range, less than 240 mOsm/L). It moves fluid from extracellular space into inside cells.

10.12   What are crystalloids?

Crystalloids are IV fluids used for replacement and maintenance of fluid therapy.

10.13   What is isotonic IV fluid?

Isotonic is IV fluid in which the concentration is the same as concentration of intracellular fluid. (Iso-osmolar range 240 to 340 mOsm/L.)

10.14   What are colloids?

Colloids are IV fluids used for volume expanders that increase the patient's fluid volume.

10.15 Name four colloids.

Four colloids are dextran, amino acids, hetastarch, and Plasmanate.

10.16 Why are lipids administered by IV?

Lipids are a fat emulsion used to provide essential fatty acids for prolonged parenteral nutrition. They are also used for IV therapy that extends longer than 5 days.

10.17 What is plasma?

Plasma is the liquid component of blood and contains mostly water, proteins, glucose, minerals, hormones, and carbon dioxide.

10.18 What is albumin?

Albumin is the protein in blood.

10.19 How much fluid per day must be taken in to maintain fluid-electrolyte balance?

A patient must take in 1900 to 2400 ml of fluid per day to maintain fluid-electrolyte balance.

10.20 What should be done before replacing fluids?

Before replacing fluids, make sure that the kidneys are properly functioning.

10.21 What causes the exchange of potassium and sodium?

The sodium-potassium pump located in cell membranes maintains the potassium and sodium balance.

10.22 What electrolyte affects water distribution inside and outside of the cells?

Sodium is the electrolyte that affects water distribution inside and outside of the cells.

10.23 Where is potassium and sodium when a muscle contracts?

When a muscle contracts, potassium is outside the cell and sodium is inside the cell.

10.24 What is the active form of calcium?

Free ionized is the active form of calcium and is half the total calcium in the body.

10.25 What regulates calcium?

The parathyroid hormone (PTH), calcitonin, and vitamin D regulate calcium.

10.26 Name one method to lower serum calcium.

One method to lower serum calcium is to administer synthetic calcitonin.

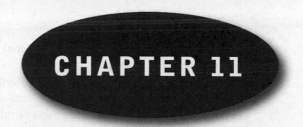

CHAPTER 11

Nutritional Support Therapies

11.1 Nutrition

Nutrition is the science that studies food composition and the way food is used by the body. Food consists of nutrients. A nutrient is a substance that is used by the body for energy and for cell growth, cell maintenance, and cell repair.

Nutrients are divided into two types:

1. Organic:
   a. Carbohydrates
   b. Fat
   c. Proteins
   d. Vitamins
2. Inorganic:
   a. Minerals
   b. Water
   c. Oxygen

11.2 Malnutrition

Malnutrition is a condition in which there are insufficient nutrients to sustain daily activities. Signs of malnutrition can appear 14 days after the patient no longer receives an adequate amount of nutrients. The patient becomes fatigued, irritable, and exhibits an abnormal appearance.

Malnutrition occurs as a result of a nutritional deficit. A nutritional deficit is the result of having a less than adequate amount of nutrients as a result of an unbalanced diet, surgery, trauma, malignancy, and other conditions that break down (catabolize) the body. A nutritional deficit prolongs healing and can prevent total recovery. A nutritional deficit is called a negative nitrogen balance. The patient lacks sufficient nitrogen to fight infectious disease.

11.3 Nutritional Support Therapy

Patients at risk for nutritional deficit are given nutritional support therapy to replace nutrients. Nutritional support therapy provides nutrients before there is a negative nitrogen balance to assure there is a positive nitrogen balance, enabling the patient to fight infectious diseases.

Nutrients are given by either the:

- *Enteral* route, in which food is administered by mouth or a feeding tube that is fed directly into the stomach or small intestine.
- *Parenteral* route, which provides high-calorie nutrients administered through large veins such as the subclavian vein. This process is called total parenteral nutrition (TPN) or hyperalimentation. Parenteral is expensive, has a high rate of infection, and does not promote GI function, liver function, or weight gain.

11.4   Enteral Nutrition Support Therapy

Enteral feeding is the preferred nutritional support therapy. The patient must have a functioning gastrointestinal (GI) tract function to digest, absorb, and excrete waste. GI motility and small bowel function must be established before beginning enteral feeding by listening to bowel sounds. If the GI tract is not functioning, then the patient may experience uncontrolled vomiting and aspiration.

Methods of enteral feeding are:

- Oral: Food is ingested naturally.
- Nasogastric tube: A tube is passed through the nose and down the esophagus, ending shortly below the xiphoid process in the stomach.
- Gastrostomy: A feeding tube is placed in a hole in the abdomen leading to the stomach.
- Nasoduodenal: A tube is passed through the nose and down the esophagus, ending in the duodenum
- Nasojejunal: A tube passed through the nose and down the esophagus, ending in the small intestine.
- Jejunostomy: A feeding tube placed in a hole in the abdomen, leading to the small intestine.

11.5   Group of Enteral Feeding Preparations

Preparation (Table 11.1) given to patients receiving enteral nutritional support therapy depends on the nutrient, caloric values, and osmolality that the patient requires. These preparations are grouped as:

- Blenderized: Liquids similar to prepared baby food based on the nutritional needs of the patient
- Polymeric:
  - Milk-based, powdered, mixed with milk or water, must be given in large amounts to provide complete nutritional requirements
  - Lactose-free, liquid for replacement feedings (Ensure, Isocal, and Osmolite), consisting of 50% carbohydrates, 15% protein, 15% fat, and 20% other nutrients in an isotonic solution (300–340 mOsm/kg H_2O). Provides 1 calorie per milliliter of feeding.
- Elemental (monomeric): Rapidly absorbed in the small intestines and used for partial GI tract dysfunction. Available in liquid and powder. More expensive enteral nutritional preparations.

11.6   Enteral Feeding Preparations

Enteral feeding preparation consists of:

- Carbohydrates: Simple sugars that are absorbed quickly in the form of dextrose, sucrose, and lactose. Starch and dextrin are also carbohydrates that may be included in the preparation.
- Protein: Protein is in the form of intact proteins, hydrolyzed proteins, or free amino acids.
- Fat: Fat is in the form of corn oil, soybean oil, or safflower oil.

TABLE 11.1 Commonly Used Preparations for Enteral Feeding

CATEGORY	MEDICATION	COMMENT
Blenderized	Compleat B (Sandox) Formula 2 (Cutter) Vitaneed (Sherwood)	Blended natural foods Ready to use
Polymeric milk-based	Meritene (Sandox) Instant Breakfast (Carnation) Sustacal Power (Mead Johnson)	Provides nutrient that are intact Pleasant tasting oral supplement
Lactose-free	Ensure, Jevity, Osmolite (Ross) Sustacal Liquid, Isocal, Ultracal (Mead Johnson) FiberSource, Resource (Sandox) Entrition, Nutren (Clinitek) Attain, Comply (Sherwood)	Used as oral supplement, tube feeding or meal replacement Ready to use Meets daily intake of vitamins and minerals
Elemental (monomeric) formulas	Vital HN (Ross) Vivonex T.E.N. (Sandox) Criticare HN (Mead Johnson) Travasorb (Clinitek) Peptamen (Clinitek) Reabilan (O'Brien)	Partially digested nutrients for feeding tube Required reconstitution except for Peptamen, Reabilan, and Criticare

Hint: Dextrose 5% in water (D5W), normal saline, and lactated Ringer's solution are not forms of nutrients. These are electrolytes and fluids.

11.7   Ways to Administer Enteral Feeding Preparations

Enteral feedings are administered as:

- Bolus: 250 to 400 ml rapidly administered four to six times each day. Each takes about 10 minutes. The patient may experience nausea, vomiting, aspiration, abdominal cramping, and diarrhea if the patient cannot tolerate the massive amount of solution given in a short time frame. Only use if the patient is ambulatory and relatively healthy.

- Intermittent drip or infusion: 300 to 400 ml given 3 to 6 hours over 30 to 60 minutes by gravity drip or infusion pump. This is an inexpensive way to administer enteral feedings.

- Continuous drip or cyclic infusion: 50 to 125 ml infused per hour at a slow rate over a 24-hour period using an infusion pump (Kangaroo set). Used for treating critically ill patients and patients who have a feeding tube in their small intestines.

11.8   Complications of Enteral Feeding

Enteral feedings complications are:

- Dehydration: Insufficient water is given or a hyperosmolar solution is given. Hyperosmolar solution draws water from the cells to maintain serum iso-osmolality (see 10.4 Fluid Concentration).

- Aspiration: When fed in a supine position or when the patient is unconscious. Prevent aspiration by raising the head of the bed 30 degrees and check for gastric residuals by gently aspirating the stomach contents before the next feeding.

- Diarrhea: Caused by
  - Rapid administration of feeding
  - High caloric solution
  - Malnutrition
  - GI bacteria (*Clostridium difficile*)
  - Antibiotics
  - Magnesium containing drugs such as antacids (Maalox) and sorbitol. Sorbitol is used as filler for certain drugs
  - Hyperosmolar fluid pulling water from the cells into the GI tract

Decreasing the infusion rate, diluting the solution, changing the solution, discontinuing the medication, or increasing daily water intake manage diarrhea.

11.9   Calculating Enteral Feedings

An enteral feeding is in a concentrated form and is diluted before being administered to the patient. There are three factors involved with dilution of enteral medication. These are:

1. Volume: There are two ways to calculate the volume of an eternal feeding.
   a. Method 1:

$$Desired\ Volume = (Desired\ dose\ /\ Dose\ On\ Hand) \cdot Volume\ On\ Hand$$

Example: The healthcare provider orders acetaminophen 650 mg, q6h, PRN for pain. You have on hand Acetaminophen elixir 65 mg/ml Average mOsm/kg = 5400.

$$Desired\ Volume = (650\ mg\ /\ 65\ mg) \times 1\ ml$$
$$Desired\ Volume = 10\ mg \times 1\ ml$$
$$Desired\ Volume = 10\ ml$$

   b. Method 2:

$$Dose\ On\ Hand : Volume\ On\ Hand = Desired\ Dose : Desired\ Volume$$

Example: Same as in Method 1

$$65\ mg : 1\ ml = 650\ mg : X$$
$$65X = 650$$
$$X = 10\ ml$$

2. Osmolality and Liquid Dilution: The feeding osmolality is found in the medication literature or provided by the pharmacist. Assume 500 mOsm is the constant for the desired osmolality. Here is how to calculate the osmolality and the total volume of liquid.

$$Total\ Volume\ of\ Liquid = (Known\ osmolality/Desired\ osmolality) \cdot Volume\ of\ Drug$$

Example: Total Volume of Liquid = $(5400\ /\ 500) \times 10$

$$Total\ Volume\ of\ Liquid = 10.8 \cdot 10$$
$$Total\ Volume\ of\ Liquid = 108\ ml$$

3. Volume of water used to dilute: The total volume of water needed to dilute the feeding is calculated by using the following method.

Volume of Water for Dilution = Total Volume of Liquid − Volume of Feeding
Example: Volume of Water for Dilution = 108 ml − 10 ml
Volume of Water for Dilution = 98 ml

11.10 Administering Enteral Feeding Preparations

Before administering enteral nutritional therapy:

- Obtain baseline laboratory values.
- Listen for bowel sounds.
- Assess placement of the feeding tube.
- Assess for gastric residual.
- Assure the tape around the feeding tube is patent.
- Plan to manage side effects.
- Dilute the medication.
- Weigh the patient.

During administering enteral nutritional therapy:

- Prevent aspiration.
- Determine if the patient can tolerate enteral feeding.
- Monitor intake and output.
- Monitor the patient for side effects.
- Manage side effects.
- Make sure that there is no skin breakdown.
- Report diarrhea, sore throat, and abdominal cramping.
- Assess continued feeding for residual every 2 to 4 hours.
- Monitor vital signs.
- Monitor the patient for hydration.
- Replace the feeding bag every 24 hours (or per healthcare facility policy).
- Make sure that the patient does not lose weight.

11.11 Parenteral Nutrition Support Therapy

Parenteral nutrition support therapy is used for disorders of the GI track, burns, and debilitating disease. Parenteral nutrition support therapy is administered through a central venous line (subclavian or internal jugular veins) to prevent irritation to the peripheral veins.

Parenteral nutrition support therapy preparation contains:

- Hyperosmolar glucose
- Amino acids
- Vitamins
- Electrolytes
- Minerals

- Trace elements
- Fat emulsion (increases calories and required for fat-soluble vitamins)

11.12   Risk of Parenteral Nutrition Support Therapy

Complications from parenteral nutrition support therapy are:

- Pneumothorax: Collapsed lung (caused by catheter insertion)
- Hemothorax: Blood accumulating in the pleural cavity (caused by catheter insertion)
- Hydrothorax: Serous fluid accumulating in the pleural cavity (caused by catheter insertion)
- Air embolism: (Caused by the infusion)
- Infection: (Caused by the infusion)
- Hyperglycemia: (Caused by the infusion)
- Hypoglycemia: (Caused by the infusion)
- Fluid overload: (Caused by the infusion)

11.13   Administering Parenteral Nutrition Support Therapy

It is critical that asepsis procedures be followed when preparing and administering parenteral nutrition preparations because the preparation is a medium that supports growth of yeast and bacteria. The pharmacy prepares parenteral nutrition preparations using a laminar airflow hood. Gloves and masks are used when changing the IV tubing and the dressing at the infusion site

Watch for hyperglycemia when initiating parenteral nutrition support therapy. The pancreas may not have time to adjust to the hypertonic dextrose solution, which is high in glucose. Hyperglycemia is usually temporary and dissipates once the pancreas adjusts. Hyperglycemia can persist if the infusion rate is too fast. Prevent hyperglycemia by beginning with 1 liter of solution for the first 24 hours, then increase by 500 to 1000 ml each day until a daily volume of 2500 ml to 3000 ml is reached.

Change the solution and tubing every 24 hours. Change the dressing every 48 to 72 hours or according to the healthcare facility's policy.

Caution: Do not suddenly interrupt parenteral nutrition support therapy. The patient can experience hypoglycemia. Discontinue gradually by decreasing the infusion rate. Monitor for hypoglycemia.

Before administering parenteral nutrition support therapy:

- Weigh the patient.
- Obtain baseline vital signs.
- Obtain baseline laboratory values.

During parenteral nutrition support therapy:

- Weigh the patient daily.
- Monitor intake and output.
- Monitor blood glucose.
- Do not use the parenteral nutritional line to draw blood, give medication, or check central venous pressure.
- Maintain asepsis when changing the solution and dressing.
- Refrigerate the parenteral nutritional preparation when not used.
- Monitor vital signs.
- Monitor catheter insertion site for infection.
- Monitor for signs of fluid volume overflow.

- Monitor for signs of dehydration.
- Monitor signs of hyperglycemia when therapy is started.
- Monitor signs for hypoglycemia after therapy is discontinued.
- Change parenteral nutritional preparation, tubing, and dressing according to the healthcare facility's policy.

Solved Problems

Nutrition

11.1 What is a nutrient?

A nutrient is a substance that is used by the body for energy, cell growth, cell maintenance, and cell repair.

11.2 Name the organic nutrients.

The organic nutrients are carbohydrates, fat, proteins, and vitamins.

11.3 What is malnutrition?

Malnutrition is a condition where there are insufficient nutrients to sustain daily activities.

11.4 What is a nutritional deficit?

A nutritional deficit is the result of having less than the adequate amount of nutrients because of an unbalanced diet, surgery, trauma, malignancy, and other conditions that breakdown (catabolize) the body.

11.5 What is another name for negative nitrogen balance?

Negative nitrogen balance is also known as nutritional deficit.

11.6 When do the first signs of malnutrition appear?

The first signs of malnutrition appear 14 days after the patient no longer receives an adequate amount of nutrients.

Nutritional Support Therapy

11.7 What is nutritional support therapy?

Nutritional support therapy provides nutrients before there is a negative nitrogen balance to assure there is a positive nitrogen balance, enabling the patient to fight infectious diseases.

11.8 What is enteral nutritional support therapy?

Enteral nutritional support therapy occurs when food is administered by mouth or a feeding tube that leads directly into the stomach or small intestine.

11.9 What is parenteral nutritional support therapy?

Parenteral nutritional support therapy is a means of providing high caloric nutrients administered through large veins such as the subclavian vein.

11.10 What is another name for parenteral nutritional support therapy?

Another name for parenteral nutritional support therapy is total parenteral nutrition (TPN) or hyperalimentation.

11.11 What does parenteral nutritional support therapy not promote?

Parenteral nutritional support therapy does not promote GI function, liver function, or weight gain.

11.12 What must be functioning before administering enteral nutritional support therapy?

GI motility and small bowel function must be established before beginning enteral feeding, by listening to bowel sounds.

11.13 Why might a patient experience uncontrolled vomiting and aspiration during enteral nutritional support therapy?

A patient might experience uncontrolled vomiting and aspiration during enteral nutritional support therapy because the GI motility and small bowel are not functioning.

11.14 What methods are used for enteral feedings?

Oral, nasogastric, gastrostomy, nasoduodenal, nasojejunal, or jejunostomy methods are used for enteral feedings.

11.15 What is the nasoduodenal method of enteral feedings?

The nasoduodenal method of enteral feedings consists of a tube passed through the nose and down the esophagus, ending in the duodenum.

11.16 What is the gastrostomy method of enteral feeding?

A feeding tube is placed in a hole in the abdomen, leading to the stomach.

11.17 What is the blenderized group of enteral nutritional support therapy preparations?

The blenderized group of enteral nutritional support therapy preparations is liquids similar to prepared baby food based on the nutritional needs of the patient.

11.18 How is the elemental group of enteral nutritional support therapy preparations used?

Elemental (monomeric) preparations are rapidly absorbed in the small intestines and used for partial GI tract dysfunction.

11.19 Name three common lactose-free liquid polymeric enteral nutritional support therapy preparations.

Three common lactose-free liquid polymeric enteral nutritional support therapy preparations are Ensure, Isocal, and Osmolite.

11.20 Name three complications of enteral nutritional support therapy.

Three complications of enteral nutritional support therapy are dehydration, aspiration, and diarrhea.

11.21 Where is parenteral nutrition support therapy administered?

Parenteral nutrition support therapy is administered through a central venous line (subclavian or internal jugular veins) to prevent irritation to the peripheral veins.

11.22 Name three elements of a parenteral nutrition support therapy preparation.

Three elements of a parenteral nutrition support therapy preparation are hyperosmolar glucose, amino acids, and vitamins.

11.23 Name three risks of a parenteral nutrition support therapy.

Three risks of a parenteral nutrition support therapy are pneumothorax, air embolism, and infection.

11.24   Why is it important to monitor for hyperglycemia when initiating parenteral nutrition support therapy?

       The pancreas may not have time to adjust to the hypertonic dextrose solution, which is high in glucose. Hyperglycemia is usually temporary and dissipates once the pancreas adjusts.

11.25   When can hyperglycemia persists in parenteral nutrition support therapy?

       Hyperglycemia can persist if the infusion rate is too fast.

11.26   How do you prevent hyperglycemia in parenteral nutrition support therapy?

       Prevent hyperglycemia by beginning with 1 liter of solution for the first 24 hours, then increase by 500 to 1000 ml each day until a daily volume of 2500 ml to 3000 ml is reached.

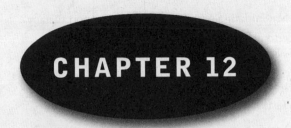

CHAPTER 12

Inflammation and Anti-Inflammatory Medication

12.1   The Inflammation Process

Inflammation is the protective response to injury to tissues. Injury causes the release of three chemicals that stimulates a vascular response forcing fluid and white blood cells (leukocytes) to flow to the injury site and stimulate nerve endings, signaling to the brain that there is an injury.

These chemicals are:

- Histamines: Histamines cause more blood and lymph fluid flow to the site.
- Kinins: Kinins are blood plasma proteins that influence smooth muscle contractions, increase blood flow, increase the permeability of small capillaries, and stimulate pain receptors.
- Prostaglandins: Prostaglandins are chemical messengers synthesized at the site in response to the white blood cells that flow to the area of injured tissue. Prostaglandins activate the inflammatory response, and produce pain and fever.

12.2   Signs of Inflammation

There are five cardinal signs of inflammation:

1. Redness
2. Swelling
3. Warmth
4. Loss of normal function
5. Pain

Hint: Inflammation is different from infection. A small percentage of infection is caused by microorganisms. Most inflammation is caused by trauma.

12.3   Phases of Inflammation

There are two phases of inflammation:

- Vascular phase: The vascular phase occurs 10 to 15 minutes after the tissue is injured. When blood vessels dilate (vasodilation), they become more permeable, enabling fluid and white blood cells to leave the plasma and flow to the injured tissue.
- Delayed phase: The delayed phase occurs when white blood cells infiltrate injured tissues to defend against infectious disease and foreign material.

12.4   Anti-Inflammatory Medication

The fever, pain, and swelling of the inflammatory response are uncomfortable for a patient. Anti-inflammatory medication reduces the inflammatory process to a more comfortable level but does not stop the inflammatory process. Anti-inflammatory medication stops the production of prostaglandins, resulting in a decrease in the inflammatory process.

12.5   Categories of Anti-Inflammatory Medication

There are three categories of anti-inflammatory medication. These are:

1. Analgesic: Relieves pain
2. Antipyretic: Reduces fever
3. Anticoagulant: Inhibits platelet aggregation

Some medications such as salicylates are anti-inflammatory medications that fall within all three categories. The most commonly used salicylate is aspirin (acetylsalicylic acid, ASA). Others fall into one or two categories such as propionic acid, which is an analgesic, antipyretic. The most common of these is ibuprofen.

12.6   Corticosteroids

Corticosteroids are hormones produced in the adrenal cortex and regulate inflammation, electrolyte levels, stress response, carbohydrate metabolism, and other physiological responses. Corticosteroids are typically prescribed for short-term treatment of inflammation.

Use of corticosteroid medication must be tapered off; otherwise, the patient risks having an adrenal crisis caused by insufficient levels of serum cortisol, a corticosteroid. The adrenal glands produce cortisol when the serum level of cortisol is low. During corticosteroid treatment there is a high level of serum cortisol, leading the adrenal glands to produce little cortisol. Stopping corticosteroid medication suddenly causes the serum level of cortisol to fall very low and does not give the adrenal glands time to resume producing cortisol. Tapering off corticosteroid medication gives the adrenal glands time to respond to the lower serum level of cortisol.

Long-term use can produced adverse side effects. These include:

- Risk of infection, since corticosteroids suppress the immune system
- Increased appetite and weight gain

- Edema (because sodium and water are retained)
- Increased blood pressure
- Stomach ulcers
- Slow-healing wounds
- Diabetes
- Mood swings

Healthcare providers manage adverse effects of corticosteroids by prescribing the lowest dose to yield the desired therapeutic effect.

12.7   Nonsteroidal Anti-Inflammatory Drugs

Nonsteroidal anti-inflammatory drugs (NSAIDs) are medications that reduce swelling, pain, and stiffness without exposing the patient to the adverse side effects that occur when using corticosteroid medication.

There are eight groups of NSAIDs. These are:

1. Salicylates (related to aspirin)
2. Parachlorobenzoic acid derivatives, or indoles
3. Pyrazolone derivatives
4. Propionic acid derivatives
5. Fenamates
6. Oxicams
7. Phenylacetic acids
8. Selective COX–2 inhibitors

SALICYLATES

Use	Anti-inflammatory, antipyretic, analgesic, transient ischemic attacks (TIAs), angina, myocardial infarction (heart attack), and rheumatological diseases such as arthritis.	Half-life: Short	Onset: 30 minutes	Peaks: 1–2 hours	Duration: 4–6 hours
Example	Aspirin	Route: PO, rectal	Pregnancy category: C	Pharmacokinetic: Absorbed from the GI tract, metabolized in the liver and primarily excreted in urine	

How it works
- Decreases inflammation
- Decrease platelet aggregation (blood clotting)

Adult dose
- Pain, fever PO/rectal: 325–600 mg q4 h as needed up to 4 g/day
- Rheumatoid arthritis, osteoarthritis, other inflammatory conditions: PO: 3.2–6 g/day in divided doses

Before administration
- Determine if there is a history of gastric upset, gastric bleeding, or liver disease.
- Determine the probability of drug interaction.

Administration
- Take with water, milk, or food; should be taken at mealtime (oral).
- The enteric-coated (EC) or buffered forms can help to decrease gastric problems.

After administration
- Monitor serum salicylate levels.
- Mild toxicity occurs at serum level of >30 mg/dl. Severe toxicity occurs at >50 mg/dl.
- Observe for signs of bleeding, such as dark (tarry) stools, bleeding bumps, petechiae (round red spots), ecchymosis (excessive bruising), and purpura (large red spots).

Contraindi- cations	• Do not give with alcohol.
	• Do not give with anticoagulant such as warfarin (Coumadin).
	• Do not give to children/teenagers who have flu or chickenpox.
Side effects/ adverse reactions	• Tinnitus (ringing in the ears), vertigo (dizziness), and bronchospasm, drowsiness, headaches, flushing, GI symptoms of heartburn, visual changes, and seizures
Patient education	• Inform the dentist before a dental procedure if taking high doses.
	• Discontinue aspirin 3 to 7 days before any surgery.
	• Patents with dysmenorrhea (painful menstruation) should take acetaminophen instead of aspirin 2 days before and 2 days during the menstrual period.
	• Take with food, at mealtime, or with a lot of fluids.
	• Salicylates are in foods such as prunes, raisins, and licorice as well as in spices such as curry powder and paprika.

PARACHLOROBENZOIC ACID

Use	Rheumatoid arthritis, osteoarthritis, and gout	Half-life: 4–11 hours	Onset: 30 minutes	Peaks: 0.5–2 hours	Duration: 4 hours
Example	Indomethacin (Indocin); sulindac (Clinoril), and tolmetin (Tolectin)	Route: PO, Indocin may be given IV	Pregnancy category: B	Pharmacokinetic: Absorbed from the GI tract, metabolized in the liver and primarily excreted in urine.	

How it works	Produces analgesic and anti-inflammatory effect by inhibiting prostaglandin synthesis, reducing inflammatory response and intensity of pain stimulus reaching sensory nerve endings
Adult dose	• Indocin: arthritis: 25 mg two to three times/day up to 1500–200 mg/day; *gout:* 100 mg than 50 mg three times/day
	• Clinoril: PO 150 mg two times/day up to 400 mg/day
	• Tolectin: 400 mg three times/day (including one dose upon rising, and one dose at bedtime) up to maintenance dose of 600–1800 mg/day in three to four divided doses
Before administration	• Assess onset, type, location, and duration of pain, fever, or inflammation.
	• Inspect affected joints for immobility, deformities, and skin condition.
Administration	• IV should be administered over 5–10 seconds; restrict fluid intake.
	• Give after meals or with food or antacids.
	• Do not crush sustained-release capsules.
After administration	• Monitor for nausea and dyspepsia (indigestion).
	• Evaluate for therapeutic response.
	• Assist patient with ambulation if dizziness occurs.
Contraindi- cations	• Do not give if there is a history of allergic reaction to aspirin or other NSAIDs.
	• Do not give if there is a history of GI lesions.
	• Use caution for patients with impaired renal/hepatic function.
	• Use caution with patients with coagulation defects.
	• Use caution with patients who have hypovolemia, heart failure, sepsis, epilepsy, parkinsonism, or psychiatric disturbances, or who are elderly.
Side effects/ adverse reactions	• Headache, nausea, vomiting, dyspepsia (heartburn, indigestion, epigastric pain), dizziness
	• Clinoril may cause a maculopapular rash or dermatitis.
	• Ulceration of GI tract mucous membranes
	• Hyperkalemia
	• May aggravate psychiatric disturbances
Patient education	• Avoid aspirin and alcohol.
	• Take with food or milk.
	• Avoid tasks requiring alertness until you determine the reaction to medication.
	• Do not crush or chew capsule.
	• Therapeutic response occurs 1–3 weeks after taking Tolectin

PROPIONIC ACID DERIVATIVES

Use	Reduces inflammation from arthritic conditions and acute injury, relieves pain associated with common cold, headache, toothache, muscular aches, backaches and menstrual cramps, and reduces fever.	Half-life: 10–15 hours	Onset: 30 minutes	Peaks: 1–2 hours	Duration: 4–6 hours
Example	Ibuprofen (Motrin, Advil, Nuprin); naproxen (Naprosyn) (Aleve is a similar OTC drug); Oxaprozin (Daypro); ketoprofen (Orudis).	Route: PO	Pregnancy category: B	Pharmacokinetic: Absorbed from the GI tract, metabolized in the liver and primarily excreted in urine	

How it works
- Produces analgesic and anti-inflammatory effect by inhibiting prostaglandin synthesis, reducing inflammatory response and intensity of pain stimulus reaching sensory nerve endings. Antipyresis produced by effect on hypothalamus, producing vasodilation, thereby decreased elevated body temperature

Adult dose
- Ibuprofen: 200–800 mg three to four time/day; maximum dose of <3.2 g/day (3200 mg/d)
- Naprosyn: 250–500 mg twice a day
- Daypro: 1200 mg/d initially with a maintenance dose of 1800 mg/d in divided doses
- Orudis: 150–300 mg/d in three to four divided doses

Before administration
- Assess onset, type, location, and duration of pain, fever, or inflammation.
- Inspect affected joints for immobility, deformities, and skin condition.

Administration
- PO: Do not crush or break enteric-coated form.
- Give with food, milk, or antacids if GI distress occurs.

After administration
- Monitor for nausea and dyspepsia (indigestion).
- Evaluate for therapeutic response.
- Assess skin for rash.

Contraindications
- Use to treat arthritis and other severe inflammatory conditions when other less toxic NSAIDs have been used unsuccessfully.
- Do not give if there is a history of active peptic ulcer, other GI ulceration, chronic inflammation of the GI tract, GI bleeding disorders, or a history of hypersensitivity to aspirin and other NSAIDs.
- Use caution with patients who have kidney, liver, GI tract disease, or a history of fluid retention.

Side effects/ adverse reactions
- Nausea, heartburn, indigestion, epigastric pain, dizziness, and rash
- Metabolic acidosis toxic reaction

Patient education
- Avoid aspirin and alcohol.
- Take with food or milk.
- Do not crush or chew capsule.

OXICAMS

Use	Long-term arthritic patients	Half-life: 30–86 hours	Onset: 2–4 hours	Peaks: 8 hours	Duration: 12 hours
Example	Piroxicam (Feldene)	Route: PO	Pregnancy category: C	Pharmacokinetic: Absorbed from the GI tract, metabolized in the liver, and primarily excreted in urine	

How it works
- Produces analgesic anti-inflammatory effect by inhibiting prostaglandin synthesis, reducing inflammatory response and intensity of pain stimulus reaching sensory nerve endings.

Adult dose
- 10 mg twice a day of 20 mg once a day

Before administration
- Assess onset, type, location, and duration of pain, fever or inflammation.
- Inspect affected joints for immobility, deformities, and skin condition.

Administration	• Do not crush or break capsule form.
	• May give with food, milk, or antacids if GI distress occurs.
After administration	• Monitor for nausea and dyspepsia (indigestion).
	• Evaluate for therapeutic response.
	• Assess skin for rash.
Contraindications	• Use to treat arthritis and other severe inflammatory conditions when other less toxic NSAIDs have been used unsuccessfully.
	• Do not give if there is a history of active peptic ulcer, other GI ulceration, chronic inflammation of the GI tract, GI bleeding disorders, or a history of hypersensitivity to aspirin and other NSAIDs.
	• Use caution with patients who have kidney, liver, GI tract disease, or a history of fluid retention.
Side effects/ adverse reactions	• Rare: nausea, heartburn, indigestion, epigastric pain, dizziness, and rash
Patient education	• Avoid aspirin and alcohol.
	• Take with food or milk.
	• Do not crush or chew capsule.

PHENYLACETIC ACID DERIVATIVES

Use	Pain and anti-inflammatory effects with patients with rheumatoid arthritis, osteoarthritis, ankylosing spondylitis, acute gout, bursitis, and tendonitis. Ophthalmic: Prophylaxis/treatment of ocular inflammation	Half-life: 2 hours	Onset: IM/IV: 10 minutes (dose dependent) PO 20–40 minutes	Peaks: 1–2 hours	Duration: 4–6 hours
Example	Diclofenac sodium (Voltaren) and Ketorolac (Toradol)	Route: PO/ IM/IV Ophthalmic	Pregnancy category: B	Pharmacokinetic: Absorbed from the GI tract, metabolized in the liver, and primarily excreted in urine; PB 99%; not removed by hemodialysis	

How It works	• Produces analgesic effect by inhibiting prostaglandin synthesis, reducing intensity of pain stimulus reaching sensory nerve endings. Reduces prostaglandin levels in aqueous humor, reducing intraocular inflammation.
Adult dose	• 25–50 mg three to four times/day or 75 mg twice a day
Before administration	• Assess onset, type, location, and duration of pain, fever, or inflammation.
	• Inspect affected joints for immobility, deformities, and skin condition.
Administration	• IM: Give deep IM slowly into large muscle mass.
	• Give undiluted as IV push over at least 15 seconds.
	• PO: Give with food, milk, or antacids if GI distress occurs.
	• Ophthalmic: Place finger on lower eyelid and pull out until pocket is formed between eye and lower lid. Hold dropper above pocket and place prescribed number of drops in pocket. Close eye gently. Apply digital pressure to lacrimal sac for 1–2 minutes to reduce the risk of systemic effects. Remove excess solution with tissue.
After administration	• Monitor for nausea and dyspepsia (indigestion).
	• Evaluate for therapeutic response.
	• Assess skin for rash.
	• Monitor stool frequency and consistency.
	• Be alert to signs of bleeding (may also occur with ophthalmic route because of systemic absorption).
Contraindications	• Use to treat arthritis and other severe inflammatory conditions when other less toxic NSAIDs have been used unsuccessfully.
	• Do not give if there is a history of active peptic ulcer, other GI ulceration, chronic inflammation of the GI tract, GI bleeding disorders, or a history of hypersensitivity to aspirin and other NSAIDs.

- Use caution with patients who have kidney, liver, GI tract disease, or a history of fluid retention.

Side effects/ adverse reactions	• Rare: nausea, heartburn, indigestion, epigastric pain, dizziness, and rash
Patient education	• Avoid aspirin and alcohol. • Take with food or milk. • Do not crush or chew capsule.

SELECTIVE COX–2 INHIBITORS

Use	Chronic inflammation	Half-life: 11.2 hours	Onset: 2 hours	Peaks: 8 hours	Duration: 12 hours
Example	celecoxib (Celebrex), Bextric and Vioxx (removed by the FDA)	Route: PO	Pregnancy category: B	Pharmacokinetic: Absorbed from the GI tract, metabolized in the liver and primarily excreted in urine; PB: 97%	

How it works	• Inhibits cyclo-oxygenase–2, the enzyme responsible for producing prostaglandins that cause pain and inflammation, producing anti-inflammatory effects.
Adult dose	• 100 mg twice a day
Before administration	• Assess onset, type, location, and duration of pain, fever, or inflammation. • Inspect affected joints for immobility, deformities, and skin condition.
Administration	• May give without regard to food. • Do not crush or break capsules.
After administration	• Monitor for nausea and dyspepsia (indigestion). • Evaluate for therapeutic response. • Assess skin for rash.
Contraindications	• Hypersensitivity to sulfonamides, NSAIDs, aspirin • Caution: Past history of peptic ulcer; >60 yr; those receiving anticoagulant therapy, steroids, alcohol consumption, smoking
Side effects/ adverse Reactions	• Abdominal pain, diarrhea, headache, indigestion, nausea, respiratory infection, sinus inflammation • Less common: back pain, dizziness, gas, insomnia, rash, runny nose, sore throat, swelling Adverse/Toxic: • None significant
Patient education	• Avoid aspirin and alcohol. • Take with food or milk. • Do not crush or chew capsule. • Possible increase in cardiac events such as a heart attack that may be common to all NSAIDs.

CORTICOSTEROIDS

Use	Treatment of chronic inflammations: allergic, neoplastic, and autoimmune diseases; management of cerebral edema, septic shock, adjuvant antiemetic in treatment of chemotherapy-induced emesis	Half-life: >24 hours	Onset: PO: — IM: — IV: rapid	Peaks: PO: 1–2 hours IM: 8 hours IV: —	Duration: PO: 66 hours IM: 6 days IV: —
Example	Dexamethasone (Decadron) and Prednisone	Route: PO/IM/IV Ophthalmic Topical Inhalation Intranasal	Pregnancy category: C	Pharmacokinetic: Absorbed from the GI tract, metabolized in the liver and primarily excreted in urine; >90%	

How it works	• Inhibits accumulation of inflammatory cells at inflammation sites, phagocytosis, lysosomal enzyme release and synthesis and/or release of mediators of inflammation. Prevents/suppresses cell and tissue immune reactions, inflammatory process
Adult dose	• Anti-inflammatory: PO: 0.75–9 mg/day in divided doses q6–12h • Cerebral edema: IV: Initially, 10 mg, then 4 mg (IM/IV) q6 hr • Chemotherapy antiemetic: IV: 8–20 mg once then (PO) 4 mg q4–6h or 8 mg q8h • Physiological replacement: PO/IM/IV: 0.03–0.15 mg/kg/day in divided doses q6–12 hours • Ophthalmic: Ointment: Thin coating three to four times/day; Suspension: Initially 2 drops q1 h while awake and q2h at night; then reduce to three to four times/day
Before administration	• Assess for hypersensitivity to any corticosteroids. • Obtain baseline height, weight, B/P, glucose, and electrolyte.
Administration	• PO: Give with milk or food. • IM: Give deep IM, preferably in gluteus maximus. Note: IV: Dexamethasone sodium phosphate may be given by IV push or IV infusion; for push, give over 1 min; for infusion, mix with 0.9% NaCl or D5W. • Ophthalmic: Place finger on lower eyelid and pull out until a pocket is formed between eye and lower lid. Hold dropper above pocket and place correct number of drops (1/4–1/2 inch ointment) into pocket; close eye gently. Solution: apply digital pressure to lacrimal sac for 1–2 min (minimizes drainage into nose and throat reducing risk of systemic effects); Ointment: Close eye for 1–2 minutes, rolling eyeball (increases contact area of drug to eye). Remove excess solution or ointment around eye with tissue; Ointment may be used at night to reduce frequency of solution administration; as with other corticosteroids, taper dosage slowly when discontinuing. • Topical: Gently cleanse area before application; use occlusive dressings only as ordered; apply sparingly and rub into area thoroughly.
After administration	• Monitor intake and output, daily weight; assess for edema. • Evaluate food tolerance and bowel activity. • Report hyperacidity promptly. • Check vitals at least two times/day. • Be alert to infection; sore throat, fever, or vague symptoms. • Monitor electrolytes. • Watch for hypercalcemia (muscle twitching, cramps) and hypokalemia (weakness and muscle cramps, numbness/tingling especially lower extremities, nausea and vomiting, irritability). • Assess emotional status and ability to sleep
Contraindi-cations	• Hypersensitivity to any corticosteroid, systemic fungal infection, peptic ulcers (except life-threatening situations). Avoid live virus vaccine such as smallpox. • Topical: Marked circulation impairment; do not instill ocular solutions when topical corticosteroids are being used on eyelids or surrounding tissues. • Cautions: Thromboembolic disorders, history of tuberculosis (may reactivate disease), hypothyroidism, cirrhosis, nonspecific ulcerative colitis, CHF, hypertension, psychosis, renal insufficiency, seizure disorders. Prolonged therapy should be discontinued slowly. • Topical: Do not apply to extensive areas.
Side effects/ adverse reactions	• Frequent: Inhalation: Cough, dry mouth, hoarseness, throat irritation. Intranasal: Burning, dryness inside nose. Ophthalmic: blurred vision. Systemic: Insomnia, facial swelling ("moon face"), moderate abdominal distention, indigestion, increased appetite, nervousness, facial flushing, increased sweating. • Occasional: Inhalation: Localized fungal infection (thrush); Intranasal: Crusting inside nose, nosebleed, sore throat, ulceration of nasal mucosa. Systemic: Dizziness, decreased/ blurred vision. Topical: Allergic contact dermatitis, purpura (blood-containing blisters), thinning of skin with easy bruising, telangiectasis (raised dark red spots on skin) • Rare: Inhalation: Increased bronchospasm, esophageal candidiasis. Intranasal: Nasal/pharyngeal candidiasis, eye pain. Systemic: General allergic reaction (rash, hives), pain, redness, swelling at injection site, psychic changes, false sense of well-being, hallucinations, depression Adverse/Toxic: • Long-term therapy: Muscle wasting (esp. arms, legs), osteoporosis, spontaneous fractures, amenorrhea, cataracts, glaucoma, peptic ulcer, CHF • Abrupt withdrawal following long-term therapy: Severe joint pain, severe headache, anorexia, nausea, fever, rebound inflammation, fatigue, weakness, lethargy, dizziness, orthostatic hypotension • Ophthalmic: Glaucoma, ocular hypertension, cataracts

| Patient education | • Do not change dose schedule or stop taking drug. MUST taper off gradually under medical supervision.
• Notify healthcare provider of fever, sore throat, muscle aches, or sudden weight gain/swelling.
• Severe stress (serious infection, surgery, or trauma) may require increased dosage.
• Inform dentist or other healthcare providers of dexamethasone therapy now or within past 12 months.
• Topical: Apply after shower or bath for best absorption. |

12.8   Arthritis Medication

Arthritis is inflammation of a joint that causes pain, stiffness, and swelling in the joint and surrounding tissue. There are two major types of arthritis.

Osteoarthritis

This type usually occurs in the later years of life when the protective cartilage that cushions the ends of the bones wears away. Bone surfaces are exposed and rub together, resulting in pain, damage to nerves and muscles, difficulty moving, and deformity. Joint stiffness usually lasts only a few minutes after initiating movement. Patients can have a genetic predisposition to arthritis. The early stage may respond to local heat and nonprescription analgesics. The later stages may require orthopedic intervention.

Rheumatoid

This usually occurs between 25 and 55 years of age. The patient feels fatigue, weakness, joint pain, and stiffness. Several weeks later, joints become inflamed, which causes a reduced range of motion and leads to joint deformity. Joint stiffness continues after initiating movement. NSAIDs and disease-modifying antirheumatic drugs (DEMARDs) are usually necessary to reduce the inflammation around the joints and inhibit the progression of the disease.

DISEASE-MODIFYING ANTIRHEUMATIC DRUGS

Use	Arrest progression of rheumatoid arthritis (RA), prevent deformities, and fight cancer	Half-life: 26 days in blood, 40–120 days in tissue	Onset: UK	Peaks: UK	Duration: 24 hours
Example	auranofin (Ridaura) (gold compound [chrysotherapy])	Route: PO/IM	Pregnancy category: C		Pharmacokinetic: Absorbed from the GI tract, metabolized in the liver, and primarily excreted in urine; PB: 60%
How it works	• Alters cellular mechanisms, enzyme systems, immune responses, collagen biosynthesis, suppressing synovitis of the active stage of rheumatoid arthritis.				
Adult dose	• PO: 6 mg/d in single or divided doses; may increase dose to 9 mg/d • IM: Initially, 10 mg, then 25 mg for 2 doses, then 50 mg weekly thereafter until total dose of 0.8–1 g given. If patient is improved and there are no signs of toxicity, may give 50 mg at 3- to 4-week intervals for many months.				
Before administration	• Assess for history of kidney or liver dysfunction, marked hypertension, heart failure, systemic lupus erythematosus (SLE), or uncontrolled diabetes mellitus. • Test for proteinuria (protein in urine) and hematuria (blood in urine).				
Administration	• Give without regard for food. • IM: Give in upper outer quadrant of gluteus.				
After administration	• Monitor patient for 30 minutes for allergic reaction. • Monitor vital signs.				

Contraindi-cations	• Do not use with patients who have renal or hepatic disease, colitis, SLE, pregnancy, or blood dyscrasias. • Use caution with patients who have diabetes mellitus or heart failure.
Side effects/ adverse reactions	• Anorexia, nausea, vomiting, diarrhea, stomatitis, abdominal cramps, pruritis, dizziness, headache, metallic taste, rash, dermatitis, and photosensitivity • Corneal gold deposits, urticaria (hives), hematuria, proteinuria, bradycardia Life-threatening: • Nephrotoxicity, agranulocytosis, thrombocytopenia, interstitial pneumonitis
Patient education	• Maintain high-fiber diet or antidiarrheal drugs to control diarrhea. • Report immediately early symptoms of gold toxicity such as a metallic taste or pruritus (itching). How to identify side effects: • Avoid direct sunlight. Use sun block. • Report any skin conditions. • Repeat bleeding gums or blood in the stool. • Adhere to scheduled blood tests. • Therapeutic effect may take 3 to 4 months.

12.9 Gout Medication

Gout is an inflammatory condition that attacks joints, tendons, and other tissues. The most common site is at the joint of the big toe. Gout is caused by problems metabolizing uric acid and purine, which is produced by proteins. The inability to metabolize uric acid and purine results in a buildup of urates (uric acid salts) and uric acid called hyperuricemia. Uric acid is also not cleared by the kidneys. Urate crystals form urate calculi known as stones that appear as tophi (bumps) in the subcutaneous tissue of earlobes, elbows, hands, and the base of the large toe.

Gout is treated with anti-inflammatory gout medication and uric acid inhibitors. Foods rich in purine should be avoided. These include wine, alcohol, organ meats, sardines, salmon, and gravy.

ANTI-INFLAMMATORY GOUT DRUG

Use	Treatment of attacks of acute gouty arthritis, prophylaxis of recurrent gouty arthritis. Reduce frequency of familial Mediterranean fever, treatment of acute attacks of calcium pyrophosphate deposition, sarcoid arthritis, amyloidosis, biliary cirrhosis, recurrent pericarditis.	Half-life: 20–30 minutes	Onset: 12 hours	Peaks: 1–2 days	Duration: 3 days
Example	Colchicine	Route: PO, IV	Pregnancy category: D	Pharmacokinetic: Absorbed from the GI tract, metabolized in the liver and primarily excreted in feces; PB: 30%–50%	
How it works	• Decreases leukocyte motility, phagocytosis, lactic acid production, resulting in decreased urate crystal deposits, inflammatory process				
Adult dose	• PO Initially: 0.5–1.2 mg; then 0.5–0.6 mg q1–2h • PO Subsequent: 0.5–0.6 mg q1–2h for pain relief for a maximum dose of mg/d • IV Initially: 2 mg • IV Subsequent: 0.5 mg q6h PRN for a maximum dose of 4 mg/day				
Before administration	• Assess drug and medical history. • Assess location of pain, joint tenderness, swelling, redness, and limitation of motion. • Baseline assessment of uric acid levels and CBC.				
Administration	• Give without regard to food for PO administration. • SC or IM administration produces severe local reaction. Use via IV route only for parenteral administration. • Administer over 2–5 minutes.				

After administration	• Instruct patient to drink 8–10 (8-oz) glasses of fluid daily while on this medication. • Discontinue medication if any GI symptoms occur. • Assess uric acid levels. • Assess for therapeutic response.
Contraindications	• Do not use with patients who have GI, renal, hepatic, or cardiac disorders or blood dyscrasias. • Use caution with elderly and debilitated patients.
Side effects/ adverse reactions	• Nausea, vomiting, abdominal discomfort • Anorexia • Bone marrow depression • Overdose first stage: burning feeling in throat/skin, severe diarrhea, abdominal pain • Overdose second stage: fever, seizures, delirium, renal damage • Overdose third stage: hair loss, leukocytosis, stomatitis
Patient education	• Encourage low-purine food intake. • Drink 8–10 (8-oz) glasses of fluid daily while on medication. • Report skin rash, sore throat, fever, unusual bruising/bleeding, weakness, tiredness, or numbness. • Stop medication as soon as gout pain is relieved or at first sign of nausea, vomiting, or diarrhea.

URIC ACID INHIBITOR

Use	Treatment of chronic gouty arthritis, uric acid nephropathy. Prevents or treats hyperuricemia secondary to blood dyscrasias, cancer chemotherapy. Prevents recurrence of uric acid or calcium stone formation.	Half-life: 2–3 hours	Onset: 2–3 days	Peaks: UK	Duration: 2–3 weeks
Example	allopurinol (Zyloprim)	Route: PO	Pregnancy category: C		Pharmacokinetic: Absorbed from the GI tract, metabolized in the liver and primarily excreted in urine

How it works	• Decreases uric acid production by inhibition of xanthine oxidase, an enzyme, reducing uric acid concentrations in both serum and urine.
Adult dose	• Mild gout: 200–300 mg/d • Severe gout: 400–600 mg/d • Neoplastic disease: PO: Initially 600–800 mg/day starting two to three days before initiation of chemotherapy or radiation therapy; IV 200–400 mg/m^2 beginning 24–48 hours before initiation of chemotherapy • Uric acid calculi: PO: 100–200 mg one to four times/day or 300 mg once daily • Calcium oxalate calculi: PO: 200–300 mg/day
Before administration	• Obtain a medical and drug history. • Develop a baseline the serum uric acid. • Develop a baseline urine output. • Develop a baseline for BUN, serum creatinine, ALP, AST, ALT, and LDH.
Administration	• Take with food.
After administration	• Monitor for side effects. • Monitor urine output. • Monitor BUN, serum creatinine, ALP, AST, ALT, and LDH.
Contraindications	• Do not use with patients who have hypersensitivity or severe renal disease. • Use caution with patients with hepatic disorders.
Side effects/ adverse reactions	• Anorexia, nausea, vomiting, diarrhea, stomatitis, dizziness, headache, rash, pruritus, malaise, and a metallic taste • Cataracts and retinopathy Life-threatening: • Bone marrow depression, aplastic anemia, thrombocytopenia, agranulocytosis, and leucopenia

| Patient education | • Maintain scheduled laboratory tests.
• Avoid alcohol and caffeine.
• Avoid large doses of vitamin C when taking medication.
• Report side effects immediately.
• Have a yearly eye examination. | | | | |

URICOSURICS

Use	Hyperuricemia in gout and gouty arthritis; adjunctive therapy with penicillins or cephalosporins to elevate and prolong antibiotic plasma levels	Half-life: 4–10 hours	Onset: 30 minutes	Peaks: 2 hours	Duration: 8 hours
Example	probenecid (Benemid)	Route: PO	Pregnancy category: B	Pharmacokinetic: Absorbed from the GI tract, metabolized in the liver and primarily excreted in urine; PB: 90%	

How it works	• Inhibits tubular reabsorption of urate at proximal renal tubule, increasing urinary excretion of uric acid
Adult dose	Gout: • Initially: 250 mg 2 time/day for 1 week • After 1 Week: 500 mg 2 times/day. May increase by 500 mg q 4 weeks to a maximum dose of 2–3 g/day. Penicillin/cephalosporin therapy: • PO: 2 g/day in divided doses Gonorrhea: • PO: 1 g 30 minutes before penicillin, ampicillin, or amoxicillin
Before administration	• Wait until acute gouty attack has subsided. • Question patient if hypersensitivity to probenecid or if taking penicillins or cephalosporins
Administration	• May be administered with antacid or food to minimize GI distress.
After administration	• If rash appears, then immediately discontinue. • 3000 mL/day fluid intake • Monitor intake and output (at least 2000 mL/day). • Monitor CBC and serum uric acid levels. • Monitor urine for cloudiness, unusual color, and odor. • Monitor for therapeutic response.
Contraindications	• Do not use in the presence of blood dyscrasias, uric acid kidney stones. • Use caution with patients with kidney problems and a history of peptic ulcer. • Do not use with penicillin in the presence of renal impairment.
Side effects/ adverse reactions	• Headache, anorexia, nausea, vomiting • Lower back/side pain, rash, hives, itching, dizziness, flushed face, frequent urge to urinate, gingivitis • Rare: severe hypersensitivity reactions, including anaphylaxis • Pruritic maculopapular rash (toxic reaction)
Patient education	• Encourage low-purine foods (eggs, cheese, and vegetables). • Drink 6–8 glasses of fluid daily. • Avoid alcohol and caffeine. • Therapeutic effect may take a week or more.

Solved Problems

The Inflammation Process

12.1   What is inflammation?

Inflammation is the protective response to injury to tissues.

12.2   What happens when tissue is injured?

Injury causes the release of three chemicals that stimulate a vascular response forcing fluid and white blood cells (leukocytes) to flow to the injury site and stimulate nerve endings, signaling the brain that there is an injury.

12.3   What do histamines do?

Histamines cause more blood and lymph fluid flow to the site.

12.4   What do kinins do?

Kinins are blood plasma proteins that influence smooth muscle contractions, increase blood flow, increase the permeability of small capillaries, and stimulate pain receptors.

12.5   What do prostaglandins do?

Prostaglandins are chemical messengers synthesized at the site in response to the white blood cells that flow to the area of injured tissue. Prostaglandins activate the inflammatory response; they produce pain and fever.

12.6   What are the signs of inflammation?

The signs of inflammation are redness, swelling, warmth, loss of normal function, and pain.

12.7   What is the difference between inflammation and infection?

Infection is caused by a microorganism. Inflammation is caused by a microorganism or trauma.

12.8   What is the vascular phase of inflammation?

The vascular phase occurs 10 to 15 minutes after the tissue is injured when blood vessels dilate (vasodilation), becoming more permeable and enabling fluid and white blood cells to leave the plasma and flow to the injured tissue.

12.9   What is the delayed phase of inflammation?

The delayed phase occurs when white blood cells infiltrate injured tissues to defend against infectious disease and foreign material.

Anti-Inflammatory Medication

12.10   What is the therapeutic response of anti-inflammatory medication?

Anti-inflammatory medication stops the production of prostaglandins, resulting in a decrease in the inflammatory process to a more comfortable level, but does not stop the inflammatory process.

12.11   What are the three categories of anti-inflammatory medication?

The three categories of anti-inflammatory medication are analgesic, antipyretic, and anticoagulant.

12.12   What is the therapeutic effect of an analgesic?

The therapeutic effect of an analgesic is relief of pain.

12.13 What is the therapeutic effect of an antipyretic?

The therapeutic effect of an antipyretic is fever reduction.

12.14 What are salicylates?

Salicylates are anti-inflammatory medications that fall within all three categories. The most commonly used salicylate is aspirin (acetylsalicylic acid, ASA).

12.15 What are corticosteroids?

Corticosteroids are hormones produced in the adrenal cortex. They regulate inflammation, electrolyte levels, stress response, carbohydrate metabolism, and other physiological responses. Corticosteroids are typically prescribed for short-term treatment of inflammation.

12.16 What can happen if the patient suddenly stops taking corticosteroids?

If the patient suddenly stops taking corticosteroids, he or she can experience adrenal crisis.

12.17 What happens when the patient tapers the use of corticosteroids?

Tapering off corticosteroids medication gives the adrenal glands time to respond to the lower serum level of cortisol.

12.18 What happens in an adrenal crisis?

Stopping corticosteroids medication suddenly causes the serum level of cortisol to fall very low and does not give the adrenal glands time to resume producing cortisol, resulting in an adrenal crisis.

12.19 Why is it that a patient on corticosteroids medication is susceptible to infection?

Corticosteroids suppress the immune system.

12.20 Name three adverse effects of taking corticosteroid medications.

Three adverse effects of taking corticosteroid medications are increased weight, increased blood pressure, and stomach ulcers.

12.21 Why do patients taking corticosteroid medications experience edema?

Corticosteroids cause the retention of sodium and water.

12.22 How do healthcare providers manage the adverse effects of corticosteroids?

Healthcare providers prescribe the lowest dose of corticosteroids to yield the desired therapeutic effect.

12.23 What are nonsteroidal anti-inflammatory drugs?

Nonsteroidal anti-inflammatory drugs are medications that reduce swelling, pain, and stiffness without exposing the patient to the adverse side effects that occur when using corticosteroids medication.

12.24 What are the eight groups of nonsteroidal anti-inflammatory drugs?

The eight groups of nonsteroidal anti-inflammatory drugs are salicylates, parachlorobenzoic acid derivatives, pyrazolone derivatives, propionic acid derivatives, fenamates, oxicams, phenylacetic acid, and selective COX–2 inhibitors.

12.25 What is the therapeutic use of DEMARDs?

Disease-modifying anti-rheumatic drugs (DEMARDs) are usually necessary to reduce the inflammation around the joints and inhibit the progression of rheumatoid arthritis.

12.26 Why are uricosurics prescribed for gout?

Uricosurics inhibit reabsorption of urate, causing an increase in excreting uric acid in urine.

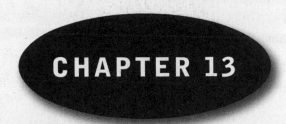

CHAPTER 13

Infection and Antimicrobials

13.1   Microorganisms

An infection occurs when microorganisms colonize inside the body and use the body's resources to grow. This process interferes with normal body functions. The body's response may be the inflammation process (see chapter 12); however, colonization does not always cause signs and symptoms of disease and may not require treatment.

Many microorganisms do not cause infection. Some microorganisms called flora help with digestion. Microorganisms that cause infections are called pathogens. An infection can be local to a site or affect an entire system of the body, which is referred to as septicemia. A body is referred to as being septic if it is infected. A body that is infection-free is called aseptic.

There are three types of microorganisms that commonly cause infection in the body:

1. Bacteria
2. Viruses
3. Fungi

13.2   Natural Defense

A pathogen is detected by the immune system as an antigen, which is a foreign substance that has entered the body. T cells, a type of white blood cell, search for antigens. When one is found, the T cell engulfs and destroys the antigen.

The T cell also signals B cells, which are another type of white blood cell, to create antibodies designed specifically to attack that antigen. Antibodies then circulate, seeking out the antigen. Once the antigen is encountered, the antibody marks the antigen for destruction. Macrophages and neutrophils, also types of white blood cells, engulf and destroy any substance marked by the antibody for destruction.

Viruses infect cells. The MHC molecule found on all cell surfaces binds to the virus until a T cell engulfs and destroys the virus.

13.3   Medication for Symptoms

A healthy immune system is able to destroy most antigens. During that time the patient experiences signs of inflammation (see 12.2 Signs of Inflammation). The inflammatory response is brought about by prostaglandins that cause vasodilatation, relax smooth muscles, and make capillaries permeable and sensitize nerve cells within the affected area to pain. Healthcare providers proscribe prostaglandins inhibitors to reduce the discomfort brought about by inflammation. Prostaglandins inhibitors do not kill the pathogen.

13.4 Antimicrobials

Antimicrobials are medications that impede the growth of or kill pathogens. An antimicrobial that impedes growth is referred to as static. For example, sulfonamides impede the growth of bacteria and are therefore called bacteriostatic. Antimicrobials that kill pathogens are called cidal. For example, penicillin (PCN) is said to be bacteriocidal because penicillin kills bacteria by using lysis, which explodes bacteria.

Some antimicrobials are both static and cidal. For example, chloramphenicol is bacteriostatic, inhibiting most bacteria from growing. In higher concentrations it is bacteriocidal and kills *S. pneumoniae* and *H. influenza* in cerebrospinal fluid. Tetracycline is also bacteriostatic and bacteriocidal.

13.5 How Antimicrobials Work

There are four ways in which antimicrobials react with pathogens. They:

1. Inhibit the pathogen from growing a cell wall.
2. Disrupt the permeability of the pathogen's membrane to prevent nutrients from entering the pathogen's cell and waste from excreting from the pathogen's cell.
3. Inhibit the pathogen's ability to make protein, resulting in the synthesis of defective proteins.
4. Inhibit the pathogen's capability to make essential metabolites. A metabolite is a substance necessary for the pathogen's metabolism.

13.6 Side Effects of Antimicrobials

Antimicrobials can have side effects that adversely affect the patient. Common adverse effects of antimicrobials are:

- Rash
- Fever
- Urticaria (hives) with pruritus (itching)
- Chills, general erythema (redness)
- Anaphylaxis (circulatory collapse)

Adverse effects of antimicrobials are treatable by using:

- Antihistamines (Benadryl)
- Epinephrine (adrenalin)
- Steroids for anti-inflammatory response

13.7 Super Infections

Antimicrobials that impede or kill bacteria are called antibiotics. Antibiotics impede or kill pathogen bacteria and flora bacteria, which are used to aid digestion. The more a bacterium is exposed to an antibiotic, the greater the chance that the bacteria can create defenses against antibiotics, making the bacteria resistant to the antibiotic. The antibiotics then no longer impede or kill the bacteria. An infection by resistant bacteria is called a super infection. Resistant bacteria can also replace the flora bacteria.

A super infection can occur when:

- A large dose of antibiotics is used.
- An antibiotic is used long term.
- Broad-spectrum antibiotics are used that can work against different strains of bacteria.

For example, the overuse of the following antibiotics can cause this bacterium to become resistant to these antibiotics:

- Cephalosporins may cause *pseudomonas*
- Tetracycline may cause *candida albicans*

Hint: Defenses against a particular antibiotic are passed down to generations of bacteria. There is a concern that over time bacteria might become resistant to known antibiotics.

13.8   Preventing Antibiotic-Resistant Bacteria

Healthcare providers take precautions to reduce the likelihood of creating antibiotic-resistant bacteria. They do so by:

- Identifying the pathogen using a culture and sensitivity study before prescribing an antimicrobial. Once the pathogen is identified, a specific—not broad-spectrum—antimicrobial is prescribed.
- Prescribing a lower dose antimicrobial (A lower dose may not impede or kill all the pathogen.)
- Prescribing a normal dose antimicrobial for a short time period (The shorter time period dose may not impede or kill all the pathogen.)
- Requiring patients to finish all the prescribed antimicrobial and to not stop taking the medication once signs and symptoms of the infection dissipate. Pathogens are still alive and growing when signs and symptoms of the infection dissipate.

13.9   Administering Antimicrobial Medication

Antimicrobial medication is administered following the same procedures as for any medication (see chapter 5). However, here are additional step to take when administering antimicrobial medication:

- Determine if the patient has allergies to drugs, food, and environmental stimuli and a family history of allergies to antibiotics.
- Display allergies in red and write clearly on the patient's record.
- Ask the patient each time if the patient has allergies before administering antimicrobial medication.
- Have emergency medication such as epinephrine, Benadryl, and steroids on hand to counteract any adverse effect of the antimicrobial medication.
- Monitor the patient for a half hour after antimicrobial medication is given to determine an adverse reaction.
- Monitor the therapeutic effect of the antimicrobial medication to determine if the medication is effective.
- Administer antimicrobials at the times specified in the medication order to maintain a therapeutic blood level of the medication.
- Expect that the first dose administered is higher than the maintenance dose to quickly achieve a therapeutic level.

- Give intramuscular (IM) injections of antibiotics deep into the muscle.
- Rotate IM injection sites if more than one injection is prescribed.
- Be aware of the healthcare facility's policy on stop orders and renewal orders. Typically antimicrobial medication orders are for 72 hours. A stop order is automatically enforced after 72 hours, requiring the healthcare provider to reassess the patient before renewing the medication order. This is to assure that the pathogen does not become resistant to the antimicrobial medication.
- Aggressive treatment requires administering an antimicrobial medication intravenously (IV). The antimicrobial medication is diluted in a neutral solution (pH 7.0 to 7.2), such as normal saline (NS), isotonic sodium chloride, or 5% dextrose and water (D5W). Antimicrobial medication can be administered as a piggyback infusion.
- Do not mix two or more antibiotics together.
- Do not administer two antibiotics simultaneously. The time period between administering two antibiotics depends on the medication.

13.10   Patient Information for Antimicrobial Medication

The patient should be informed that antimicrobial medication may expose the patient to:

- Sepsis
- Ototoxicity (ears)
- Blood dyscrasias
- Nephrotoxicity (kidney)

The patient must be told:

- To take all the medication even after the symptoms subside.
- Not to take medication left over from a previous illness. The medication may not treat the patient's condition or may have lost its therapeutic capabilities.
- Not to share drinks, food, and utensils until the healthcare provider determines that the patient is no longer infected.
- How to recognize the therapeutic effects, side effects, and adverse reactions that might occur as a result of taking the medication.
- To call the healthcare provider if the patient experience side effects or adverse reactions to the medication.
- To wear a med-alert bracelet if the patient has allergies to medication.

13.11   Penicillin

Penicillin (PCN), discovered in 1940, is derived from molds and is the most effective and least toxic antimicrobial medication. Penicillin weakens the cell wall of a bacterium, rupturing and destroying the cell in a process called lysis. Penicillin is most active against gram-positive bacteria and some gram-negative bacteria. Penicillin is not active against bacteria that contain enzymes that destroy penicillin.
There are four types of penicillin:

1. Basic (natural)
2. Penicillinase-resistant (resistant to beta-lactamase inactivation)
3. Aminopenicillins (broad-spectrum)
4. Extended-spectrum

- After administering PCN, monitor for:
  - Serum electrolytes for hyperkalemia (elevated potassium) and/or hypernatremia (elevated sodium)
  - Unusual weight loss (especially in the elderly)
  - Vital signs
  - White blood cells (WBCs)
  - Cultures
  - Prothrombin time (PT) (bleeding times)

Basic (Natural) Penicillin

Pregnancy Category: B

Protein-Binding: 65%

Half-Life: 0.5 hour

ROUTE	DOSE	TIME
Penicillin G		
PO	200,000–500,000	Every 4–6 hours
IV	1–5 mu	Every 4–6 hours
IM	1.2–2.4 micro units	Single dose
Penicillin V (take on empty stomach)		
PO	125–500 mg	Every 8 hours

Penicillinase-Resistant Penicillin

Pregnancy Category: B

Half-Life: 0.5–1 hour

ROUTE	DOSE	TIME
Cloxacillin (Tegopen)		
Protein-Binding: 90%		
PO	2–6 g/day	Every 6 hours
IV	250–500 mg	Every 4–6 hours
Dicloxacillin (Dynapen)		
Protein-Binding: 90%		
PO	125–250 mg	Every 6 hours
Methicillin (Staphcillin)		
Protein-Binding: 25%–40%		
IV	1 g	Every 6 hours
IM	1 g	Every 4–6 hours
Nafcillin (Unipen)		
Protein-Binding: 90%		
PO	250 mg–1 g	Every 4–6 hours
IV	0.5–1.5 g	Every 4 hours
IM	500 mg	Every 4–6 hours
Oxacillin (Prostaphlin)		
Protein-Binding: 95%		
PO	0.5–1 g	Every 4–6 hours
IV	250–1 g	Every 6 hours
IM	250–1 g	Every 4–6 hours

Aminopenicillins (Broad-Spectrum) Penicillin

Pregnancy Category: B

ROUTE	DOSE	TIME
Amoxicillin, (Amoxil)		
Protein-Binding: 20%		
Half-Life: 1–1.3 hours		
PO	250–500 mg	Every 8 hours
Amoxicillin + Potassium Clavulanate (Augmentin, Clavulin)		
Protein-Binding: 25%		
Half-Life: 1–1.5 hours		
PO	5000 mg	Every 8 hours
Ampicillin (Polycillin, Omnipen)		
Protein-Binding: 15%–28%		
Half-Life: 1–2 hours		
PO	250–500 mg	Every 6 hours
IV	250–500 mg	Every 8 hours
IM	250–500 mg	Every 8 hours
Ampicillin and sulbactam (Unasyn)		
Protein-Binding: 28–38%		
Half-Life: 1–2 hours		
IV	1.5–3 g	Every 6 hours
IM	1.5–3 g	Every 6 hours
Bacampicillin (Spectrobid)		
Protein-Binding: 17%–20%		
Half-Life: 1 hour		
PO	499–800 mg	Every 12 hours

Extended-Spectrum Penicillin

Pregnancy Category: B

ROUTE	DOSE	TIME
Carbenicillin (Geocillin)		
Protein-Binding: 50%		
Half-Life 1–1.5 hours		
PO	0.5–1 g	Every 6 hours
IV	50–83.3 mg/kg	Every 4 hours
IM	50–83.3 mg/kg	Every 4 hours
Mezlocillin (Mezlin)		
Protein-Binding: 30%–40%		
Half-Life: 0.5–1 hour		
IV	33.3–58.3 mg/kg	Every 4 hours
IM	33.3–58.3 mg/kg	Every 4 hours
Piperacillin (Pipracil)		
Protein-Binding: 16%–22%		
Half-Life: 0.6–1.5 hours		

(Continued)

(Continued from previous page)

IV		3–4 g	Every 4–6 hours
IM		3–4 g	Every 4–6 hours

Piperacillin + tazobactam (Zosyn, Tazocin)
Protein-Binding: Unknown
Half-Life: 0.7–1.2 hours

IV		3.375–4 .5 g	Every 6–8 hours

Ticarcillin (Ticar)
Pregnancy Category: C
Protein-Binding: 45%–65%
Half-Life: 0.5–1.5 hours

IV		1–4 g	Every 6 hours
IM		1 g	Every 6 hours

Ticarcillin + clavulanate (Timentin)
Protein-Binding: 45%–65%
Half-Life: 1–1.5 hours

IV		33.3–50 mg	Every 4 hours

13.12 Classification of Penicillin

Penicillin is categorized by its usefulness against bacterial enzymes capable of destroying the medication. Table 13.1 contains abbreviations commonly used to describe medication. Four classifications used for all antibiotics are:

1. Pregnancy category: The pregnancy category determines how safe the antibiotic is to take when pregnant (see 1.14 Pregnancy Categories).
2. Beta-lactam ring: A beta-lactam ring makes the antibiotic less susceptible to bacteria enzymes that inactivate the antibiotic. Beta-lactam ring antibiotics are more active against gram-negative cell wall bacteria than antibiotics that do not contain the beta-lactam ring.
3. Protein-binding: Protein-binding occurs when a medication binds to plasma proteins. Medication bound to protein is not available for therapeutic use. The medication must be free and not bound to protein to be available for therapeutic use. Medications are measured as the percent of protein binding. The higher the percentage, the lower the amount of medication there is for therapeutic use.
4. Half-life: Half-life is the time for half the medication to be eliminated from the body.

TABLE 13.1 Common Abbreviations Used to Describe Medication

ABBREVIATION	DESCRIPTION
PB	Protein-binding
$t_{1/2}$	Half-life
UK	Unknown
PO	By mouth
IV	Intravenous
IM	Intramuscular
A	Adult
C	Child

13.13 Precautions When Administering Penicillin

There are several precautions that must be taken when administering penicillin. These are:

- Avoid giving PCN orally an hour before and an hour after eating.
- Give PCN orally with a full glass of water.
- Do not give PCN orally with acidic fruit juices.
- Administer PCN IV slowly. Penicillin contains potassium. Administering PCN IV quickly risk heart failure if the patient has renal insufficiency.
- Assess for allergies before administering PCN.
- Assess if the patient is allergic to cephalosporins, cephamycins, griseofulvin, or penicillamine. Penicillin has a cross-sensitivity to these medications.
- Assess for allergic reactions after administering PCN. Reactions can be a mild rash or anaphylactic shock.
- Do not administer PCN to patients who have:
  - Bleeding tendency
  - Ulcerative colitis and other gastrointestinal GI diseases
  - Mononucleosis
  - A low-salt diet
  - Impaired renal function

13.14 Penicillin and Drug–Drug Interactions

Adverse effects might be produced when PCN is administered with other medications. Here are potential adverse reactions:

- Hyperkalemia
  - Monitor serum potassium levels
  - PCN given with:
    - Aldactone (potassium-sparing diuretic)
    - Captopril (ACE inhibitor antihypertensive)
    - Kay Ciel (potassium supplement)
- Increased risk of bleeding
  - PCN given with:
    - Parenteral carbenicillin (inhibits platelet aggregation)
    - Ticarcillin (inhibits platelet aggregation)
    - Streptokinase (thrombolytic agent)
- Decreased absorption of Penicillin G
  - PCN given with:
    - Cholestyramine (Questran)
    - Colestipol (Colestid)
- Decreased effectiveness of contraceptives
  - PCN given with:
    - Estrogen contraceptives
- Risk of methotrexate (Folex) toxicity because of decreased ability to excrete methotrexate (Folex)
  - PCN given with:
    - Methotrexate (Folex)
- Increased serum level of Penicillin by decreasing renal excretion of Penicillin
  - PCN given with:
    - Probenecid (Benemid)

13.15   Penicillin and Patient Education

The patient must be instructed to:

- Expect improvement in his or her condition in 48 hours.
- Call the healthcare provider if the symptoms do not improve.
- Expect a longer time period to see improvement for patients with diabetes, immunosuppressed conditions, and cancer.
- Use alternate means of birth control other than estrogen-based contraceptives.
- Expect that he or she might have a discolored tongue or a sore mouth.
- Be alert to signs of allergic reaction and call the healthcare provider immediately if a rash develops and call 911 at the first sign of difficulty breathing.

13.16   Cephalosporin

Cephalosporin is a family of chemically modified versions of penicillin that stops growth and kills a broad spectrum of bacteria by making it impossible for bacteria to create a cell wall. Cephalosporin is commonly used as a prophylaxis before surgery to prevent postsurgical infections. Cephalosporin is prescribed for patients who are allergic to PCN but do not experience an anaphylaxis from it. Ten percent of patients allergic to PCN are also allergic to cephalosporin.

The side effects of cephalosporin are:

- Diarrhea
- Abdominal cramps
- Oral and/or vaginal candidiasis
- Rash
- Pruritus
- Redness
- Edema
- Increased bleeding and bruising (with cefamandole, cefmetazole, cefoperazone, and cefotetan)

Caution: Cephalosporin can exacerbate existing bleeding disorders. Assess the patient for such disorders before administering cephalosporin.

13.17   Before Administering Cephalosporin

Before administering cephalosporins to the patient, you must:

- Assess for allergies.
- Assess vital signs.
- Assess urine output.
- Review renal and liver function labs (AST, ALT, ALP, and bilirubin, BUN, serum creatinine).
- Assess bleeding time (PT and PTT).
- Obtain culture and sensitivity to determine if cephalosporins are effective against the bacteria.
- Administer cephalosporins using the same methods as used for penicillin.
- Provide the same instructions to a patient as with penicillin.

13.18 Generations of Cephalosporins

There are four generations of cephalosporins:

1. First generation: Effective against gram-positive bacteria
2. Second generation: Increased activity against gram-negative microorganisms
3. Third generation: More active against gram($-$); ceftazidime and cefoperazone are also effective against *Pseudomonas aeruginosa* (gram–) and β-lactamase–producing microbial strains; less effective against gram (+) cocci
4. Fourth generation: Same as third generation, but is more resistant to β-lactamases

First Generation: Effective against gram (+) bacteria

Pregnancy Category: B

ROUTE	DOSE	TIME
Cefadroxil (Duricef)		
Protein-Binding: 20%		
Half-Life 0.5–2 hours		
PO	500 mg	Every 12 hours
Cefazolin (Ancef, Kefzol)		
Protein-Binding: 75%–85%		
Half-Life: 0.5–2.5 hours		
IV	0.25–1.5 g	Every 6–8 hours
IM	1 g	Presurgery
Cephalexin (Keflex)		
Protein-Binding: 65%–80%		
Half-Life: 0.5–1 hour		
PO	250–500 mg	Every 6 hours
Cephalothin (Keflin)		
Protein-Binding: 10%–15%		
Half-Life: 0.5–1.2 hours		
IM/IV	0.5–1 g	Every 4 to 6 hours
Cephapirin (Cefadyl)		
Protein-Binding: 40%–50%		
Half-Life: 0.5–1 hours		
IM /IV	0.5–1 g	Every 4 to 6 hours
Cephradine (Velosef, Anspor)		
Protein-Binding: 20%		
Half-Life: 1–2 hours		
PO	250–500 mg	Every 8 hours
IM/IV	0.5–1 g	Every 6 hours

(*Continued*)

(Continued from previous page)

Second Generation: Increased activity against gram(−) microorganisms

Pregnancy Category: B

ROUTE	DOSE	TIME
Cefaclor (Ceclor)		
Protein-Binding: 25%		
Half-Life 0.5–2 hours		
PO	250–500 mg	Every 8 hours
IM/IV	500 g	Every 6 hours
Cefamandole (Mandol)		
Protein-Binding: 60%–75%		
Half-Life: 0.5–1 hour		
IM/IV	500 mg	Every 6–8 hours
Cefmetazole (Zefazone)		
Protein-Binding: 68%		
Half-Life: 2.5–3 hours		
IV	2 g	Every 12 hours
Cefonicid (Monocid)		
Protein-Binding: 98%		
Half-Life: 0.5–1.2 hours		
IM/IV	0.5–1 g	Every 24 hours
Cefotetan (Cefotan)		
Protein-Binding: 85%		
Half-Life: 3–5 hours		
IM/IV	102 g	Every 12 hours
Cefoxitin (Mefoxin)		
Protein-Binding: 70%		
Half-Life: 45 minutes–1 hour		
IV	102 g	Every 6 to 8 hours
Cefprozil (Cefzil)		
Protein-Binding: 99%		
Half-Life: 1–2 hours		
PO	500 mg	Every 12 hours
Cefuroxime (Ceftin, Zinacef)		
Protein-Binding: 50%		
Half-Life: 1.5–2 hours		
PO	250–500 mg	Every 12 hours
IM/IV	0.75–1.5 g	Every 8 hours
Loracarbef (Lorabid)		
Protein-Binding: Unknown		
Half-Life: 1 hour		
PO	200–400 mg	Every 12 hours

Third Generation: More active against gram($-$); ceftazidime and cefoperazone are also effective against *Pseudomonas aeruginosa* (gram$-$) and β-lactamase–producing microbial strains; less effective against gram($+$) cocci

Pregnancy Category: B

ROUTE	DOSE	TIME
Cefixime (Suprax)		
Protein-Binding: 65%		
Half-Life 2.5–4 hours		
PO	200 mg	Every 12 hours
Cefoperazone (Cefobid)		
Protein-Binding: 70%–80%		
Half-Life: 2.5 hours		
IV	1–2 g	Every 12 hours
Cefotaxime (Claforan)		
Protein-Binding: 30%–40%		
Half-Life: 1–1.5–3 hours		
IV	1–2 g	Every 12 hours
Cefpodoxime (Vantin, Proxetil)		
Protein-Binding: 20%–40%		
Half-Life: 2–3 hours		
PO	200 mg	Every 12 hours
Ceftazidime (Fortaz)		
Protein-Binding: 10%–17%		
Half-Life: 1–2 hours		
IM / IV	0.5–2 g	Every 8–12 hours
Ceftibuten (Cedax)		
Protein-Binding: Unknown		
Half-Life: 1.5–3 hours		
PO	400 mg	Once per day
Ceftriaxone (Rocephin)		
Protein-Binding: 85%–95%		
Half-Life: 8 hours		
IV	1–2 g	Every 24 hours
Ceftizoxime (Cefizox)		
Protein-Binding: 30%–60%		
Half-Life: 2 hours		
IM/IV	500 mg	Every 8–12 hours
Cefdinir (Omnicef)		
Protein-Binding: Unknown		
Half-Life: 1.7 hours		
PO	300 mg or 600 mg/d	Every 12 hours

(Continued)

(Continued from previous page)

Fourth Generation: Cefepime same as third generation + more resistant to β-lactamases

Pregnancy Category: B

ROUTE	DOSE	TIME
Cefepime (Maxipime)		
Protein-Binding: Unknown		
Half-Life 0.5–2 hours		
IM.IV	0.5–1 g	Every 12 hours

13.19 Cephalosporin and Drug–Drug Interactions

Adverse effects might be produced when cephalosporin is administered with other medications. Here are potential adverse reactions:

- Risk for nausea, vomiting, hypotension, headaches, sweating, difficulty breathing, flushed face, tachycardia
  - Cefamandole, cefoperazone, or moxalactam given with:
    - Alcohol
- Risk of hemorrhage:
  - Cefamandole, cefmetazole, cefoperazone, or cefotetan given with:
    - Coumarin (anticoagulant)
    - Indanedione (anticoagulant)
    - Heparin (anticoagulant)
    - Thrombolytic (clot buster)
    - NSAIDs (reduce platelet aggregation)
    - Aspirin (reduce platelet aggregation)
    - Sulfinpyrazone (Anturane) (reduce platelet aggregation)
- Extends the half-life of cephalosporin
  - Cephalosporin given with:
    - Probenecid (Benemid) (increases excretion of uric acid)

13.20 Cephalosporin and Patient Education

The patient must be instructed to:

- Avoid medications that counteract with cephalosporin.
- Remember that Cephalosporin decreases the effects of birth control pills.
- Understand that the healthcare provider might prescribe that probenecid (Benemid) and cephalosporin are to be taken together. The goal is to extend the half-life of cephalosporin without having to increase the dose.
- Monitor for adverse effects (see 13.19 Cephalosporin and Drug–Drug Interactions) and to call the healthcare provider immediately if any are present.

13.21   Macrolide Antibiotics

Macrolide antibiotics are bacteriostatic for gram-positive and -negative bacteria; therefore, they inhibit bacteria reproduction but do not kill the bacteria. Bacteria are killed by the immune system. Macrolide antibiotics are prescribed for soft tissue, skin, respiratory, and gastrointestinal tract infections.

Common side effects are:

- Nausea
- Vomiting
- Stomach pain
- Stomach cramps

13.22   Administering Macrolide Antibiotics

Before administering macrolides to the patient:

- Assess the patient for the same conditions as for cephalosporin (see 13.17 Before Administering Cephalosporin).
- Determine if the patient has a history of cardiac arrhythmias or liver disease. Those patients should not take erythromycin.

Administering macrolides to the patient:

- Take macrolides with a full glass of water
- Administer macrolide an hour before meals or two hours after meals. This reduces gastric distress.
- Macrolides administered via IV must be diluted in 100 to 200 ml of 0.9% solution or 5% dextrose solution (D5W) and infused over a period of 20 to 60 minutes.

13.23   Macrolides and Drug–Drug Interactions

Adverse effects might be produced when macrolides are administered with other medications. Here are potential adverse reactions:

- Risk for increasing the therapeutic levels of other medications
  - Macrolides given with:
    - Alfentanil (Alfenta) (opioid analgesic)
    - Carbamazepine (Tegretol) (seizures, nerve pain, and bipolar disorder)
    - Cyclosporine (Sandimmune) (prevents transplant rejection)
- Risk for cardiac toxicity
  - Macrolides given with:
    - Terfenadine (Seldane) (antihistamine)
    - Astemizole (Hismanal) (antihistamine)
- Risk for hemorrhage
  - Macrolides given with:
    - Warfarin (Coumadin) (anticoagulant)
- Risk for increasing the therapeutic level
  - Theophylline given with:
    - Caffeine

13.24 Macrolides and Patient Education

The patient must be instructed to:

- Provide their healthcare provider with a complete history of over-the-counter medications, prescribed medications, and herbal therapies to identify contraindications for macrolides.
- Explain that there might be a chance of hearing loss as an adverse side effect of macrolides.
- Monitor for adverse effects (see 13.21 Macrolide Antibiotics), and call the healthcare provider immediately if one is present.

Macrolide Antibiotics

Pregnancy Category: B

ROUTE	DOSE	TIME
Erythromycin (E-Mycin, Erythrocin, Erythrocin Lactobionate)		
Protein-Binding: 65%		
Half-Life: PO 1–2 hours IV 3–5 hours		
PO	250–500 mg	Every 6 hours
IV	1–4 g/d	Divided doses
Azithromycin (Zithromax)		
Protein-Binding: 50%		
Half-Life: 11–55 hours		
PO	500 mg	First day
	250 mg	Daily thereafter
Clarithromycin (Biaxin)		
Protein-Binding: 65%–75%		
Half-Life: 3–6 hours		
Pregnancy Category C		
PO	250–500 mg	Every 12 hours
Erythromycin, dirithromycin (Dynabac)		
Protein-Binding: Unknown		
Half-Life: 20–50 hours		
Pregnancy Category: C		
PO	250 mg (erythromycin)	Every 6 hours
		Once a day
	500 mg (dirithromycin)	
IV	250–500 mg	Every 6 hours

13.25 Lincomycins

Lincomycin (Lincocin) is bacteriostatic in lower doses and bacteriocidal in larger doses and is used to treat serous streptococci, pneumococci, and staphylococci infections. It is prescribed for infections of bone, joint, pelvic (female), intraabdominal, skin, and soft tissue.

Lincomycin has generally been replaced by Clindamycin (Cleocin) because there are significant occurrences of pseudomembranous colitis in patients who use lincomycins. Clindamycin is a semisynthetic derivative of lincomycin that is safer and more effective than lincomycin.

Common side effects are:

- Abdominal cramps
- Diarrhea
- Weight loss
- Weakness

13.26   Administering Lincomycin Antibiotics

Before administering lincomycin to the patient:

- Assess the patient for the same conditions as for cephalosporin (see 13.17 Before Administering Cephalosporin).
- Determine if the patient has a history of GI, kidney, or liver disease. Those patients should not take lincomycin.

Administering lyncomycins to the patient:

- Remember that lyncomycins should be taken with a full glass of water.
- Monitor for side effects (see 13.25 Lincomycins).

After administering lyncomycins to the patient:

- Request a white blood cell count to determine if the lyncomycins are effective.

13.27   Lincomycins and Drug–Drug Interactions

Adverse effects might be produced when lincomycins are administered with other medications. The potential adverse reaction is:

- Risk of enhanced neuromuscular blockage, skeletal muscle weakness, respiratory depression and even paralysis
  - Lincomycin is given with:
    - Anesthetic agent

13.28   Lincomycins and Patient Education

The patient must be instructed to:

- Monitor for hypersensitivity.
- Monitor for adverse effects (see 13.25 Lincomycins) and to call the healthcare provider immediately if one is present.

Lincomycins

Pregnancy Category: B

ROUTE	DOSE	TIME
Clindamycin (Cleocin, Dalacin) semisynthetic		
Protein-Binding: 94%		
Half-Life: 2–3 hours		
PO/IM/IV	150–300 mg	Every 6 hours
Lincomycin (Lincorex)		
Protein-Binding: 70%–75%		
Half-Life: 4–6 hours		
PO	500 mg	Every 6–8 hours Max 8 g/d
IM	600 mg	Every day
IV	Dilute in 100 cc fluid	Every day

13.29 Vancomycin

Vancomycin is an antibiotic used to treat *Staphylococcus* and *Clostridium difficile.* These bacteria infect bones and joints and cause endocarditis and enterocolitis. Vancomycin is commonly prescribed to patients who are susceptible to endocarditis to prevent this infection from occurring. Vancomycin is particularly successful in treating methicillin-resistant strains of bacteria. However, parenteral vancomycin is not used to treat antibiotic-associated pseudomembranous colitis.

13.30 Administering Vancomycin Antibiotics

Before administering vancomycin to the patient:

- Assess the patient for the same conditions as for cephalosporin (see 13.17 Before Administering Cephalosporin).
- Assess if the patient has hearing loss. Do not administer vancomycin if there is hearing loss.
- Assess if the patient has kidney problems. Administer a low dose of vancomycin if the patient has kidney problems.
- Assess if the patient has an inflammatory intestinal disorder. Monitor the patient after administering vancomycin for toxicity.

Administering vancomycin to the patient:

- Do not administer vancomycin as a bolus IV.
- Infuse over 24 hours or infuse intermittently over 60 minutes.
- Dilute 1 to 2 g of vancomycin in a sufficient amount of 0.9% sodium chloride (normal saline) or D5W if infused over 24 hours.
- Dilute the dose in 100 ml of 09% sodium chloride (normal saline) or dilute in 100 ml of 5% dextrose solution (D5W) if infused intermittently over 60 minutes.
- Rotate the IV sites to prevent local irritation.

After administering vancomycin to the patient:

- Monitor renal output to assure there is adequate volume of urine to excrete vancomycin.
- Monitor the white blood count to determine if vancomycin is effective.

13.31   Vancomycin and Drug–Drug Interactions

Adverse effects might be produced when vancomycin is administered with other medications. Here are potential adverse reactions:

- Risk of lower therapeutic effect of vancomycin
  - Vancomycin given with:
    - Cholestyramine (Questran) (oral) (reduces cholesterol)
    - Colestipol (Colestid) (oral) (reduces cholesterol)
- Risk of ototoxicity and nephrotoxicity
  - Vancomycin given with:
    - Aminoglycosides (antibiotic)
- Risk of toxicity
  - Vancomycin given with:
    - Amphotericin B (antifungal)
    - Aspirin
    - Bacitracin (antibiotic)
    - Parenteral bumetanide (Bumex) (loop diuretic)
    - Capreomycin (Capastat) (antibiotic)
    - Cisplatin (Platinol) (chemotherapy)
    - Cyclosporine (Sandimmune) (prevents rejection)
    - Ethacrynate parenteral (Edecrin) (loop diuretics)
    - Furosemide parenteral (Lasix) (loop diuretics)
    - Paromomycin (Humatin) (antibiotic)
    - Polymyxins (antibiotic)
    - Streptozocin (Zanosar) (pancreatic islet cell cancer)

13.32   Vancomycins and Patient Education

The patient must be instructed to:

- Monitor for adverse effects (see 13.25 Lyncomycins) and to call the healthcare provider immediately is one is present.
- Monitor the volume of urine output. Notify the healthcare provider if urine output is less than 30 cc per hour.
- Monitor for loss of hearing and ringing in the ears. Call the healthcare provider immediately if these occur.

Vancomycin

Pregnancy Category: C

ROUTE	DOSE	TIME
Vancomycin (Vancocin)		
Protein-Binding: 10%		
Half-Life 5–11 hours		
IV	500 mg	Every 6 hours

13.33　Aminoglycosides

Aminoglycosides are antibiotics that are effective against gram-positive and -negative bacteria but are commonly prescribed for gram-negative bacteria. Aminoglycosides are primarily used to treat life-threatening infections because they have significant side effects. In life-threatening infections, healthcare providers prescribe aminoglycosides with penicillin, cephalosporins, or vancomycin to assure that the bacteria are killed.

Common adverse effects are:

- Nephrotoxicity
- Neurotoxicity
- Hypersensitivity
- Ototoxicity
- Muscle weakness if patient has myasthenia gravis, parkinsonism, or is an infant with botulism

13.34　Administering Aminoglycosides

Before administering aminoglycosides to the patient:

- Assess the patient for the same conditions as for cephalosporin (see 13.17 Before Administering Cephalosporin).
- Assess for kidney function as a baseline.
- Assess for hearing problems as a baseline.
- Assess for allergies.

Administering aminoglycosides to the patient:

- For administering aminoglycosides IV, dilute the medication in the solution as per the package insert and infuse it over a 30- to 60-minute period.
- Use a smaller than normal dose for elderly patients who are at greater risk for kidney and ear toxicity.
- For administering aminoglycosides IM, give the injection deep into the upper outer quadrant of the gluteal muscle.

After administering aminoglycosides to the patient:

- Keep the patient well hydrated.
- Monitor intake and output. (Determine if there is nephrotoxicity.)
- Monitor temperature, cultures, and white blood cell count to determine if the infection is resolved.
- Monitor daily urinalysis (for signs of kidney irritation).

13.35　Aminoglycosides and Drug–Drug Interactions

Adverse effects might be produced when aminoglycosides are administered with other medications. Here are potential adverse reactions:

- Risk for hearing, kidney, and neuromuscular problems long after treatment stops
  - Aminoglycosides given with:
    - Capreomycin (Capastat) (antibiotic)
- Risk for neuromuscular blockage
  - Aminoglycosides given with:
    - Halogenated hydrocarbon (anesthetics)
    - Citrate-anticoagulated blood
    - Methoxyflurane (Penthrane) (anesthetics)
    - Polymyxins (antibiotic)

- Risk for adverse reaction
  - Aminoglycosides given with:
    - Amphotericin B parenteral (Fungizone) (antifungal)
    - Aspirin
    - Bacitracin parenteral (antibiotic)
    - Parenteral bumetanide [Bumex] (loop diuretic)
    - Cephalothin (Keflin) (antibiotic)
    - Cisplatin (Platinol) (chemotherapy)
    - Cyclosporine (Sandimmune) (prevents rejection)
    - Ethacrynate parenteral (Edecrin) (loop diuretics)
    - Furosemide parenteral (Lasix) (loop diuretics)
    - Paromomycin (Humatin) (antibiotic)
    - Polymyxins (antibiotic)
    - Streptozocin (Zanosar) (pancreatic islet cell cancer)
    - Vancomycin (Vancocin) (antibiotic)

13.36   Aminoglycosides and Patient Education

The patient must be instructed to monitor for:

- Kidney problems (nephrotoxicity)
- Twitching, numbness, or seizures (neurotoxicity)
- Hypersensitivity
- Loss of hearing and ringing in the ear
- Dizziness and loss of balance (ototoxicity)
- Tingling in fingers and toes (peripheral neuritis)

Aminoglycosides

Pregnancy Category: C

ROUTE	DOSE	TIME
Amikacin (Amikin)		
Protein-Binding: 4%–11%		
Half-Life: 2–3 hours		
IM/IV	5 mg/kg	Every 8 hours
Gentamicin (Garamycin)		
Protein-Binding: Unknown		
Half-Life: 2 hours		
IM/IV	1–1.7 mg/kg	Infusion every 8 hours
Kanamycin (Kantrex)		
Protein-Binding: 10%		
Half-Life: 2–3 hours		
Pregnancy Category: D		
IM	3.75 mg/kg	Every 6 hours

(Continued)

(Continued from previous page)

ROUTE	DOSE	TIME
Neomycin SO$_4$ (Mycifradin)		
Protein-Binding: 10%		
Half-Life: 2–3 hours		
PO (GI Surgery)	1 g	Every hour for four doses
	1g	
(Hepatic coma)		Every 4 hours thereafter
	4–12 g/d	for 24 hours or other
		regimens
		Divided doses
IM	15 mg/kg/d	Every 6 h for four doses
		Max 1 g/d
Netilmicin (Netromycin)		
Protein-Binding: 10%		
Half-Life: 2–3 hours		
Pregnancy Category: D		
IM/IV	1.3–2.2 mg/kg	Every 8 hours
Streptomycin S O$_4$		
Protein-Binding: 30%		
Half-Life: 2–3 hours		
IM (tuberculosis)	1 g	Every day with
(Endocarditis)	1 g	antimycobacterials
		Every 12 hours for 1 week.
		Dose may be decreased
Tobramycin SO4 (Nebcin)		
Protein-Binding: 10%		
Half-Life: 2–3 hours		
IM/IV	0.75 mg to 1.25 mg/kg	Every 6 hours

13.37   Tetracyclines

Tetracyclines are the first broad-spectrum antibiotic used to impede the growth of gram-positive and -negative bacteria. Tetracyclines are prescribed for acne vulgaris, actinomycosis, anthrax, bronchitis, and urinary tract infections. Demeclocycline, a member of the tetracycline family, is also prescribed for syndrome of inappropriate antidiuretic hormone (SIADH). Demeclocycline inhibits water-induced reabsorption in the kidneys.

Restrictions for using tetracyclines are:

* Not for patients who are pregnant or breastfeeding
* Not for children under 8 years of age. Tetracyclines can permanently mottle and discolor the teeth and decrease linear skeletal growth in both children and the fetus
* Not for patients who are hypersensitive to lidocaine, procaine, and other caine medication because IM injection of tetracyclines contains caine medication
* Not for patients who have renal problems except for doxycycline and minocycline, which are members of the tetracyclines family

13.38   Administering Tetracyclines

Before administering tetracyclines to the patient:

- Assess the patient for the same conditions as for cephalosporin (see 13.17 Before Administering Cephalosporin).
- Assess if the patient is pregnant.
- Assess if the patient is hypersensitive to lidocaine, procaine, and other caine medication.
- Assess if the patient has renal problems.

Administering tetracyclines to the patient:

- Have the patient take with a full glass of water on an empty stomach.
- Do not administer an hour before meals or two hours after meals except for doxycycline and minocycline.
- Do not give antacids and laxatives containing aluminum, calcium, magnesium, or iron products.
- Do not give food, milk, or other daily products for 1 hour before or 2 hours after tetracyclines are administered.
- Doxycycline and oxytetracycline can be administered through IV. Doxycycline is given in concentrations not less than 100 mcg or greater than 1 mg/ml. Oxytetracycline is diluted in at least 100 ml of appropriate IV solution.
- Do not infuse rapidly.
- Do not administer doxycycline IM or SC.
- Each IM injection site should not exceed 2 ml of the medication.
- Do not administer tetracycline IV except for doxycycline and oxytetracycline.

After administering tetracyclines to the patient:

- Have the patient avoid direct sunlight and ultraviolet. Tetracyclines might cause sensitivity to sunlight.
- Make sure the patient knows to use sunscreen in the sun.
- Remind the patient to discard unused tetracyclines. Tetracycline becomes toxic as it decomposes.

13.39   Tetracyclines and Drug–Drug Interactions

Adverse effects might be produced when tetracyclines are administered with other medications. Here are potential adverse reactions:

- Risk of decreased absorption
  - Tetracyclines given with:
    - Colestipol (Colestid) (reduces cholesterol)
    - Cholestyramine (Questran) (reduces cholesterol)
    - Antacids
    - Calcium supplements
    - Magnesium salicylates (analgesic NSAIDs)
    - Iron supplements
    - Magnesium laxatives
- Risk of reducing contraceptive effectiveness and breakthrough bleeding
  - Tetracyclines given with:
    - Estrogen-containing oral contraceptives

13.40 Tetracyclines and Patient Education

The patient must be instructed to monitor for:

- Nephrogenic diabetes insipidus
- Hepatotoxicity
- Pancreatitis
- Dizziness
- Syncope
- Increase sensitivity to sunlight
- Use of alternative methods of birth control if taking estrogen-containing oral contraceptives while on antibiotics

Tetracyclines

Pregnancy Category: D

ROUTE	DOSE	TIME
Tetracycline: Short-acting		
Protein-Binding: 20%–60%		
Half-Life: 6–12 hours		
PO	250–500 mg	Every 6 hours
IM	150 mg	Every 12 hours
Oxytetracycline (Terramycin): Short-acting		
Protein-Binding: 20%–40%		
Half-Life: 6–10 hours		
PO	250–500 mg	Every 6 hours
IV	250–500 mg	Infusion every 12 hours
Demeclocycline (Declomycin): Intermediate-acting		
Protein-Binding: 35%–90%		
Half-Life: 10–17 hours		
PO	150 mg	Every 6 hours
	300 mg	Every 12 hours
Doxycycline (Vibramycin): Long-acting		
Protein-Binding: 25%–92%		
Half-Life: 20 hours		
PO	100 mg	Twice the first day
	100–200 mg	Once a day thereafter
Minocycline (Minocin): Long-acting		
Protein-Binding: 55%–88%		
Half-Life: 11–20 hours		
PO	200 mg	First dose
	100 mg	Every 12 hours

13.41   Chloramphenicol (Chloromycetin)

Chloramphenicol is a broad-spectrum antibiotic. In low doses, chloramphenicol slows the growth of gram-positive and -negative bacteria. Chloramphenicol kills gram-positive and -negative bacteria in high doses.

Chloramphenicol is prescribed to treat meningitis (*H. influenzae, S. pneumoniae,* and *N. meningitides*), parathyroid fever, Q fever, Rocky Mountain spotted fever, typhoid fever, typhus infections, brain abscesses, and bacterial septicemia.

Restrictions for using chloramphenicol are:

- Not for use in patients who are pregnant or are breastfeeding. Neonates may develop gray syndrome (blue-gray skin, hypothermia, irregular breathing, coma, and cardiovascular collapse).
- Not for use in patients who are undergoing radiation therapy or who have bone marrow depression.
- Not for use in patients who have bone marrow depression.

Chloramphenicol adverse effects are:

- Diarrhea
- Nausea
- Vomiting
- Blood dyscrasias
- Optic neuritis
- Irreversible bone marrow depression
- Aplastic anemia

13.42   Chloramphenicol and Drug–Drug Interactions

Adverse effects might be produced when chloramphenicol is administered with other medications. Here are potential adverse reactions:

- Risk for increasing serum level of other medications
  - Chloramphenicol given with:
    - Alfentanil (Alfenta)
    - Phenobarbital (luminal)
    - Phenytoin (Dilantin)
    - Warfarin (Coumadin)
- Risk for bone marrow depression
  - Chloramphenicol given with:
    - Anticonvulsants
- Risk for hypoglycemia
  - Chloramphenicol given with:
    - Antidiabetic medication
- Risk for decreasing therapeutic effect of other medications
  - Chloramphenicol given with:
    - Clindamycin
    - Erythromycin
    - Lincomycin

13.43　Chloramphenicol and Patient Education

The patient must be instructed to monitor for:

- Rash
- Fever
- Dyspnea
- Blurred vision, loss of vision, eye pain (neuritis)
- Tingling, numbness, and burning pain of the hands and feet (neuritis)
- Confusion, delirium (neurotoxic reaction)
- Hypoglycemia if taking diabetic medication

Chloramphenicol (Chloromycetin)
Pregnancy Category: C

ROUTE	DOSE	TIME
Chloramphenicol (Chloromycetin)		
Protein-Binding: 50%–60%		
Half-Life: 4 hours		
PO/IV	12.5 mg/kg	Every 6 hours

13.44　Fluoroquinolones

Fluoroquinolones are a synthetic broad spectrum antibiotic that stops the growth of bacteria in bones and joints. Fluoroquinolones are also prescribed for bronchitis, gastroenteritis, gonorrhea, pneumonia, and urinary tract infections. Restriction for fluoroquinolones: *Not used for infants or children.*

Fluoroquinolones' adverse effects are:

- Dizziness
- Drowsiness
- Restlessness
- Stomach distress
- Diarrhea
- Nausea
- Vomiting
- Psychosis
- Confusion
- Hallucinations
- Tremors
- Hypersensitivity
- Interstitial nephritis

13.45　Administering Fluoroquinolones

Before administering fluoroquinolones to the patient:

- Assess for allergies.
- Assess hepatic and renal problems.

Administering fluoroquinolones to the patient:

- Give with full glass of water to minimize possibility of crystalluria.
- Give a reduced dose if hepatic or renal problems exist.
- Monitor the serum level of fluoroquinolones for patients who have CNS disorders. They are at risk for CNS toxicity.
- If given IV, infuse slowly.
- If given Ofloxacin IV, a member of the fluoroquinolones family, then infuse into a large vein over 60 minutes to minimize discomfort and venous irritation

After administering fluoroquinolones to the patient:

- Monitor urinary output. The patient should void at least 1200 to 1500 ml daily.
- Monitor the pH of the urine. The pH should be 7.0 or less.

13.46   Fluoroquinolones and Drug–Drug Interactions

Adverse effects might be produced when fluoroquinolones are administered with other medications. Here are potential adverse reactions:

- Risk of decreasing absorption
  - Ciprofloxacin, a member of the fluoroquinolones family, given with:
    - Antacids
    - Ferrous sulfate (iron supplement)
    - Sucralfate (treatment of peptic ulcer disease)
- Risk for bleeding
  - Fluoroquinolones given with:
    - Warfarin (anticoagulant)

13.47   Fluoroquinolones and Patient Education

The patient must be instructed to monitor for:

- Rash
- Fever
- Dyspnea nephritis (blood in the urine and lower back pain, edema)
- Increased sensitivity of skin to sunlight
- Dizziness, headache, insomnia (CNS toxicity)
- Confusion, hallucinations, blurry or double vision, sensitivity to light, dizziness, lightheadedness, or depression (CNS stimulation)
- Joint discomfort and stiffness (arthralgia)
- Prothrombin time (PT) if taking warfarin

The patient must remember to:

- Avoid taking fluoroquinolones within two hours of taking an antacid.
- Wear sunglasses and avoid bright lights, sunlight, and sunlamps.

Fluoroquinolones

Pregnancy Category: C

ROUTE	DOSE	TIME
Ciprofloxacin (Cipro)		
Protein-Binding: 20%		
Half-Life: 3–4 hours		
PO	250–500 mg	Every 12 hours
Fluoroquinolone server infections	500–750 mg	Every 12 hours
IV Mild to moderate infections	400 mg	Every 12 hours
Enoxacin (Penetrex)		
Protein-Binding: 40%		
Half-Life: 3–6 hours		
PO	200–400 mg	Every 12 hours 1–2 weeks
Levofloxacin (Levaquin)		
Protein-Binding: 50%		
Half-Life: 6 hours		
IV	500 mg/d	7–14 days
Lomefloxacin (Maxaquin)		
Protein-Binding: Unknown		
Half-Life: 6–8 hours		
PO	400 mg	10–14 days
Norfloxacin (Noroxin)		
Protein-Binding: 10%–11%		
Half-Life: 3–4 hours		
PO	400 mg	Every 12 hours for 72 hours
Ofloxacin (Floxin)		
Protein-Binding: 20%		
Half-Life: 5–8 hours		
PO/IV	300–400 mg	Every 12 hours for 10 days

13.48   Miscellaneous Antibiotics

The following are other antibiotics prescribed to treat microbial infections.

ANTIBIOTIC	DESCRIPTION
Aztreonam (Azactam)	Synthetic bactericidal activity similar to PCN
	Use: treats urinary tract, bronchitis, intraabdominal, gynecologic, and skin infections
	Route: IV
	Dose: 0.5–2 g
	Time: q8–12 h

Protein-Binding: 56%

Half-Life: 1.7–2.1 hours

Pregnancy Category: B

Side Effects: Gastric distress, diarrhea, nausea, vomiting, hypersensitivity and thrombophlebitis at the site of injection

Drug interaction: None

Imipenem-cilastatin (Primaxin IM, Primaxin IV)

Use: treats bone, joint, skin, and soft tissue infections, bacterial endocarditis, intra-abdominal bacteria infections, pneumonia, and gram-positive gram-aerobic and anaerobic organisms

Route: IV, IM

Dose: IV 250–500 mg q6h for mild infections to 500 mg for moderate to severe infections. Maximum dose is 50 mg/kg daily.

IM 500–750 mg up to a maximum of 1500 mg/day

Time: IV q6–8 h

IM q12h

Protein-Binding: 20%

Half-Life: 1 hour

Pregnancy Category: C

Side Effects: Gastric distress, diarrhea, nausea, vomiting, allergic type reactions, confusion, lightheadedness, convulsions, and tremor

Drug interaction: None

Contraindication: Not for use in children less than 12 years old

Meropenem (Merrem IV)

Use: treats susceptible intraabdominal infections (complicated appendicitis and peritonitis) and bacterial meningitis

Route: IV, IM

Dose: IV 1 g over 40–60 minutes

Time: q8h

Protein-Binding: 20%

Half-Life: 1 hour

Pregnancy Category: C

Side Effects: Pseudomembranous colitis, hypersensitivity, diarrhea, nausea, vomiting, headache, and rash

Drug interaction: None

Contraindication: Use with caution with clients with allergy to imipenem, cilastin, or other beta-lactams. Kidney problems require a reduced dosage. If given more than 2 g daily, patients are at high risk for seizures.

13.49 Sulfonamides

Sulfonamides stop the growth of *E. coli* and *Pseudomonas aeruginosa, Serratia, Enterobacter*. Sulfonamides are prescribed for urinary tract infections.

Restrictions for using fluoroquinolones are:

- Not used if the patient is allergic to a member of the sulfonamides family of medication
- Not used for neonates

13.50   Administering Sulfonamides

Before administering sulfonamides to the patient:

- Assess for allergies.

Administering sulfonamides to the patient:

- Have the patient take at least 3000 ml of fluids each day to flush the urinary tract.
- Remember that sulfonamides should be taken on an empty stomach.
- Remember that the patient should avoid antacids (which decrease absorption of sulfonamides).
- Remember that the patient should avoid coffee, tea, citric acid juices, cola, alcohol, chocolate, and spices.

After administering sulfonamides to the patient:

- Have the patient drink water daily to flush the urinary tract.
- Advise the patient to follow good hygiene to reduce risk of acquiring infection again.

13.51   Sulfonamides and Drug–Drug Interactions

Adverse effects might be produced when sulfonamides are administered with other medications. Here are potential adverse reactions:

- Risk of toxic effect by adversely affecting serum levels of other medication
  - Sulfonamides given with:
    - Coumarin (anticoagulants)
    - Indanedione (anticoagulants)
    - Anticonvulsants
    - Oral antidiabetic agents
    - Methotrexate (chemotherapy)

13.52   Sulfonamides and Patient Education

The patient must be instructed to:

- Watch for an allergic reaction.
- Drink water daily to flush the urinary tract.
- Follow good hygiene.

Sulfonamides
Pregnancy Category: C

ROUTE	DOSE	TIME
Sulfadiazine (Microsulfon)		
Protein-Binding: 20%–30%		
Half-Life: 8–12 hours		
PO	4 g First	7–10 days
Increase fluid intake to greater than 2000 ml/d	2–4 g subsequent	

Sulfamethizole (Sulfosol, Thiosulfil Forte)
Protein-Binding: 90%
Half-Life: 1.5 hours
PO

	0.5–1 g in three to four divided doses	7–10 days

Sulfisoxazole (Gantrisin):
Protein-Binding: 60%–70%
Half-Life: 7–12 hours
PO

	2–3 g/d in two to three divided doses	7–10 days

Sulfasalazine (Azulfidine; Salazopyrin)
Protein-Binding: 99%
Half-Life: 5.5 hours
PO

	Initially 1 g	q6–8h
	maintenance 2 g	q6h

Trimethoprim-sulfamethoxazole
Protein-Binding: 50%–65%
Half-Life: 8–12 hours
Most widely used antibacterial agent in the world
PO

	160/800 mg	q12h

Solved Problems

Microorganisms

13.1   What is an infection?

An infection occurs when microorganisms colonize inside the body and use the body's resources to grow. This process interferes with normal body functions. The body response is the inflammation process.

13.2   What are flora?

Flora are microorganisms that help with digestion.

13.3   What is a pathogen?

A pathogen is a microorganism that causes infection.

13.4   What is sepsis?

Sepsis is a body that is infected.

13.5   Name three types of microorganisms.

Three types of microorganisms are bacteria, viruses, and fungi.

Natural Defense

13.6   What are T cells?

T cells are a type of white blood cell that searches for antigens.

13.7   What is an antigen?

An antigen is a foreign substance that enters the body.

13.8   How does a T cell destroy an antigen?

The T cell engulfs the antigen.

13.9   What is a B cell?

B cells are another type of white blood cell that creates antibodies designed specifically to attack a particular antigen.

Antimicrobials

13.10   What are antimicrobials?

Antimicrobials are medication that impedes the growth of or kills pathogens.

13.11   What is bacteriostatic?

Bacteriostatic is an antimicrobial that impedes the growth of bacteria, giving time for the immune system to kill the bacteria.

13.12   What is bacteriocidal?

Bacteriocidal is an antimicrobial agent that kills bacteria.

13.13   What is lysis?

Lysis is a method of killing bacteria by exploding bacteria.

13.14   Name two ways in which antimicrobials react with pathogens.

1. Inhibit the pathogen from growing a cell wall.
2. Disrupt the permeability of the pathogen's membrane to prevent nutrients from entering the pathogen's cell and prevent waste from excreting from the pathogen's cell.

13.15   How are adverse effects of antimicrobials treated?

Adverse effects of antimicrobials are treated with antihistamines (Benadryl), epinephrine (adrenalin), and steroids for anti-inflammatory response.

13.16   What is the name of antimicrobials that impede or kill bacteria?

The name of antimicrobials that impede or kill bacteria is antibiotics.

13.17   What is a super infection?

A super infection is an infection caused by bacteria that is resistant to antibiotics.

13.18   Name two ways that a super infection can occur.

1. A large antibiotic dose is used.
2. An antibiotic is used for a long period.

13.19   Name one way to reduce the likelihood of developing antibiotic-resistant bacteria.

One way to reduce the likelihood of developing antibiotic-resistant bacteria is to use culture and sensitivity to identify the bacteria causing the infection and then use only the appropriate antibiotic to treat the infection.

13.20 What question is important to ask the patient each time before administering an antibiotic?

Do you have allergies?

13.21 What should be available when administering antibiotics?

Emergency medication such as epinephrine, Benadryl, and steroids should be available to counteract any adverse effect of the antibiotic.

13.22 What is a stop order?

Typically antimicrobial medication orders are for 72 hours. A stop order is automatically enforced after 72 hours, requiring the healthcare provider to reassess the patient before renewing the medication order. This is to ensure that the pathogen does not become resistant to the antimicrobial medication.

13.23 Why is it important for the patient to take all the prescribed antibiotic even after the symptoms subside?

Bacteria is alive and growing even when symptoms subside. Taking the all the prescribed antibiotic ensures that bacteria are killed.

13.24 How does penicillin kill bacteria?

Penicillin weakens the cell wall of bacteria, rupturing and destroying the cell in a process called lysis.

13.25 How should penicillin be administered orally?

Penicillin should be given with a full glass of water. Do not give with acidic fruit juices.

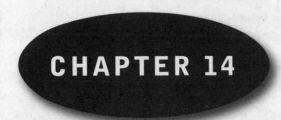

CHAPTER 14

Respiratory Diseases and Medication

14.1   Respiration

The respiratory tract is divided into the upper and lower tracts. The upper respiratory tract contains the nares, nasal cavity, pharynx, and larynx and the lower tract consists of the trachea, bronchi, bronchioles, alveoli, and alveolar-capillary membrane.

Air is inhaled during respiration and passes through the upper respiratory tract and to the alveoli capillary membrane in the lower respiratory tract. The lower respiratory tract is the site of gas exchange. Oxygen attaches to hemoglobin in blood. Carbon dioxide leaves the blood and is expelled through the lower and upper respiratory tracts during expiration.

There are three phases of respiration:

1. Ventilation: Ventilation is the process by which oxygenated air passes through the respiratory tract during inspiration.
2. Perfusion: Perfusion occurs when blood from the pulmonary circulation is sufficient at the alveolar-capillary bed to conduct diffusion. For perfusion to occur, the alveolar pressure must be matched by adequate ventilation. Mucosal edema, secretions, and bronchospasm increase resistance to the airflow, resulting in decreased ventilation and decreased diffusion.
3. Diffusion: Diffusion is the process by which oxygen moves into the capillary bed and carbon dioxide leaves the capillary bed.

14.2   Compliance

Compliance is the ability of the lungs to be distended. Compliance is expressed as a change in volume per unit change in pressure—how well the lungs can stretch when filling with air.

Two factors affect compliance:

1. Connective tissue: Connective tissue consists of collagen and elastin.
2. Surface tension: Surface tension in the alveoli is controlled by surfactant. Surfactant lowers surface tension in the alveoli, preventing interstitial fluid from entering the alveoli.

Compliance increases lung volume in patients who have chronic obstructive pulmonary disease (COPD). Compliance decreases lung volume in patients who have restrictive pulmonary disease. Lungs are stiff, requiring increased pressure to expand because of either an increase in connective tissue or an increase in surface tension in the alveoli.

14.3 Controlling Respiration

Respiration is controlled by three factors. These are the blood concentrations of:

1. Oxygen (O_2)
2. Carbon dioxide (CO_2)
3. Hydrogen (H+) ion

Chemoreceptors sense concentrations of oxygen, carbon, and carbon dioxide in the blood. A change in concentration causes the chemoreceptors to send a message to the central chemoreceptors located in the medulla. The medulla then sends the necessary physiological response through cerebrospinal fluid.

For example, chemoreceptors, called peripheral chemoreceptors, located in carotid arteries and aortic arteries, monitor changes in oxygen pressure in the arteries. If oxygen pressure falls below 60 mm Hg, the peripheral chemoreceptors send a message to the respiratory center in the medulla to increase ventilation.

14.4 The Tracheobronchial Tube

The tracheobronchial tube is a fibrous spiral of smooth muscles connecting the pharynx to the bronchial tree. The bronchial tree extends to terminal bronchioles in the lungs, providing an unobstructed airway to exchange gases. The size of the airway increases or decreases by relaxing or contracting the bronchial smooth muscle, which is controlled by the vagus nerve of the parasympathetic nervous systems.

Acetylcholine is released when the vagus nerve is stimulated, causing contraction of the tracheobronchial tube. This is called *bronchoconstriction*. Epinephrine is released when the sympathetic nervous system is stimulated, causing the beta$_2$ receptor in the bronchial smooth muscle to relax, resulting in dilation of the tracheobronchial tube. This is called *bronchodilation*.

14.5 Respiratory Tract Disorders

Respiratory disorders are divided into two groups.

Upper Respiratory Tract Disorders

Upper respiratory tract disorders are diagnosed as upper respiratory infections (URIs) and include acute rhinitis, sinusitis, acute tonsillitis, and acute laryngitis. Do not confuse acute rhinitis with allergic rhinitis.

Lower Respiratory Tract Disorders

Lower respiratory disorders are conditions that obstruct or restrict tracheobronchial tubes, preventing exchange of gases. These conditions are called chronic obstructive pulmonary disease (COPD), and include bronchitis, chronic bronchitis, bronchiectasis, emphysema, asthma, and chronic asthma.

14.6   Acute Rhinitis (the Common Cold)

Acute rhinitis, known as the common cold, occurs when a rhinovirus invades the nasopharyngeal tract, causing acute inflammation of the mucous membranes of the nose and increased nasal secretions. Acute rhinitis is seasonable—half occur in the winter, one fourth in the summer, and the rest any time throughout the year. Acute rhinitis is contagious 1 to 4 days before symptoms present; this is called the *incubation period*. During the incubation period the rhinovirus can be transmitted by touching contaminated surfaces and from contact with droplets from an infected patient who sneezes and coughs. After the incubation period, the patient experiences a watery nasal discharge called rhinorrhea, nasal congestion, cough, and mucosal secretions.

14.7   Home Remedies for Acute Rhinitis

Home remedies ease the symptoms of acute rhinitis, but do not impede the growth of the rhinovirus or kill it. Home remedies are:

- Rest
- Vitamin C (not proved effective against the rhinovirus)
- Megadoses of other vitamins (not proved effective against the rhinovirus)
- Chicken soup

14.8   Medications for Acute Rhinitis

Commonly prescribed medications and over-the-counter medications used for acute rhinitis follow.

Antihistamines (H_1 Blocker)

Antihistamines reduce the production of histamines. Histamines are vasodilators that react to a foreign substance, including the rhinovirus, and cause redness, itching, and swelling to defend against the foreign substance. Antihistamines compete for the same receptor sites as histamines. An antihistamine latches to the site, blocking the histamine from latching to the site and therefore preventing histamine action, and resulting in a reduction of redness, itching, and swelling. There are two types of histamine receptors, H_1 and H_2. Antihistamines are named according to which histamine receptor site it blocks.

Decongestants (Sympathomimetic Amines)

Decongestants reduce nasal congestion. Nasal congestion occurs when the nasal mucous membranes swell in response to the presence of the rhinovirus. This is commonly referred to as a runny nose. Decongestants stimulate the alpha-adrenergic receptors, causing constriction of the capillaries within the nasal mucosa. This results in shrinking the swelling of the nasal mucous membranes, reducing secretions from the nose. Decongestants should not be used for more than 5 days, otherwise the patient may become tolerant of the medication and experience rebound nasal congestion. There are three types of decongestants:

- Nasal decongestants: Provide quick relief
- Systemic decongestants: Provide longer-lasting relief
- Intranasal glucocorticoids: Used to treat seasonal and perennial rhinitis

Antitussives

Antitussives suppress the cough center in the medulla. A cough from acute rhinitis is caused by nasal mucous draining into the respiratory tract. There are two types of antitussives, non-narcotic and narcotic.

Expectorants

Expectorants are medications that loosen viscous (thick) mucous secretions, making it easy to cough and expel the mucous. Expectorants increase fluid output of the respiratory tract and decrease the respiratory tract's adhesiveness and surface tension.

ANTIHISTAMINE (H₁ BLOCKER)

Use	Treats common cold, allergic rhinitis, itching; prevents motion sickness; sleep aid; antitussive	Half-life: 2–7 hours	Onset: PO: 15–45 minutes IM: 15–30 minutes IV: Immediate	Peaks: PO: 4–8 hours IM: 4–7 hours IV: 4–7 hours
Example	Diphenhydramine HCl (Benadryl), astemizole (Hismanal), cetirizine (Zyrtec) chlorpheniramine maleate (Chlor-Trimeton, Kolomnin, Phenetron, Techlor, Teldrin); loratadine (Claritin)	Route: PO, IM, IV	Pregnancy category: B	Pharmacokinetic: Absorbed from GI tract. Metabolized by the liver and excreted in urine.

How it works	• Competes with histamine for receptor sites, thus preventing a histamine response • Causes the extravascular smooth muscles, including those lining the nasal cavity, to constrict
Adult dose	• PO: 25–50 mg q6 h • IM/IV: 10–50 mg as single dose q4–6h, maximum dose of 400 mg/day
Before administration	• Obtain baseline vital signs. • Obtain drug history. • Assess cardiac and respiratory status including rate, depth, rhythm, type of respirations, and quality and rate of pulse. Assess lung sounds for rhonchi, wheezing, and rales.
Administration	• Take with food to avoid gastric distress. • Administer IM in large muscle. • Do not give as SC injection.
After administration	• Monitor blood pressure for hypotension. • Maintain safe environment. Causes drowsiness. • Hydrate patient.
Contraindi-cation	• Do not give to a patient who is having an acute asthma attack. • Do not give to a patient who is receiving MAO inhibitors. • Do not give to a patient who is breastfeeding. • Use caution when giving to a patient who has one of the following conditions: narrow-angle glaucoma, peptic ulcer, prostatic hypertrophy, pyloroduodenal or bladder neck obstruction, chronic asthma, COPD.
Side effects/ adverse reactions	• Children and elderly people are more susceptible to side effects. • Drowsiness, dizziness, fatigue, nausea, vomiting, urinary retention, constipation, blurred vision, dry mouth and throat, reduced secretions, hypotension, epigastric distress, hearing disturbances, excitation in children, and photosensitivity • Hypersensitivity reactions: Eczema, pruritus, rash, and cardiac disturbances Life-threatening side effects: • Agranulocytosis, hemolytic anemia, and thrombocytopenia
Patient education	• Avoid driving a motor vehicle. • Avoid performing dangerous activities. • Avoid alcohol and other central nervous system (CNS) depressants. • If used for motion sickness, take at least 30 minutes before traveling, before meals, and at bedtime during travel.

ANTIHISTAMINE USED TO TREAT ALLERGIC RHINITIS

Phenothiazines (antihistamine action) Promethazine HCl (Phenergan)	• PO/IM: 12.5–25 mg q4–6h PRN • Maximum dose: 150 mg/d • Before meals and bedtime • Pregnancy category: C • Protein bound: Unknown • Half-life: Unknown
Piperazine derivative—hydroxyzine (Atarax, Vistaril)	• PO 25–100 mg TID/QID • Pregnancy category: C • Protein bound: Unknown • Half-life: 3 hours
Butyrophenone derivative (terfenadine, Seldane)	• PO 60 mg BID • Pregnancy category: C • Protein bound: 97% • Half-life: 20 hours
Ethanolamine derivative—carbinoxamine and pseudoephedrine (Rondec)	• PO: 5 ml QID or 1 tab QID • Pregnancy category: C • Protein bound: Unknown • Half-life: Unknown
Clemastine fumarate (Tavist)	• PO: 1.34–2.68 mg BID, TID • Maximum dose: 8 mg/d • Pregnancy category: C • Protein bound: Unknown • Half-life: Unknown
Propylamine derivatives—brompheniramine maleate (Bromphen, Dimetane, Histaject, Nasahist B, Oraminic II)	• PO: 4 mg q4 h–6h or SR: 8 mg q8–12h maximum dose 24 mg/d • IM/IV/SC: 10 mg q8–12h; max: 40 mg/d • Pregnancy category: C • Protein bound: Unknown • Half-life: 25–36 hours
Triprolidine and pseudoephedrine (Actifed)	• PO: 2.5 mg q6–8h; max: 10 mg/d • Pregnancy category: B • Protein bound: Unknown • Half-life: 3 hours

ALPHA-ADRENERGIC AGONIST
Nasal Decongestant

Use	Nasal congestion	Half-life: Unknown	Onset: 2 minutes	Peaks: 8 hours
Example	Oxymetazoline HCl (Afrin)	Route: Intranasal spray	Pregnancy category: C	Pharmacokinetics: Topical; absorbed via mucous membranes
How it works	• Stimulates alpha-adrenergic receptors, producing vascular constriction of the capillaries within the nasal mucosa			
Adult dose	• Intranasal: 0.05% gtt q nostril BID. Use only 3–5 days • Spray: 1–2 sprays q nostril BID. Use only 3–5 days			
Before administration	• Obtain baseline vital signs. • Obtain drug history.			

Administration	To use the *nose drops:*
	• Blow the nose gently. Tilt the head back while standing or sitting up, or lie down on a bed and hang the head over the side. Place the drops into each nostril and keep the head tilted back for a few minutes to allow the medicine to spread throughout the nose.
	• Rinse the dropper with hot water and dry with a clean tissue. Replace the cap right after use.
	• To avoid spreading the infection, do not use the container for more than one person.
	To use the *nose spray:*
	• Blow the nose gently. With the head upright, spray the medicine into each nostril. Sniff briskly while squeezing the bottle quickly and firmly. For best results, spray once into each nostril, wait 3 to 5 minutes to allow the medicine to work, then blow the nose gently and thoroughly. Repeat until the complete dose is used.
	• Rinse the tip of the spray bottle with hot water, taking care not to suck water into the bottle, and dry with a clean tissue. Replace the cap right after use.
	• To avoid spreading the infection, do not use the container for more than one person.
After administration	• Monitor blood pressure for a possible increase.
	• Monitor blood glucose in diabetics for a possible increase.
	• Monitor the duration that the patient is being treated with the medication.
Contraindication	• Use caution when giving to a patient who has hypertension, cardiac disease, hyperthyroidism, or diabetes mellitus.
Side effects/ adverse reactions	• There is a rebound effect if used for more than 3–5 days.
Patient education	• Avoid alcohol.
	• Avoid caffeine.
	• *Use this medicine only as directed.* Do not use more of it, do not use it more often, and do not use it for longer than 3 days without first checking with your doctor. To do so may make your runny or stuffy nose worse and may also increase the chance of side effects.
	• Do not share this medication with family or friends to avoid spreading the infection.

SYSTEMIC DECONGESTANT

Use	Allergic rhinitis, including hay fever and acute coryza (profuse nasal discharge). Provides longer-lasting relief than nasal decongestants	Half-life: 9–15 hours	Onset: 15–30 minutes	Peaks: 30–60 minutes
Example	Pseudoephedrine hydrochloride (Actifed, Sudafed), phenylpropanolamine (Allerest, Dimetapp), phenylephrine HCK (Neo-Synephrine, Sinex), and pseudoephedrine (Actifed, Sudafed); frequently combined with an antihistamine, analgesic, or antitussive (anticough) in oral cold remedies	Route: Tablet, capsule, liquid	Pregnancy category: C	Pharmacokinetic: Absorbed by the GI tract, metabolized in liver and excreted in urine. Not removed by hemodialysis
How it works	• Acts directly on alpha-adrenergic receptors and to a lesser extent on beta-adrenergic receptors, producing vasoconstriction of respiratory tract mucosa, which causes shrinkage of nasal mucous membranes, edema, and nasal congestion			
Adult dose	• PO: 60 mg q4–6 h; maximum dose 240 mg/day, extended release 120 mg q12 hours			
Before administration	• Obtain baseline vital signs.			
	• Obtain drug history.			
Administration	• Do not crush or chew extended-release tablets. Swallow whole.			
After administration	• Monitor blood pressure for a possible increase.			
	• Monitor blood glucose in diabetics for a possible increase.			
Contraindications	• Use caution when giving to a patient who has hypertension, cardiac disease, hyperthyroidism, or diabetes mellitus.			

Side effects/ adverse reactions	• Jitters, nervousness, restlessness; symptoms disappear as the body adjusts. • Raises blood pressure • Increases blood glucose • Large dose: Tachycardia, palpitations, lightheadedness, nausea, and vomiting • Overdose: Hallucinations in patients greater than 60 years old; can cause CNS depression and seizures
Patient education	• Do not crush or chew extended-release tablets. • Avoid caffeine. • Avoid alcohol. • Discontinue if the patient continues to experience side effects.

INTRANASAL GLUCOCORTICOIDS

Use	Inhibits early-phase allergic reaction and migration of inflammatory cells into nasal tissue and decreases response to seasonal and perennial rhinitis. Inhalation: Control of bronchial asthma in those requiring chronic steroid therapy. Intranasal: Relief of seasonal/perennial rhinitis; prevention of nasal polyps from recurring after surgical removal; treatment of nonallergic rhinitis. Nasal: Prophylaxis of seasonal rhinitis.	Half-life: 3–15 hours	Onset: Immediate	Peaks: 2 hours
Example	Beclomethasone dipropionate (Vanceril)	Route: Inhalation/ intranasal	Pregnancy category: C	Pharmacokinetic: Rapidly absorbed from pulmonary, nasal, and GI tissue. PB: 87%; metabolized in liver; excreted in feces.

How it works	• Inhalation: Decreases number and activity of inflammatory cells into bronchial wall, inhibits bronchoconstriction; produces smooth muscle relaxation; decreases mucus secretions. • Intranasal: Inhibits early phase allergic reaction, migration of inflammatory cells into nasal tissue, decreasing response to seasonal and perennial rhinitis.
Adult dose	• Inhalation: 42 mcg; two inhalations 304 times/day; maximum 20 inhalations/day (84 mcg) • Intranasal: One to two sprays in each nostril one to two times/day; maximum 12 sprays/day
Before administration	• Obtain history of hypersensitivity to any corticosteroids.
Administration	• Intranasal: Clear nasal passages before use; insert spray up into nostril, pointing toward nasal passages away from nasal septum; spray into nostril while holding other nostril closed and concurrently inspire through nose to permit medication as high into nasal passages as possible. • Inhalation: Shake container well, exhale completely, place mouthpiece between lips, inhale, and hold breath as long as possible before exhaling; allow at least 1 min between inhalations; rinse mouth after each use to decrease dry mouth and hoarseness.
After administration	Intranasal: • Monitor for nasal-crusting. • Monitor for nosebleeds. • Monitor for sore throat. • Monitor for nasal ulceration. Inhalation: • In those receiving bronchodilators by inhalation concomitantly with inhalation of steroid therapy, advise the patient to use bronchodilator several minutes before corticosteroid aerosol (enhances penetration of the steroid into bronchial tree).
Contraindi- cations	• Do not administer if there is an untreated localized infection involving nasal mucosa.

- Hypersensitivity to any corticocosteroid; primary treatment of status asthmaticus, systemic fungal infections, persistently positive sputum cultures for *Candida albicans.*
- *Caution:* Adrenal insufficiency, cirrhosis, glaucoma, hypothyroidism, untreated infection, osteoporosis, tuberculosis, sensitivity to beclomethasone

Side effects/ adverse reactions	Intranasal: • Frequent: Burning, dryness inside nose • Occasional: Nasal crusting, nosebleeds, sore throat, or nasal ulceration after prolonged use • Rare: Nasal/pharyngeal candidiasis, eye pain Inhalation: • Frequent: Throat irritation, dry mouth, hoarseness, cough • Occasional: Localized fungal infection (thrush) • Rare: Transient bronchospasm, esophageal candidiasis Adverse/Toxic • Acute hypersensitivity reaction; occurs rarely • Transfer from systemic to local steroid therapy may unmask previously suppressed bronchial asthma condition
Patient education	• Improvement should be in 2–3 days. • Clear nasal passages before use. • Contact healthcare provider if symptoms persist. • Instruct on proper installation of nasal spray or use of inhaler. • Do not change dose schedule or stop taking drug; must taper off gradually under medical supervision. • Inhalation: Maintain careful mouth hygiene. Rinse mouth with water immediately after inhalation. Contact health care provider if sore throat or mouth occurs.

ANTITUSSIVES

Use	Provide temporary suppression of a nonproductive cough to reduce viscosity of tenacious secretions	Half-life: Unknown	Onset: 15–30 minutes	Peaks: 3–6 hours
Example	Dextromethorphan hydrobromide (Robitussin DM, Romilar, PediaCare, Benylin DM), benzonatate (Tessalon), diphenhydramine (Benadryl); promethazine with dextromethorphan [combination of a phenothiazine and nonnarcotic antitussive]	Route: PO	Pregnancy category: C	Pharmacokinetic: Absorbed in GI tract, metabolized in liver and excreted in urine
How it works	• Non-narcotic antitussive suppresses the cough center in the medulla • Does not cause physical dependence, tolerance, or depress respirations			
Adult dose	• PO: 10–30 mg q4–8h; maximum 120 mg/24 h; sustained action 60 mg q12 h			
Before administration	• Obtain medical history. • Obtain medication history. • Assess type, severity, frequency of cough, and productions. • Increase fluid intake and environmental humidity to lower viscosity of lung secretions.			
Administration	• Give without regard to meals. • Do not crush or break sustained-release capsule. May sprinkle contents on soft food, then swallow without crushing or chewing.			
After administration	• Monitor for side effects. • Provide a safe environment. • Initiate deep breathing and coughing exercises, particularly in a patient with impaired pulmonary function. • Assess for clinical improvement and record onset of relief of cough.			
Contraindication	• Do not administer if the patient has COPD, chronic productive cough; hypersensitivity; or is taking monoamine oxidase inhibitors			
Side effects/ adverse reactions	• Nausea, dizziness, drowsiness, sedation • Hallucinations at high doses			

Patient education	• Avoid alcohol. • Avoid driving or operating machinery until response to drug is known. • Be alert for side effects. • Give without regard to meals. • Perform coughing and deep breathing exercises.

EXPECTORANTS

Use	Loosens bronchial secretions so they can be eliminated with coughing	Half-life: Unknown	Onset: 15–30 minutes	Peaks: 2 hours
Example	Guaifenesin (Robitussin)	Route: PO, syrup, liquid or capsules	Pregnancy category: C	Pharmacokinetic: Absorbed in GI tract, metabolized in liver, and excreted in urine

How it works	• Enhances fluid output of respiratory tract by decreasing adhesiveness and surface tension and promotes removal of viscous mucus
Adult dose	• PO: 200–400 mg q4h; maximum dose 2.4 g/day
Before administration	• Assess type, severity, frequency of cough, and productions of mucous or other materials. • Increase fluid intake and environmental humidity.
Administration	• Give with a full glass of water.
After administration	• Initiate deep breathing and coughing exercises. • Assess for clinical improvement and mucous production. • Obtain mucous specimens if ordered.
Contraindication	• Not for use with persistent cough because of smoking, asthma, emphysema, or cough accompanied by excessive secretions.
Side effects/ adverse reactions	• Rare: Dizziness, headache, rash, diarrhea, nausea, vomiting, stomach pain • An excessive dose may produce nausea and vomiting.
Patient education	• Maintain good hydration. • Avoid driving or operating machinery until a response to the drug is known. • Use a humidifier to increase environmental hydration. • Take with a full glass of water. • Do not crush or break sustained-release capsule. • Can sprinkle contents on soft food and swallow without crushing or chewing. • Contact healthcare provider if cough is persistent or the nature of production changes.

14.9 Sinusitis

Sinusitis is the inflammation of the sinuses' mucous membranes. Commonly affected sinuses are the:

- Maxillary
- Frontal
- Ethmoid
- Sphenoid

The treatment for sinusitis is:

- Systemic decongestants or nasal decongestants for the reduction of the congestion that accompanies sinusitis
- Acetaminophen (Tylenol) or ibuprofen for discomfort
- Antibiotics (if infection is suspected)
- Increased fluids
- Rest

14.10   Acute Pharyngitis (Sore Throat)

Acute pharyngitis is inflammation of the throat that results in coughing, an elevated temperature, and pain when swallowing. Acute pharyngitis can lead to other upper respiratory tract diseases, such as acute rhinitis or acute sinusitis.

    There are two types of acute pharyngitis.

Viral Pharyngitis

Viral pharyngitis is caused by a virus. Antibiotics are not used to treat viral pharyngitis. Medication is given to treat the symptoms of viral pharyngitis, but not to impede or kill the virus. Acetaminophen or ibuprofen is given to reduce body temperature and ease discomfort. Saline gargles, lozenges, and increased fluid help soothe the throat.

Bacterial Pharyngitis

Bacteria pharyngitis can be caused by the beta-hemolytic streptococci bacteria, which is known as strep throat. A throat culture and sensitivity is performed to determine the bacteria causing the infection and the antibiotic to treat the infection. Saline gargles, lozenges, and increased fluid help soothe the throat.

14.11   Acute Tonsillitis

Acute tonsillitis is the inflammation of the tonsils commonly caused by streptococcus bacteria, which results in a sore throat, chills, fever, aching muscles, and pain when swallowing. A throat culture and sensitivity is performed to determine the bacteria causing the infection and the antibiotic to treat the infection. Acute tonsillitis also can be caused by a virus. Saline gargles, lozenges, and increased fluid help soothe the throat.

14.12   Acute Laryngitis

Acute laryngitis is an inflammation of the vocal cords that causes swelling of the vocal cords and results in a weak or hoarse voice. Acute laryngitis can be caused by a viral infection or overuse of the vocal cords. Acute laryngitis is treated by refraining from speaking and avoiding substances that irritate the vocal cords, such as smoking.

14.13   Lower Respiratory Disorders

Lower respiratory disorders, called COPD, are conditions that obstruct or restrict tracheobronchial tubes, which prevent the exchange of gases. These conditions include bronchitis, chronic bronchitis, bronchiectasis, emphysema, and chronic asthma. Lower respiratory disorders constrict bronchioles (bronchospasm) and increase mucous secretions, resulting in increased resistance of airflow during inspiration and expiration. This airflow causes impaired oxygen flow to lung tissue and the patient has breathing difficulties (dyspnea). In some cases this damage is irreversible.

14.14   Pneumonia

Pneumonia is an infection in the lungs caused by viruses, bacteria, fungi, or chemical irritants. Pneumonia starts as an upper respiratory infection as a result of acute pharyngitis or acute rhinitis and leads to a lower respiratory infection. Pneumonia is contagious and spreads via droplets in the air from coughing and sneezing. Symptoms of pneumonia can occur 3 days after the upper respiratory infection.

Symptoms of pneumonia are:

- Fever
- Chills
- Cough
- Rapid breathing
- Wheezing
- Grunting respirations
- Labored breathing
- Vomiting
- Chest pain
- Abdominal pain
- Loss of appetite
- Decreased activity
- Hypoxia (cyanosis)

There are two kinds of pneumonia.

Viral Pneumonia

Viral pneumonia is treated symptomatically with bronchodilators, antipyretics, analgesics, expectorants and mucolytics, and cough suppressants.

Bacterial and Fungal Pneumonia

Bacterial and fungal pneumonias are treated with antimicrobials (see chapter 12) and with bronchodilators, antipyretics, analgesics, expectorants and mucolytics, and cough suppressants.

14.15   Tuberculosis

Tuberculosis (TB) is a lower respiratory infection caused by bacillus *Mycobacterium tuberculosis*, which is commonly called tubercle bacillus and is an acid-fast bacillus (AFB). Tuberculosis is transmitted by droplets dispersed in the air through coughing and sneezing and inhaled into the alveoli of the lung. Tuberculosis spreads from the lungs to other organs via the blood and lymphatic system in patients with a compromised immune system.

Symptoms of tuberculosis are:

- Anorexia
- Cough
- Sputum production
- Increased fever
- Night sweats
- Weight loss
- Positive acid-fast bacilli (AFB) in the sputum

Tuberculosis can be prevented by using the Bacillus Calmette-Guerin (BCG) tuberculosis vaccine, a weakened form of the tuberculosis bacterium that does not cause a tuberculosis infection. The vaccine enables the immune system to create antibodies for tuberculosis bacterium.

Tuberculosis is treated with antibiotics (see chapter 13).

14.16 Chronic Bronchitis

Chronic bronchitis is a persistent inflammation of the bronchi because of excess mucous production that irritates the bronchial and results in a persistent productive cough. Smoking is a common cause of chronic bronchitis and is aggravated by air pollution, infection, and allergies. Patients with chronic bronchitis have rhonchi (a gurgling sound) on inspiration and expiration, caused by airway blockage from excess mucus. This excess results in hypercapnia (buildup of carbon dioxide in the blood) and hypoxemia (decreased oxygen in the blood). The patient experiences respiratory acidosis.

Chronic bronchitis is treated with bronchodilator medication that dilates the bronchi. Antibiotics are not used to treat chronic bronchitis except if a subsequent lung infection develops.

14.17 Bronchiectasis

Bronchiectasis is the irreversible dilation of parts of the bronchi that results in the formation of pockets where secretions can accumulate. These pockets create an environment that fosters the growth of bacteria and infection. Bacteria commonly found in bronchiectasis are *Staphylococcus*, Klebsiella, and Bordetella pertussis. These are treated with antibiotics (see chapter 13).

14.18 Emphysema

Emphysema occurs when the alveoli enlarge, trapping air and preventing an adequate gas exchange. Excess mucus, residue from cigarette smoking, and airborne pollutants block the terminal bronchioles, which results in alveoli losing fiber, becoming inelastic and unable to adequately contract after expanding during inspiration. Emphysema also occurs when there is a lack of alpha$_1$-antitrypsin protein. Alpha$_1$-antitrypsin protein inhibits proteolytic enzymes and protects the alveoli from proteolytic enzymes released by bacteria in the lungs.

Emphysema is treated by using bronchodilators such as anticholinergic and beta$_2$-agonists (ipratropium bromide, theophylline) to open the airway by relaxing muscles around the bronchi. Corticosteroids are used to reduce the inflammation that is associated with emphysema.

14.19 Acute Asthma

Acute asthma is a reactive airway disease (RAD) occurring when extrinsic (environmental) or intrinsic (internal) allergens stimulate bronchoconstriction, causing bronchospasms that result in wheezing and difficulty breathing.

An allergen is something that causes an allergic reaction. Common allergens that can trigger an asthmatic attack are:

- Humidity
- Air pressure changes
- Temperature changes
- Smoke
- Fumes (exhaust, perfume)
- Stress
- Emotional upset
- Animal dander
- Dust mites
- Aspirin
- Indomethacin
- Ibuprofen

Allergens attach to mast cells and basophils in connective tissues, causing an antigen–antibody reaction. Mast cells stimulate the release of chemical mediators that constrict the bronchi, increase mucous secretions, stimulate the inflammatory response, and cause pulmonary congestion.

Chemical mediators are:

- Histamines (vasodilator)
- Cytokines (regulate inflammatory response)
- Eosinophil chemotactic factor (ECF-A) (bronchoconstrictors, factor of anaphylaxis)
- Leukotrienes (bronchoconstrictors)

Treat acute asthma by:

- Administering sympathomimetics (beta-adrenergic agonists): Sympathomimetics promote the production of cyclic AMP, which cause bronchodilation.
- Identifying extrinsic allergens that trigger an asthmatic attack, then avoiding those allergens.

14.20   Medications to Treat Chronic Obstructive Pulmonary Disease

There are five types of medication used to treat chronic obstructive pulmonary disease. They are:

- Bronchodilators: Bronchodilators relax smooth muscles around the bronchioles.
  - *Sympathomimetics*: Sympathomimetics are bronchodilators that increase the production of cyclic AMP, causing dilation of the bronchioles by acting as an adrenergic agonistic. Sympathomimetics are either selective or nonselective. Sympathomimetics are selective to particular adrenergic receptors. These are referred to as alpha$_1$-, beta$_2$-, and beta$_2$-adrenergic. Nonselective sympathomimetics affect all types of adrenergic receptor sites.
    - Epinephrine (adrenalin): Epinephrine is a nonselective sympathomimetic given subcutaneously, IV, or via an endotracheal tube in emergency to restore circulation and increase airway patency.
    - Selective beta$_2$-adrenergic agonists: Selective beta$_2$-adrenergic agonists have fewer side effects than epinephrine (adrenalin). They are given by aerosol or as a tablet. Selective beta$_2$-adrenergic agonists include:
      - Albuterol (Proventil, Ventolin)
      - Isoetharine HCl (Bronkosol)
      - Metaproterenol sulfate (Alupent)
      - Salmeterol (Serevent)
      - Terbutaline SO$_4$ (Brethine)
  - *Ipratropium bromide (Atrovent)*: Ipratropium bromide is an anticholinergic that inhibits vagal mediated response by reversing the action of acetylcholine. This reversal results in the relaxation of smooth muscle, causing bronchodilating. Administer ipratropium bromide (Atrovent) 5 minutes before administering glucocorticoid (steroid) or cromolyn via inhalation to assure bronchioles dilate so steroids can be delivered to the bronchioles. Ipratropium bromide, when administered with albuterol sulfate (Combivent), creates a longer dilation effect and is used to treat chronic bronchitis.
  - *Methylxanthine (xanthine)*: Methylxanthine is a bronchodilator that stimulates the central nervous system to increase respirations, dilate coronary and pulmonary vessels, and increase urination (diuresis).
- Bronchoconstrictors: Bronchoconstrictors contract smooth muscles around the bronchi, resulting in restricted airflow to the lungs.
  - *Leukotriene (LK)*: Leukotriene is the primary bronchoconstrictor. This increases migration of eosinophil, increases mucous production and increases edema in the bronchi, resulting in bronchoconstriction. There are two types of leukotriene modifiers: LT receptor antagonists and LT synthesis inhibitors. Both reduce inflammatory symptoms of asthma. Leukotriene modifiers include:

- Zafirlukast (Accolate)
- Zileuton (Zyflo)
- Montelukast sodium (Singulair)

- Anti-inflammatories: Anti-inflammatories reduces respiratory tract inflammation.
  - *Glucocorticoids* (see chapter 19) are given to reduce the inflammation. Glucocorticoids are administered orally, via aerosol inhalation, intramuscularly, and intravenously.
    - Aerosol inhalation glucocorticoids are:
      — Beclomethasone (Beconase, Vanceril)
      — Dexamethasone (Decadron)
      — Flunisolide (AeroBid, Nasalide)
      — Triamcinolone (Azmacort, Kenalog, Nasacort)
    - Glucocorticoids (steroids) used for other routes are:
      — Betamethasone (Celestone)
      — Cortisone acetate (Cortone acetate, Cortistan)
      — Dexamethasone (Decadron)
      — Hydrocortisone (Cortef, Hydrocortone)
      — Methylprednisolone (Medrol, Solu-Medrol, Depo-Medrol)
      — Prednisolone
      — Prednisone
      — Triamcinolone (Aristocort, Kenacort, Azmacort)

- Expectorants: Expectorants, called mucolytics, liquefy and loosen viscous mucous secretions so the secretions can be removed by coughing.
  - *Acetylcysteine (Mucomyst)*: Acetylcysteine is the expectorant prescribed for chronic obstructive pulmonary disease. Acetylcysteine is administered by nebulizer 5 minutes after bronchodilators are administered. Acetylcysteine should not be mixed with other medication. Acetylcysteine is also an antidote for acetaminophen overdose if given within 12 to 24 hours after the overdose.

- Mast Cell Stabilizer: A mast cell stabilizer prevents bronchospasms and inhibits asthmatic response by blocking the release of histamine, leukotrienes, and other mediators from the mast cell that cause the inflammatory process. A mast cell stabilizer does not have an effect on inflammatory mediators that were already released. Mast cell stabilizers are administered by aerosol inhalation. The most common mast stabilizers are:
  - Cromolyn (Intal)
  - Nedocromil (Tilade)

BETA-ADRENERGIC

Use	Acute and chronic asthma, bronchitis, and exercise-induced bronchospasm	Half-life: 4–5 hours	Onset: PO: 30 minutes Aerosol	Peaks: PO: 4–6 Aerosol
Example	Albuterol (Proventil, Ventolin)	Route: PO, Aerosol	Pregnancy category: C	Pharmacokinetic: Absorbed in GI tract, gradual absorption from bronchi after inhalation; metabolized in liver and excreted in urine
How it works	• Stimulates beta$_2$-adrenergic receptor sites			
Adult dose	• PO: Tablets: 2–4 mg three to four times/day; gradually increased to maximum dose of 8 mg five times/day • PO: Syrup: 2–4 mg three to four times/day; maximum 32 mg/day			

- PO: Extended-release: 4 or 8 mg q 12h; may be gradually increased to 16 mg/daily.
- Inhalation (aerosol): Two inhalations q4–6 h; wait 1–2 min. before administering second inhalation
- Inhalation (capsules): 200–400 mcg q4–6h
- Inhalation (solution): 2.5 mg three to four times/day by nebulization

Before administration	• Assess and monitor rate, depth, rhythm, and type of respiration.
Administration	• If using an inhaler, shake container well and use a spacer if available. • If PO do not crush or break ER tablets. • If PO give with or without food. • If nebulizer dilutes 0.5 ml of 0.5% solution to final volume of 3 ml with 0.9% NaCl to provide 2.5 mg, administer over 5–15 min; use with compressed air or oxygen at rate of 6–10 L/min
After administration	• Assess and monitor blood pressure because it may cause increase. • Assess and monitor quality and rate of pulse because it may cause tachycardia. • Assess and monitor adventitious breath sounds because they may cause rales and wheezing. • Monitor ECG, serum potassium, and arterial blood gases. • If using an inhaler, rinse the mouth well after use. • Assess to determine if the medication is having a therapeutic effect.
Contraindications	• Use caution with a patient who has hypersensitivity, cardiovascular disease, hyperthyroidism, or diabetes mellitus.
Side effects/ adverse reactions	• Headache, nausea, restlessness, nervousness, trembling, dizziness, throat dryness, throat irritation, pharyngitis, blood pressure changes, hypertension; heartburn, transient wheezing • Insomnia, weakness, unusual/bad taste or taste/smell changes; with inhalation • Excessive sympathomimetic stimulation may produce palpitations, extrasystoles tachycardia, chest pain, slight increase in blood pressure followed by substantial decrease; chills, sweating, blanching of skin • Excessive use leads to loss of bronchodilating effectiveness and/or severe paradoxic bronchoconstriction.
Patient education	• Avoid excessive use of caffeine. • Know the proper use of the inhaler. • Do not take more than two inhalations at any one time. • Rinse mouth immediately after inhalation. • Increase fluid intake.

ADRENERGIC AGONIST

Use	Bronchoconstriction and reversible obstructive pulmonary disease	Half-life: Unknown	Onset: 1–5 minutes	Peaks: 1–4 hours
Example	Isoetharine HCl (Bronkosol)	Route: Aerosol	Pregnancy category: C	Pharmacokinetic: Absorbed in GI tract, gradual absorption from bronchi after inhalation, metabolized in liver, and excreted in urine

How it works	• Stimulates beta$_1$- and some beta$_2$-adrenergic receptor sites
Adult dose	• Inhalation: one to two puffs; aerosol nebulizer: 0.5–1.0 ml of 5% solution of 0.5 ml of 1% solution diluted in 3 ml of NSS
Before administration	• Assess and monitor rate, depth, rhythm, and type of respiration
Administration	• If using inhaler, shake container well and use a spacer if available • If nebulizer dilutes 0.5 ml of 0.5% solution to a final volume of 3 ml with 0.9% NaCl to provide 2.5 mg, administer over 5–15 min.; use with compressed air or oxygen at rate of 6–10 L/min
After	• Assess and monitor blood pressure because it may cause increase.

administration	• Assess and monitor the quality and rate of pulse because it may cause tachycardia. • Assess and monitor adventitious breath sounds because they may cause rales and wheezing. • Monitor ECG, serum potassium, and arterial blood gases. • If using an inhaler, rinse the mouth well after use. • Assess to determine if the medication is having a therapeutic effect.
Contraindications	• Use caution with a patient who has hypersensitivity, cardiovascular disease, hyperthyroidism, or diabetes mellitus.
Side effects/ adverse reactions	• Headache, nausea, restlessness, nervousness, trembling, dizziness, throat dryness, throat irritation, pharyngitis, blood pressure changes, hypertension; heartburn, transient wheezing • Insomnia, weakness, unusual/bad taste or taste/smell changes; with inhalation • Excessive sympathomimetic stimulation may produce palpitations, extrasystoles tachycardia, chest pain, slight increase in blood pressure followed by substantial decrease; chills, sweating, blanching of skin. • Excessive use leads to loss of bronchodilating effectiveness and/or severe paradoxic bronchoconstriction.
Patient education	• Avoid excessive use of caffeine. • Know the proper use of the inhaler. • Do not take more than two inhalations at any one time. • Rinse mouth immediately after inhalation. • Increase fluid intake.

ANTICHOLINERGICS

Use	Maintenance treatment of bronchospasm because of chronic obstructive airway disease, including bronchitis, emphysema. Adjunct to bronchodilators for maintenance treatment of bronchial asthma. Not to be used for immediate bronchospasm relief. Nasal spray: Rhinorrhea associated with perineal rhinitis (0.03%) and with common cold (0.06%).	Half-life: 1.5–4 hours	Onset: Inhalation: Less than 15 minutes	Peaks: 1–2 hours
Example	Ipratropium bromide (Atrovent) and ipratropium with albuterol (Combivent)	Route: Aerosol/ nasal spray	Pregnancy category: B	Pharmacokinetic: Minimal systemic absorption; metabolized in liver if systemically absorbed; eliminated in feces
How it works	• Inhibits vagally mediated response by reversing action of acetylcholine, producing smooth muscle relaxation, bronchodilating response. Produces significant increased in forced vital lung capacity			
Adult dose	• Inhalation: COPD: 2 puffs TID, QID greater than 4-hr intervals; maximum 12 inhal/day • Nebulization: 500 mcg three to four times/day • Intranasal: 0.03% two sprays two to three times/day; 0.06% two sprays three to four times/day			
Before administration	• Assess and monitor rate, depth, rhythm, and type of respiration.			
Administration	• If using inhaler, shake container well and use a spacer if available If nebulizer dilutes 0.5 ml of 0.5% solution to final volume of 3 ml with 0.9% NaCl to provide 2.5 mg, administer over 5–15 min, use with compressed air or oxygen at rate of 6–10 L/min			
After	• Assess and monitor blood pressure because it may cause an increase.			

administration	• Assess and monitor quality and rate of pulse because it may cause tachycardia.
	• Assess and monitor adventitious breath sounds because they may cause rales and wheezing.
	• Monitor ECG, serum potassium, and arterial blood gases.
	• If using an inhaler, rinse the mouth well after use.
	• Assess to determine if medication is having a therapeutic effect.
Contraindi-cation	• Use caution with a patient who has narrow-angle glaucoma, hypersensitivity, cardiovascular disease, hyperthyroidism, or diabetes mellitus.
Side effects/ adverse reactions	• Headache, nausea, restlessness, nervousness, trembling, dizziness, throat dryness, throat irritation, pharyngitis, blood pressure changes, hypertension, heartburn, transient wheezing
	• Insomnia, weakness, unusual/bad taste or taste/smell changes; with inhalation
	• Excessive sympathomimetic stimulation may produce palpitations, extrasystole tachycardia, chest pain, a slight increase in blood pressure followed by substantial decrease; chills, sweating, and blanching of skin.
	• Excessive use leads to loss of bronchodilating effectiveness and/or severe paradoxic bronchoconstriction.
Patient education	• Avoid excessive use of caffeine.
	• Know the proper use of the inhaler.
	• Do not take more than two inhalations at any one time.
	• Rinse the mouth immediately after inhalation.
	• Increase fluid intake.

METHYLXANTHINE

Use	Promotes bronchodilation; to treat asthma and COPD	Half-life: 7–9 hours nonsmokers 4–5 hours smokers	Onset: 30 minutes	Peaks: 6 hours
Example	Theophylline (Theo-Dur, Theophyllines, Kl, Slo-Phyllin, Slo-BID; Aminophyllin)	Route: PO	Pregnancy category: C	Pharmacokinetic: Metabolized by liver and 90% excreted in urine

How it works	• Directly relaxes smooth muscle of bronchial airway, pulmonary blood vessels, relieving bronchospasm, increasing vital capacity. Produces cardiac and skeletal muscle stimulation.
Adult dose	• PO: 250–500 mg q8 h–12h. Dosing is highly individualized based on therapeutic serum levels 10–20 mcg/ml.
Before administration	• Obtain baseline testing to include pulmonary function tests, chest x-ray, liver enzyme tests, SGOT, SGPT, alkaline phosphatase
Administration	• Administer after meals to reduce GI distress.
	• Do not crush sustained-release or enteric-coated tablets.
After administration	• Assess and monitor serum levels. Normal is 10–20 mcg/ml. Toxicity occurs with levels greater than 20 mcg/ml.
	• Provide adequate hydration.
	• Assess and monitor vital signs including blood pressure.
	• Assess and monitor pulse rate and quality and ECG.
	• Assess and monitor respiratory rate, depth, rhythm, quality, breath sounds, and oxygenation.
	• Provide pulmonary therapy by chest clapping and postural drainage as ordered.
	• Assess patient response to medication.
Contraindi-cation	• Do not use with patients who have hypersensitivity to xanthine and caffeine.
	• Use caution with patients who have impaired cardiac, renal or hepatic function, hypertension, hyperthyroidism, diabetes mellitus, peptic ulcer, glaucoma, severe hypoxemia, or underlying seizure disorder.
Side effects/ adverse reactions	• Momentary change in sense, heartburn, vomiting, headache, mild diuresis, insomnia, nausea, hyperglycemia, decreased clotting time and, rarely, increased white blood cell count (leukocytosis).
	• IV administration: shakiness, restlessness, tachycardia, trembling
	• Too rapid rate of IV administration may produce marked fall in B/P with accompanying faintness and lightheadedness, palpitations, tachycardia, hyperventilation, nausea, vomiting, angina-like pain,

seizures, ventricular fibrillation, cardiac standstill

Patient education	• Increase fluid intake.
	• Monitor pulse before and after taking medication.
	• Do not stop taking medication suddenly.
	• Report side effects to health care provider.
	• Have laboratory tests done as ordered.
	• Have regular eye exams and report any vision changes.
	• Restrict salt, caffeine, and alcohol intake.

LEUKOTRIENE MODIFIERS AND LT SYNTHESIS INHIBITORS

Use	For prophylaxis and maintenance therapy for chronic asthma	Half-life: Accolate: 10 hours Singulair: 2.5–5.5 hours Leutrol, Zyflo: 2.5 hours	Onset: Immediate	Peaks: Accolate: 4 hours Singulair: 1 hour Leutrol, Zyflo: 1.5 hours
Example	Zafirlukast (Accolate), montelukast (Singulair) are LT modifiers; Zileuton (Leutrol, Zyflo) is an LT inhibitor	Route: PO	Pregnancy category: Accolate: B Singulair: C Leutrol, Zyflo: C	Pharmacokinetic: Absorbed in GI tract and excreted in the urine

How it works	• Reduces airway inflammation and decreases bronchoconstriction; rapidly absorbed after PO administration.
Adult dose	• Accolate: PO: 20 mg BID 1 h before or 2 h after meals. • Singulair PO: 10 mg daily in evening without food. • Leutrol, Zyflo: PO: 600 mg QID
Before administration	• Obtain medication history. • Assess and monitor liver function lab values.
Administration	• Accolate: before or 2 h after meals. • Singulair: Daily in evening without food.
After administration	• Assess and monitor respiration status. • Monitor liver function lab values.
Contraindications	• Use caution with patients who have impaired hepatic function.
Side effects/ adverse reactions	• Headache, nausea, diarrhea • Singulair is better tolerated than Accolate, Leutrol, and Zyflo • Coadministration of inhaled corticosteroids increases risk of UTI. Hepatotoxicity may result from the use of zileuton.
Patient education	• Increase fluid intake. • Take all medication. Do not stop after symptoms subside. • Do not use for severe asthma attacks. • Do not change or stop taking other asthma medications. • Report nausea, jaundice, abdominal pain, flulike symptoms, or worsening of asthma.

MAST CELL STABILIZER

Use	Prophylactic management of severe bronchial asthma and exercise-induced bronchospasm. Perennial or seasonal allergic rhinitis. Mastocytosis, food allergy, treatment of	Half-life: 5 hours	Onset: Immediate	Peaks: 3 hours

	inflammatory bowel disease (IBD). Conjunctivitis

Example	Cromolyn sodium (Intal)	Route: PO/Inhalation	Pregnancy category: B	Pharmacokinetic: Minimal absorption following PO, inhalation, or nasal administration. Absorbed portion excreted in the urine or via biliary elimination

How it works	• Inhibits degranulation of mast cells; also inhibits release of histamine and SRS-A (a leukotriene) from the mast cell. This inhibits the early asthmatic response by stabilizing the mast cell; also inhibits the late asthmatic response. It has no intrinsic bronchodilator, antihistaminic, anticholinergic, vasoconstrictor, or anti-inflammatory activity.
Adult dose	• Inhalation powder: 20 mg q 6 h; nebulization 20 mg (1.2 ml amp) q 6–8 h • Nasal solution each nostril TID to QID • MDI two puffs QID; food allergy • IBD 200–400 mg four time/day • Systemic 200 mg four times/day
Before administration	• Assess lung sounds.
Administration	• Rinse mouth immediately after inhalation.
After administration	• Monitor rate, depth, rhythm, type of respiration. • Monitor quality and rate of pulse.
Contraindication	• Use caution with patients who have impaired renal and hepatic function.
Side effects/ adverse reactions	• Inhalation: Cough, dry mouth/throat, stuffy nose, throat irritation, unpleasant taste • Nasal: Burning, stinging, irritation of nose, increased sneezing • Ophthalmic: Burning, stinging of eye • PO: Headache, diarrhea
Patient education	• Increase fluid intake. • Rinse mouth immediately after inhalation. • Administer as prescribed at regular intervals. • Report side effects to healthcare provider.

Solved Problems

Respiration

14.1   What happens in the ventilation phase of respiration?

Ventilation is the process by which oxygenated air passes through the respiratory tract during inspiration.

14.2   What is compliance?

Compliance is the ability of the lungs to be distended.

14.3   What controls surface tension in the alveoli?

Surface tension in the alveoli is controlled by surfactant.

14.4   Does compliance increase or decrease in chronic obstructive pulmonary disease (COPD)?

Compliance increases (increases lung volume) in patients who have chronic obstructive pulmonary disease.

14.5   What role do chemoreceptors have in respiration?

Chemoreceptors sense concentrations of oxygen, carbon, and carbon dioxide in the blood. A change in concentration causes the chemoreceptors to send a message to the central chemoreceptors located in the medulla. The medulla then signals the necessary physiological response through cerebrospinal fluid.

14.6   What role does acetylcholine have in respiration?

Acetylcholine is released when the vagus nerve is stimulated, causing the contraction of the tracheobronchial tube called bronchoconstriction.

Respiratory Tract Disorders

14.7   What causes acute rhinitis?

Acute rhinitis, known as the common cold, is caused by the rhinovirus.

14.8   What effect do home remedies have on acute rhinitis?

Home remedies ease the symptoms of acute rhinitis, but do not impede the growth of or kill the rhinovirus.

14.9   What effect do antihistamines have on acute rhinitis?

Antihistamines reduce the production of histamines. Histamines are vasodilators that react to a foreign substance, including the rhinovirus. These reactions cause redness, itching, and swelling to defend against the foreign substance.

14.10   How do antihistamines work?

Antihistamines compete for the same receptor sites as histamines. An antihistamine latches to the site, blocking the histamine from latching to the site and therefore preventing the histamine action. This results in a reduction of redness, itching, and swelling.

14.11   How do decongestants work?

Decongestants stimulate the alpha-adrenergic receptors, causing constriction of the capillaries within the nasal mucosa. This constriction results in shrinking the swelling of the nasal mucous membranes and reducing secretion from the nose.

14.12   What is rebound nasal congestion?

Rebound nasal congestion occurs when decongestants are used for more than 5 days and the patient becomes tolerant of the medication.

14.13   Name three types of decongestants.

Three types of decongestants are nasal decongestants, systemic decongestants, and intranasal glucocorticoids.

14.14   What decongestants provide quick relief?

Nasal decongestants provide quick relief.

14.15 What do antitussives treat?

Antitussives suppress the cough center in the medulla.

14.16 Are antibiotic prescribed for viral pharyngitis?

Antibiotics are not used to treat viral pharyngitis because pharyngitis is caused by a virus.

14.17 What bacteria commonly cause acute tonsillitis?

Streptococcus are the bacteria that commonly cause acute tonsillitis.

14.18 How would you prevent tuberculosis?

Tuberculosis can be prevented by using the Bacillus Calmette-Guerin (BCG) tuberculosis vaccine, a weakened form of the tuberculosis bacterium, which does not cause a tuberculosis infection.

14.19 What is the function of bronchodilators?

Bronchodilators relax smooth muscles around the bronchioles.

14.20 How does leukotriene work?

Leukotriene is the primary bronchoconstrictor. This increases migration of eosinophil, increases mucous production, and increases edema in the bronchi, resulting in bronchoconstriction. There are two types of leukotriene modifiers, LT receptor antagonists and LT synthesis inhibitors. Both reduce the inflammatory symptoms of asthma.

14.21 When is acetylcysteine administered?

Acetylcysteine is administered by nebulizer 5 minutes after bronchodilators are administered.

14.22 How does a mast cell stabilizer work?

Mast cell stabilizers prevent bronchospasms and inhibit asthmatic response by blocking the release of histamines, leukotrienes, and other mediators from the mast cell that cause the inflammatory process.

14.23 What is a limitation of a mast cell stabilizer?

A mast cell stabilizer does not have an effect on inflammatory mediators that were already released before administering the mast cell stabilizer.

14.24 What is the function of sympathomimetics?

Sympathomimetics promote the production of cyclic AMP, which causes bronchodilation.

14.25 What medications are prescribed to treat emphysema?

Emphysema is treated by using bronchodilators such as anticholinergic and beta$_2$ agonists (ipratropium bromide, theophylline) to open the airway by relaxing muscles around the bronchi. Corticosteroids are used to reduce the inflammation associated with emphysema.

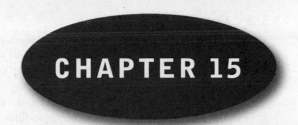

CHAPTER 15

The Neurologic System and Medication

15.1 The Nervous System

The nervous system is comprised of the brain, spinal cord, nerves, and ganglia. They collectively receive stimuli and transmit information.

The nervous system is divided into two types:

1. Central nervous system (CNS): The central nervous system consists of the brain and spinal cord. A message is received from the peripheral nervous system to the central nervous system where the message is interpreted. The appropriate message is sent to the peripheral nervous system to stimulate cellular activity, which either increases or blocks neuron activity. Neurons are nerve cells.

2. Peripheral nervous system (PNS): The peripheral nervous system has two divisions.

    a. Somatic nervous system (SNS): The somatic nervous system acts on skeletal muscles to produce voluntary movement and respiration.

    b. Autonomic nervous system (ANS): The autonomic nervous system, known as the visceral system, is responsible for involuntary movement and controls the heart, respiratory system, gastrointestinal system, and endocrine system (glands). The autonomic nervous system is organized into two divisions:

       i. Sympathetic nervous systems: The sympathetic nervous system is called the adrenergic system and uses the norepinephrine neurotransmitter to send information. It is also referred to as the thoracolumbar division of the autonomic nervous system. The sympathetic system excites organs (increases heart rate).

       ii. Parasympathetic nervous systems: The parasympathetic system, called the cholinergic system, uses the acetylcholine neurotransmitter to transmit information. It is also known as the craniosacral division of the autonomic nervous system. The parasympathetic system inhibits the organs (decreases heart rate).

15.2   Neurologic Pathways

Neurologic pathways extend from the spinal cord to parts of the body. These pathways contain two types of nerve fibers that are connected together by a ganglion:

- Preganglionic fibers: The preganglionic nerve fiber carries messages from the central nervous system to the ganglion. A preganglionic nerve fiber is long—from the spinal cord to the ganglion.
- Postganglionic fibers: The postganglionic nerve fiber transmits messages from the ganglion to specific tissues and organs. A postganglionic nerve fiber is relatively short—from the ganglion to the cells of the body.

Neurologic pathways in the sympathetic nervous system originate from the thoracic (T1 to T12) and the upper lumbar segments (L1 and L2) of the spinal cord. Neurologic pathways in the parasympathetic nervous system originate from cranial nerves III, VII, IX, and X, from the brainstem, and the sacral segments S2, S3, and S4 from the spinal cord. This is why the parasympathetic nervous system is also known as the craniosacral division of the autonomic nervous system.

15.3   Central Nervous System Stimulants

Medication stimulates the central nervous system to induce a therapeutic response. There are four major groups of medication that stimulate the central nervous system. They are:

- *Amphetamines:* Amphetamines stimulate the cerebral cortex of the brain. Amphetamines are also taken to decrease weight and increase energy, enabling performing work quickly without rest.
- *Caffeine:* Caffeine stimulates the cerebral cortex and stimulates respiration by acting on the brainstem and medulla. Caffeine is found in many beverages, foods, over-the-counter medication, and prescription medications. Caffeine is found in Anacin, Excedrin, Cafergot, Fiorinal, and Midol.
- *Analeptics:* Analeptics have a similar effect on the brain stem and medulla as caffeine.
- *Anorexiants:* Anorexiants inhibit appetite by stimulating the cerebral cortex and the hypothalamus. Anorexiants can produce psychological dependence. A patient can build a tolerance to the therapeutic effect of anorexiants, which may result in withdrawal symptoms if discontinuing anorexiant use abruptly.

Amphetamines, analeptics, and anorexiants stimulate the release of neurotransmitters, norepinephrine, and dopamine from the brain and from the peripheral nerve terminals of the sympathetic nervous system, resulting in euphoria and increase alertness. Patients can experience sleeplessness, restlessness, tremors, irritability, and cardiovascular problems (increase heart rate, palpitations, dysrhythmias, and hypertension).

Anorexiants and analeptics include:

- Benzphetamine (Didrex)
- Diethylpropion (Tenuate)
- Fenfluramine (Pondimin)
- Phentermine (Pheneturide)

AMPHETAMINE-LIKE DRUGS

Use	For ADD and ADHD; for narcolepsy and treatment of secondary depression	Half-life: 2–4 hours	Onset: 2 hours	Peaks: 3 hours	Duration: 8–12 hours
Example	Methylphenidate HCl (Ritalin, Concerta) CSS II	Route: PO, IV	Pregnancy category: C	Pharmacokinetic: Incompletely absorbed from GI tract; metabolized in liver; excreted in urine and feces via biliary system	

How it works	• Blocks reuptake mechanisms of dopaminergic neurons. Decreases motor restlessness, enhances ability to pay attention; increases motor activity, mental alertness, diminishes sense of fatigue, enhances spirit, produces mild euphoria.
Adult dose	• Ritalin PO 2.5–5 mg before breakfast and lunch; may increase by 5–10 mg/day at weekly intervals for a maximum dose of 60 mg/day • Concerta: Initially, PO 18 mg once daily; may increase by 18/mg/day at weekly intervals to maximum dose of 54 mg/day • Narcolepsy: PO 10 mg two to three times/day; range of 10–60 mg/day
Before administration	• Obtain medical and drug history. • Assess vital signs for baselines.
Administration	• Administer before meals.
After administration	• Monitor vital signs. • Assess and monitor client's mental status. • Assess and monitor height (in children) and weight. • Assess and monitor CBC with differential and platelets. • Monitor for side effects.
Contraindications	• Hypersensitivity; hyperthyroidism, history of marked anxiety, tension, agitation; glaucoma; those with motor tics; family history of Tourette's disorder • *Caution:* In patients with hypertension, depression, alcoholism, and who are pregnant
Side effects/ adverse reactions	• Frequent nervousness, insomnia, anorexia • Occasional dizziness, drowsiness, headache, nausea, stomach pain, fever, rash, joint pain, irritability Adverse effects: • Tachycardia, growth suppression, palpitations, transient loss of weight, increased hyperactivity, dyskinetic movements (face, lips, tongue), hepatitis, jaundice • Life-threatening: Exfoliative dermatitis, uremia, thrombocytopenia
Patient education	• Take drug before meals. • Avoid alcohol consumption. • Use sugarless gum to relieve dry mouth. • Monitor weight. • Avoid driving and using hazardous equipment when experiencing tremors, nervousness, or increased heart rate. • Avoid caffeine. Read labels on over-the-counter (OTC) products because many contain caffeine. • Do not abruptly discontinue the drug; it must be tapered off to avoid. Withdrawal symptoms; consult healthcare provider before adjusting the dose. • Maintain a well-balanced diet.

15.4   Migraine Headaches

A migraine is a debilitating neurovascular disorder that is not clearly understood. Research indicates blood vessels expand and release abnormal amounts of dopamine and serotonin, resulting in inflammation and pain. Research also indicates that in some patients blood vessels are unusually sensitive to dopamine and serotonin, which are normally found in the brain.

Signs and symptoms of a migraine are:

- Intense throbbing/pulsating headache pain
- Nausea
- Photophobia (sensitivity to light)
- Phonophobia (sensitivity to sound)
- Temporary disability
- Preceded by an aura (breeze, odor, beam of light, a spectrum of colors)
- Can occur on one side of the head (unilateral)

15.5 Treatment for Migraine Headaches

Treatment is divided into prevention and symptom management.

Prevention

There are six medication categories prescribed to prevent migraines:

1. Blood vessel constrictors (see chapter 19)
   a. Methysergide—Methysergide is particularly effective, however there are side effects that might make this drug less tolerable.
2. Blood vessel dilators (see chapter 19)
3. Antiseizure (see 15.29 Epilepsy)
   a. Divalproex sodium
   b. Topiramate
4. Antidepressants (see 15.33 Antidepressants)
   a. Amitriptyline
   b. Bupropion
   c. Cyproheptadine
   d. Fluvoxamine
   e. Imipramine
5. Beta-blockers (see chapter 19)
   a. Propranolol
   b. Timolol
   c. Diltiazem
6. Analgesics (see chapter 16)
   a. Ibuprofen

Symptom Management

- Antiemetics (see chapter 18)
- Ergot alkaloids
- Nonsteroidal anti-inflammatory drugs (NSAIDs) (see chapter 12)
- Analgesics
- Nonopioids
- Opioids
- Triptans

ERGOT ALKALOIDS AND RELATED COMPOUNDS

Use	A first-line drug for treatment of an acute migraine attack.	Half-life: 21 hours	Onset: 1.5 hours	Peaks: 2 hours	Duration: 8 hours
Example	Dihydroergotamine (DHE, Ergomar; with caffeine Cafergot)	Route: IM, SC, Intranasal	Pregnancy category: C	Pharmacokinetic: Slow incomplete absorption from GI tract; metabolized in liver; excreted in feces.	
How it works	• May have agonist/antagonist actions with alpha adrenergic, serotonergic, dopaminergic receptors. Directly stimulates vascular smooth muscle, constricting arteries and veins. May inhibit reuptake of norepinephrine.				

Adult dose	• The IM or subcutaneous dose is 1 mg at onset and may repeat at hourly intervals, up to three injections daily.
	• Intranasal dose is 2 mg, one spray in each nostril; repeat in 15 minutes, up to 3 mg daily
Before administration	• Obtain medical and drug history.
	• Obtain pregnancy test.
	• Assess and monitor migraine onset, location, and duration.
Administration	• Administer at first sign of migraine.
After administration	• Assess pain.
Contraindica-tions	• Peripheral vascular disease, impaired renal/hepatic function, severe pruritus, coronary artery disease, hypertension, sepsis, malnutrition
Side effects/ adverse reactions	• Cough and dizziness
	• Adverse effects: Prolonged administration or excessive dosage may produce ergotamine poisoning—nausea, vomiting, weakness of legs, pain in limb muscles, numbness and tingling of fingers/toes, precordial pain, tachycardia or bradycardia, hyper/hypotension. Localized edema itching because of vasoconstriction of peripheral arteries and arterioles. Feet, hands will become cold, pale, and numb. Muscle pain occurs when walking and later even at rest. Gangrene may occur. Occasionally confusion, depression, drowsiness, and convulsions appear.
Patient education	• Start medication at first sign of migraine.
	• Report if there is a need to progressively increase the dose.
	• Report any signs and symptoms of overdose or toxicity.
	• Use contraception (report suspected pregnancy immediately) before adjusting the dose.

SEROTONIN AGONISTS: TRIPTANS

Use	Relief of migraine pain	Half-life: 2 hours	Onset: 1 hour	Peaks: 2 hours	Duration: 12 hours
Example	Sumatriptan (Imitrex)	Route: PO, SC, Intranasal	Pregnancy category: C	Pharmacokinetic: metabolized in liver and excreted in the urine	

How it works	• Binds selectively to vascular receptors producing a vasoconstrictive effect on cranial blood vessels
Adult dose	• SC: 6 mg no more than two 6 mg injections within a 24-hour period and separated by at least 1 hour between injections
	• PO: 50 mg maximum single dose 100 mg; may repeat no sooner than 2 hours with a maximum of 200 mg/24 hours
	• Nasal: 5–20 mg may repeat in 2 hours; maximum 40 mg/24 hours
Before administration	• Obtain medical and drug history.
	• Obtain pregnancy test.
	• Assess and monitor migraine onset, location, and duration.
Administration	• Administer at first sign of migraine
After administration	• Assess pain.
	• Monitor side effects.
Contraindications	• IV use; ischemic heart disease; silent ischemia, Prinzmetal's angina, uncontrolled hypertension, concurrent ergotamine-containing preparations, hemiplegic or basilar migraine
	• Caution with liver and kidney problems
Side effects/ adverse reactions	• Frequent: Oral—tingling, nasal discomfort; SC—injection site reactions, tingling, warm, hot sensation, dizziness, vertigo; Nasal—bad, unusual taste, nausea and vomiting
	• Occasional: Flushing, weakness, visual disturbances; SC—burning sensation, numbness, chest discomfort, drowsiness, weakness; Nasal—discomfort of nasal cavity/throat, dizziness
	• Adverse effects: Excessive dosage may produce tremor, redness of extremities, reduced respirations, cyanosis, convulsions, paralysis. Serious arrhythmias occur rarely but particularly in those with hypertension, obesity, smokers, diabetes, and those with strong family history of coronary artery disease.

(Continued)

(Continued from previous page)

SEROTONIN AGONISTS: TRIPTANS

Patient education	• Teach patient how to properly use the autoinjection and injection techniques. • Discuss proper discarding of used syringes. • Do not use more frequently than ordered. • Report any side effects immediately.

OTHER TRIPTANS

Almotriptan	6.25–12.5 mg and repeat one dose if necessary; use with greater caution in patients with liver and kidney impairment; fewer side effects reported.
Eletriptan	20–40 mg tablets repeated in 2 hours; high drug–drug interaction
Frovatriptan	2.5 mg at onset and may repeat after 2 hours; has longest half-life with a slow onset of action
Naratriptan	1–2.5 mg tablets and repeat after 4 hours; onset of action is slower but has the second longest half-life; has less side effects
Rizatriptan	5–10 mg repeated in 2 hours; fast acting
Zolmitriptan	2.5–5 mg dose with 2-hour repeats available PO and nasal spray; increased risk of drug–drug interaction

15.6   Central Nervous System Depressants

Central nervous system depressants are medications that suppress the transmission of information throughout the central nervous system. There are seven classifications of central nervous system depressants.
They are:

1. Sedative-hypnotics
2. General and local anesthetics
3. Analgesics (see chapter 16)
4. Narcotic analgesics (see chapter 16)
5. Anticonvulsants
6. Antipsychotics
7. Antidepressants

15.7   Sedative-Hypnotics

Sedative-hypnotics, the mildest form of central nervous system depressant, are given in low doses to diminish physical and mental responses without affecting consciousness. Short-acting sedative-hypnotics are prescribed to help fall asleep, allowing the patient to awake early without a lingering after effect. Intermediate-acting sedative-hypnotics are used for sustaining sleep and have residual drowsiness after waking. Sedative-hypnotics are not prescribed for patients who have severe respiratory disorders or who are pregnant.

Sedative-hypnotics are prescribed for short-term use because the patient can develop a tolerance of and dependency on the medication. Avoid chronic use of sedative-hypnotics. Nonpharmacological methods that promote sleep should be tried before prescribing sedative-hypnotics to aid with sleep.
These methods are:

• Arise at the same hour in the morning.
• No daytime naps
• No heavy meals or strenuous exercise before bed
• Relax before bed (warm bath, read, listen to music, drink warm milk).
• No loud noises
• Do not watch disturbing television before bed.
• Do not drink a lot of fluids before bed.

Administer sedative-hypnotics during the day and with increased doses to cause the patient to fall asleep. High doses anesthetize the patient. Gradually discontinue high doses of sedative-hypnotics to minimize withdrawal symptoms

Hint: Over-the-counter sleep medications contain antihistamine and not sedative-hypnotics.

SEDATIVE–HYPNOTIC–BENZODIAZEPINE–SCHEDULE IV

Use	Short-term treatment of insomnia (up to 4 weeks); reduces sleep induction time and number of nocturnal awakenings; increases length of sleep.	Half-life: Dalmane: 2.3 hours Benadryl: 2–8 hours Restoril: 9.5–12.4 hours Halcion: 1.7–5 hours Ambien: 1.4–4.5 hours	Onset: 15–45 minutes 1–3 hours 2–2.5 hours 15–30 minutes 30 minutes	Peaks: 3–6 hours 2–4 hours 2–3 hours 0.5 hours 30–120 minutes	Duration: 7–8 hours 4–7 hours 3–18 hours 1.5–5.5 hours 6–8 hours
Example	flurazepam hydrochloride (Dalmane) Diphenhydramine (Benadryl) Temazepam (Restoril) Triazolam (Halcion) Zolpidem (Ambien)	Route: PO	Pregnancy category: X	Pharmacokinetic: Absorbed from GI tract; crosses blood–brain barrier; metabolized in liver, and excreted in urine	

How it works
- Enhances action of inhibitory neurotransmitter gamma-aminobutyric acid (GABA), producing hypnotic effect caused by CNS depression

Adult dose
- Flurazepam hydrochloride (Dalmane) 15–30 mg at bedtime (15 mg for elderly)
- Zolpidem (Ambien): PO 10 mg at bedtime (elderly, debilitated 5 mg)
- Triazolam (Halcion): PO 0.125–0.5 mg at bedtime (elderly 0.0625–0.125 mg)
- Temazepam (Restoril): PO 15–30 mg at bedtime (elderly 7.5–15 mg)

Before administration
- Obtain pregnancy test.

Administration
- Give without regard to meals.
- Capsules may be emptied and mixed with food.
- Triazolam (Halcion): Tablets may be crushed and grapefruit juice may alter absorption.
- Zolpidem (Ambien): For faster sleep onset, do not give with or immediately after a meal.

After administration
- Assess and monitor vital signs.
- Provide a safe environment (raised side rails; adequate lighting if at home).
- Provide a quiet environment conducive to sleep (soft music, back rub).
- Assess for paradoxical reaction.
- Evaluate for therapeutic response.

Contraindications
- Narrow-angle glaucoma, acute alcohol intoxication, and pregnancy. Use with caution with impaired liver or kidney function.

Side effects/ adverse reactions
- Drowsiness, dizziness, ataxia, sedation. Morning drowsiness may occur initially. Occasionally GI disturbances, nervousness, blurred vision, dry mouth, headache, confusion, skin rash, irritability, and slurred speech
- Hangover, REM Rebound, dependence, tolerance, excessive depression, respiratory depression, hypersensitivity

Patient education
- Smoking reduces drug effectiveness.
- Do not abruptly stop after long-term use.
- Notify if become pregnant.
- Give without regard to meals.
- Capsules may be emptied and mixed with food.

15.8　Barbiturates

Barbiturates are a type of sedative-hypnotic used to induce sleep and as an anesthetic. In high doses barbiturates control epileptic seizures. Barbiturates are Class II controlled substances prescribed for no more than two weeks because of adverse side effect such as CNS depression in the elderly.

Barbiturates are classified by duration of action. These are:

- Ultrashort-acting: Ultra–short-acting barbiturates (thiopental sodium; Pentothal) are an anesthetic
- Short-acting: Short-acting barbiturates (Secobarbital; Seconal), pentobarbital (Nembutal) induce sleep
- Intermediate-acting: Intermediate-acting barbiturates (amobarbital; Amytal), aprobarbital (Alurate) and butabarbital (Butisol)) induce longer sleep periods
- Long-acting: Long-acting barbiturates (phenobarbital and mephobarbital) control epileptic seizures

SEDATIVE-HYPNOTIC: BARBITURATES AND OTHERS

Use	Treat insomnia; use for sedation, preoperative medication, barbiturate coma (for controlled increased intracranial pressure)	Half-life: 4 hours (first phase); 30–50 hours (second phase)	Onset: PO: 15–30 minutes IM: 10–15 minutes IV: Immediate	Peaks: PO: 1 hour IM: 1 hour IV: 2–3 minutes	Duration: PO: 3–6 hours IM: 3–6 hours IV: 15–60 minutes
Example	pentobarbital sodium (Nembutal Sodium) short-acting barbiturate	Route: PO, IM, IV	Pregnancy category: D	Pharmacokinetic: Excreted in the urine	
How it works Adult dose	• Depression of the CNS, including the motor and sensory activities • PO 20–30 mg TID • Hypnotic: PO 100–200 mg • Preoperative PO/IM/IV: 100 mg, repeat if needed				
Before administration	• Assess medical and drug history (interacts with alcohol, narcotics, and other sedative-hypnotics)				
Administration	• IV pentobarbital at a rate of less than 50 mg/min • Do NOT mix with other medications. • IM should be given into a large muscle. • PO give 30 minutes before bedtime				
After administration	• Maintain a safe environment after administration (side rails up; proper lighting; toileting before medicating). • Monitor vital signs. • Observe for adverse reactions. • Observe for signs of withdrawal if taken over a prolonged period of time and then abruptly discontinued.				
Contraindications Side effects/ adverse reactions	• Respiration depression, severe liver disease, pregnancy (fetal immaturity), nephrosis • Nausea, vomiting, diarrhea, lethargy, drowsiness, hangover, dizziness, rash • Drug dependence or tolerance, urticaria (hives), hypotension if given rapidly IV • Respiratory distress, laryngospasm				
Patient education	• Use nonpharmacological ways to induce sleep such as enjoying a warm bath, listening to music, drinking warm fluids, and avoiding drinks with caffeine for 6 hours before bedtime. • Do not drive a motor vehicle or operate machinery. • Take 30 minutes before bedtime. • Report side affects such as hangover because prescribed drug dose may need to be changed.				

OTHER BARBITURATES

Short-acting	Secobarbital sodium (Seconal Sodium) class II	Preoperative sedation Used to induce sleep	PO 100–200 mg before surgery; hypnotic PO/IM 100–200 mg

			h.s.; Status epilepticus: IV; 5.5 mg/kg; reappear in 3–4 hours; with spinal anesthesia IV; 50–100 mg.; infused over 30 seconds; maximum dose of 250/mg
Intermediate-acting	Amobarbital sodium (Amytal Sodium)	Sleep sustainers	PB 50%–60%; half-life 20–40 hours; Sedative: PO 30–50 mg BID-TID; Hypnotic PO/IM 65–200 mg/h, IV: 65–200 mg
Other	Chloral hydrate Class IV	No hangover and less respiratory depression; give with meals or fluids to prevent gastric irritation	Pregnancy category: C; PB 70%–80%; half-life 8–10 hours; PO 250 mg TID before meals; Hypnotic: PO 500 mg to 1 g/h.
Other	Paraldehyde Class IV	Exhaled via the lungs; strong odor and disagreeable taste; seldom used; has been used to control delirium tremens (DTS) in alcoholics; can be used for drug poisoning	Status epilepticus and tetanus to control convulsions; Pregnancy category: C; PB UK; half-life 7.5 hours; Sedative PO 5–10 ml q4–6h PRN in water or juice; maximum dose of 30 ml; Hypnotic: PO 10–30 ml/h

15.9　Anesthetic Agents

Anesthetic agents depress the central nervous system, causing a loss of consciousness (except for local and regional anesthetic agents) and relieving pain. Anesthetic agents are classified as:

- *Local Anesthetic*: Block specific nerve pathways in a region and result in temporary analgesia and paralysis but no loss of consciousness.
- *General Anesthetic*: A general anesthetic used for surgery consists of one medication or a combination that causes a temporary loss of consciousness.

15.10　Administering General Anesthetic Agents

The combination of general anesthetic medication is called a balance based on the patient's age, weight, medical history, health, and allergies. The balanced approach administers the general anesthetic in phases to:

- Minimize cardiovascular adverse effects.
- Decrease the amount of general anesthetic.
- Reduce postanesthetic nausea and vomiting.
- Minimize disturbance of organ function.
- Increase recovery time.

A sedative-hypnotic is administered the night before surgery to assist with sleep. An hour before the surgery, premedications are administered to sedate and decrease anxiety. Premedications are an anticholinergic (atropine) to decrease secretions and either a narcotic analgesic or benzodiazepine.

　　In the operating room, the patient is given a short-acting barbiturate (thiopental sodium; Pentothal) to induce anesthesia. A general anesthetic agent is then given either by IV or combined with oxygen as an inhaled gas delivered through a mask or breathing tube. A muscle relaxant may also be administered depending on the surgery.

15.11   Four Stages of Anesthesia

There are four stages of anesthesia that occur rapidly. These stages are:

1. Analgesia: The patient is conscious and able to converse, but has lost the sense of pain.
2. Excitement: Breathing increases, blood pressure increases and become irregular. Delirium sets in and the patient may become violent. This stage is shortened by administering a barbiturate (sodium pentothal) before administering the anesthesia.
3. Surgical Anesthesia: Eye movement slows then stops as breathing becomes regular. Skeletal muscles relax and surgery begins.
4. Medullary Paralysis: The respiratory center (medulla oblongata) becomes paralyzed. Breathing and vital functions cease. Death occurs. However, the anesthetist adjusts the general anesthetic to prevent the patient from reaching this stage.

INHALATION AND INTRAVENOUS ANESTHETICS

Use	Depress the CNS, alleviate pain, and cause a loss of consciousness	Half-life: UK	Onset: 1.5–3 minutes	Peaks: Dose dependent 2 days	Duration: Dose dependent 8 days
Example	Inhalation: Volatile liquids: halothane (Fluothane),	Route: Inhalation	Pregnancy category: C	Pharmacokinetic: Metabolized in liver; eliminated via respiratory methoxyflurane within 24 hours as exhaled gas	

How it works	• See stages of anesthesia
Adult dose	• Response to anesthesia may differ based on age, current health problems, pregnancy, history of heavy smoking, obesity, and frequent use of alcohol and drugs. The dose of anesthesia is based on all of these factors.
Before administration	• Assess patient's medical and drug history.
	• Assess use of drugs, alcohol, and other such medications (such as antihistamines, sedatives, tranquilizers, sleep aids, certain pain relievers, muscle relaxants, and antiseizure medication) for at least 24 hours, except as prescribed by the patient's healthcare provider.
	• Notify anesthesiologist/anesthetist if any of the above medications were taken or if the patient has any respiratory difficulties, fever, or other acute medical conditions.
	• Determine if the patient has any allergies or has had any hypersensitivities to barbiturates or benzodiazepine in the past.
	• Determine if the patient has any blood relatives who have had reactions to anesthesia such as malignant hyperthermia.
	• Obtain a pregnancy test.
	• Determine if the patient has any dentures, dental bridges, or loose teeth.
	• Complete any other preoperative procedures required by the agency.
Administration	• Determine medical and drug history.
	• Determine if any relatives experienced an adverse response to anesthetic agents.
After administration	• Assess and maintain a patent airway.
	• Provide oxygen as necessary.
	• Monitor vital signs frequently.
	• Monitor oxygen levels.
	• Maintain a safe environment.
	• Keep the patient warm (postoperative shivering is a common response to anesthesia).
	• Maintain the patient NPO until the patient has a gag reflex and can swallow.
	• Assess for side effects and provide medication if necessary.
Contraindications	• Hypersensitivity to halothane or components
Side effects/ adverse reactions	• Most side effects usually disappear as the anesthetic wears off.
	• Patients may feel drowsy, weak, or tired and experience fuzzy thinking, blurred vision, and coordination problems for as long as a few days after having general anesthesia.
	• Headache, shivering or trembling, muscle pain, dizziness, lightheadedness or faintness, mood or mental changes, nausea or vomiting, sore throat, and nightmares or unusual dreams.

Patient education
- Patients should not drive, operate machinery, or perform other activities that could endanger themselves or others for at least 24 hours or longer if necessary.
- Notify healthcare provider if these symptoms occur within two weeks of having general anesthesia.
- Severe headache, pain in the stomach or abdomen, back or leg pain, severe nausea, black or bloody vomit, unusual tiredness or weakness, weakness in the wrist and fingers, weight loss or loss of appetite, increase or decrease in amount of urine, pale skin, yellow eyes or skin

COMMONLY ADMINISTERED INTRAVENOUS ANESTHETIC AGENTS

Ketamine (Ketalar)	Affects the senses, and produces a dissociative anesthesia (catatonia, amnesia, analgesia) in which the patient may appear awake and reactive, but cannot respond to sensory stimuli. These properties make it especially useful for use in developing countries and during warfare medical treatment. Ketamine is frequently used in pediatric patients because anesthesia and analgesia can be achieved with an intramuscular injection. It is also used in high-risk geriatric patients and shock cases, because it also provides cardiac stimulation.
Thiopental (Pentothal)	A barbiturate that induces a rapid hypnotic state of short duration. Because thiopental is slowly metabolized by the liver, toxic accumulation can occur. Therefore, it should not be continuously infused. Side effects include nausea and vomiting on awakening.
Opioids	Fentanyl, sufentanil, and alfentanil are frequently used before anesthesia and surgery as a sedative and analgesic, as well as a continuous infusion for primary anesthesia. Because opioids rarely affect the cardiovascular system, they are particularly useful for cardiac surgery and other high-risk cases. Opioids act directly on spinal cord receptors, and are frequently used in epidurals for spinal anesthesia. Side effects may include nausea and vomiting, itching, and respiratory depression.
Propofol (Diprivan)	Propofol is a nonbarbiturate hypnotic agent and the most recently developed intravenous anesthetic. Its rapid induction and short duration of action are identical to thiopental, but recovery occurs more quickly and with much less nausea and vomiting. Also, propofol is rapidly metabolized in the liver and excreted in the urine, so it can be used for long durations of anesthesia, unlike thiopental. Hence, propofol is rapidly replacing thiopental as an anesthetic agent.

15.12   Topical Anesthetic Agents

Topical anesthetic agents decrease the sensitivity of nerve endings on skin surfaces. Topical anesthetic agents are in the form of solutions, liquid spray, ointment, creams, and gels.

Commonly used topical anesthetic agents are:

- LET: LET is a combination of lidocaine, epinephrine, and tetracaine.
- EMLA: EMLA anesthetizes skin before IM injections, venipuncture curettage, and biopsy. EMLA is administered 90 minutes before the procedure.
- ELA-Max: ELA-Max is an OTC medication that anesthetizes skin faster than EMLA. ELA-Max uses the liposomal delivery system where tiny lipid balls provide moisture to the skin and penetrate the cell wall.

TOPICAL ANESTHETIC AGENTS (TAC)

TAC (0.5% tetracaine, 1:2000 epinephrine, and 11.8% cocaine)	2–5 ml (1 ml per cm of laceration) applied to wound with cotton or gauze for 10–30 minutes; Onset: effective 10–30 minutes after application; Duration: not established; May be as effective as lidocaine for lacerations on face and scalp. Rare severe toxicity, including seizures and sudden cardiac death.
LET (4% lidocaine, 1:2000 and 0.5% tetracaine)	1–3 ml directly applied to wound for 15–30 minutes Onset: 20–30 minutes Duration: not epinephrine, established; Similar to TAC for face and scalp lacerations; less effective on extremities; no severe adverse effects reported
EMLA (2.5% lidocaine and 2.5% prilocaine)	Thick layer (1–2 g per 10 cm^2) applied to intact skin with covering patch of Tegaderm; Onset: must be left on for 1–2 hours. Duration: 0.5 to 2 hours; Variable, depending on duration of application; Contact dermatitis, methemoglobinemia (very rare)

(Continued)

(Continued from previous page)

TOPICAL ANESTHETIC AGENTS (TAC)

Iontophoresis	Small current applied to lidocaine-soaked sponges on intact skin; Onset: 10 minutes Duration: 10–20 minutes. Good for small procedures, depth of anesthesia greater than EMLA; Stinging sensation; may burn skin if high current

15.13   Local Anesthesia

A local anesthetic agent blocks pain at the site where the medication is administered. It is used for:

- Suturing lacerations
- Short-term localized surgery
- Spinal anesthesia
- Diagnostic producers

There are two groups of local anesthetics:

1. Esters: A chemical compound formed from the reaction between an acid and an alcohol
2. Amides: An organic chemical compound formed by reaction of an acid chloride, acid anhydride, or ester with an amine; are hypoallergenic

LOCAL ANESTHETICS

Use	For nerve block, infiltration, epidural (also called saddle block) and spinal anesthesias. Also used to treat cardiac dysthymias	Half-life: 2–10 minutes	Onset: 1.5–5 minutes	Peaks: 0.5–2 hours	Duration: 1–4 hours, depending on location
Example	Lidocaine (Xylocaine): Moderate-acting amide (1–3 hours)	Route: IM/SC/I V Topical	Pregnancy category: B	Pharmacokinetic: Metabolized in liver; PB: 60%–80%	
How it works	• Most local anesthetics are vasodilators therefore they increase blood flow to the area of administration and increase their own absorption. To decrease absorption, epinephrine (1:200,000 to 1:50,000) or other vasoconstrictors are often added to local anesthetic solutions. Block action by blocking Na+ channels				
Adult dose	• Local anesthetic: Injectable dose dependent on procedure; maximum dose: 4.5 mg/kg. Do not repeat within 2 hours • IM: 300 mg (or 4.3 mg/kd). May repeat in 60–90 min • IV: Initially 50–100 mg (1 mg/kg) IV bolus at rate of 25–50 mg/min. May repeat in 5 min. Give no more than 200–300 mg in 1 hr. Maintenance: 20–50 mcg/kg/min (1–4 mcg/min) as IV infusion • Topical: Apply to affected areas as needed • Dermal patch: Apply to intact skin over most painful area (up to three patches once for up to 12 hours in a 24-hour period)				
Before administration	• Obtain medical and drug history. • Assess for hypersensitivity to lidocaine, amide anesthetics. • Obtain baseline B/P, pulse, respirations, ECG, and electrolytes.				
Administration	• Resuscitative equipment and drugs (including oxygen) should always be readily available when administering lidocaine by any route • IM: Use 10% (100 mg/ml); clearly identify lidocaine that is for IM use; give in deltoid muscle (blood level is significantly higher than if injection is given in gluteus muscle or lateral thigh) • Instruct patient that local infiltration may burn and sting briefly				

- IV: Use only clearly marked for IV use; infusion solution should be 1 g to 1 liter D5W to provide concentration of 1 mg/ml; IV push use 1% (10 mg/ml) or 2% (20 mg/ml); administer IV push at rate of 25–50 mg/min; administer IV infusion at rate of 1–4 mg/min (1–4 ml); use volume control IV set.
- Topical: Not for ophthalmic use; for skin disorders apply directly to affected area or put on gauze or bandage, which is then applied to the skin; for mucous membrane use apply to desired area using manufacturer's insert; administer the lowest dose possible that still provides anesthesia.

After administration	• Assess and monitor vital signs.
	• Maintain patient safety if patient is receiving spinal or epidural anesthesia.
	• Monitor ECG if given for cardiac dysrhythmias; assess pulse for irregularity, strength/weakness, bradycardia.
	• Assess B/P for evidence of hypotension.
	• Monitor for therapeutic serum level (1.5–6 mcg/ml).
	• Drowsiness should be considered a warning sign of high blood levels of lidocaine.
Contraindications	• Do not use a vasoconstrictor on appendages such as fingers, toes, earlobes, and penis.
	• Use with caution with cardiac patients.
	• Hypersensitivity to amide-type local anesthetics, Adams-Stoke syndrome, supraventricular arrhythmias, Wolf-Parkinson-White syndrome. Spinal anesthesia contraindicated in septicemia.
	• *Caution:* Dosage should be reduced for elderly, debilitated, acutely ill; safety in children has not been established. Severe renal/hepatic disease, hypovolemia, CHF, shock, heart block, marked hypoxia, severe respiratory depression, bradycardia, incomplete heart block. Anesthetic solutions containing epinephrine should be used with caution in peripheral or hypertensive vascular disease and during or following potent general anesthesia. Sulfite sensitivity or asthma for some local and topical anesthetic preparations. Tartrazine or aspirin sensitivity with some topical preparations.
Side effects/ adverse reactions	• Anxiety, insomnia, apprehension, blurred vision, loss of hearing acuity, and nausea
	• CNS depression, convulsion and respiratory depression
	• Cardiovascular effects. Main toxic actions are in the heart. These may cause arrhythmias, decreased contraction, hypotension, cardiovascular collapse.
Patient education	• Explain possible side effects.
	• Advise patient to take an analgesic drug as ordered, such as ibuprofen or acetaminophen before these anesthetic agents wear off.
	• Report any side effects immediately to the healthcare provider

OTHER LOCAL ANESTHETIC AGENTS

Procaine (Novocaine)	Short-acting (0.5 to 1 hour)—ester, first synthetic local anesthetic, relatively safe because of rapid metabolism in the plasma, fast onset–short duration, not good for topical anesthesia
Cocaine	Ester, only local anesthetic that is a vasoconstrictor, only local anesthetic that produces euphoria, used by ENTs for surgical procedures because it reduces pain and controls bleeding
Tetracaine (Pontocaine)	Long-acting—Ester, used for spinal anesthesia and topical
Bupivacaine	Long-acting—Amide, can be cardiotoxic at high concentrations, used for infiltration, epidural, and nerve blocks.

15.14 Spinal Anesthesia

Spinal anesthesia is a local anesthetic injected into the spinal column to produce a regional neural block. The injection is in the third or fourth lumbar space. Headaches and hypotension are common side effects of spinal anesthesia because of changes in cerebrospinal fluid pressure caused by the injection. Side effects are reduced by reaming in the supine position and increasing fluids.

There are four types of spinal anesthesia:

1. Subarachnoid block: The injection is into the subarachnoid space in the third or fourth lumbar space.
2. Epidural block: The injection is into the outer covering (dura mater) of the spinal cord near the sacrum.
3. Saddle block: The injection is given into the lower end of the spinal column to block the perineal area.
4. Caudal block: The injection is near the sacrum.

15.15   Autonomic Nervous System and Adrenergic Blockers

The autonomic nervous system (visceral system) regulates smooth muscles and glands (heart, respiratory system, GI tract, eyes), involuntarily using two sets of nerves.

- Sensory (afferent) neurons transmit impulses to the brain via the central nervous system where impulses are interpreted by the brain.
- Motor (efferent) neutrons transmit impulses from the brain to specific organ cells via the spinal cord in response to impulses received from sensory neurons.

The sympathetic branch of the autonomic nervous system (see 15.1 The Nervous System) stimulates cells using the neurotransmitter norepinephrine. Adrenergics (sympathomimetics) mimic actions (Table 15.1) of the sympathetic nervous system. These are referred to as adrenergic agonists because it starts a response at the adrenergic receptor sites.

There are four types of adrenergic receptors: alpha$_1$, alpha$_2$, beta$_1$, and beta$_2$ (Table 15.2).

The parasympathetic branch of the autonomic nervous system (see 15.1 The Nervous System) depresses a response using adrenergic blockers (sympatholytics) that block the norepinephrine response at the adrenergic receptor sites (see Table 15.2).

Hint: The cholinergic system is another name for the parasympathetic branch because an acetylcholine neurotransmitter stimulates receptor cells to produce a response. The enzyme acetylcholinesterase inactivates the acetylcholine before it reaches the receptor cell.

Cholinergic (parasympathomimetics) medications mimic acetylcholine. They initiate a response and inhibit the effect of acetylcholine. Medications that block the effect of acetylcholine are called anticholinergic (parasympatholytics) or cholinergic antagonists because they inhibit the effect of acetylcholine.

Two types of cholinergic receptors are:

- Nicotinic: Stimulated by alkaloids nicotine
- Muscarinic: Stimulated by muscarine

TABLE 15.1   Actions of Sympathetic and Parasympathetic Medication

SYMPATHETIC STIMULANTS	PARASYMPATHETIC STIMULANTS
Sympathomimetics (adrenergics, adrenomimetics, or adrenergic agonists)	**Parasympathomimetics (cholinergics or cholinergic agonists)**
Increase blood pressure	Decrease blood pressure
Increase pulse rate	Decrease pulse rate
Relax bronchioles	Constrict bronchioles
Dilate pupils of eyes	Construct pupils of eyes
Uterine relaxation	Increase urinary contraction
Increase blood sugar	Increase peristalsis
	Indirect-acting
	Cholinesterase
	Inhibitors (anticholinesterase)
	Increase muscle tone
SYMPATHETIC DEPRESSANTS	**PARASYMPATHETIC DEPRESSANTS**
Sympatholytics (adrenergic blockers, adrenolytics, or adrenergic antagonists)	**Parasympatholytics (anticholinergics, cholinergics or adrenergic antagonists)**
Decrease blood pressure	Increase pulse rate
Decrease pulse rate	Decrease mucus secretions
Constrict bronchioles	Decrease gastrointestinal motility
	Increase urinary retention
	Dilate pupils of eyesInsert

TABLE 15.2 Adrenergic Receptors

RECEPTOR	PHYSIOLOGIC RESPONSES
Alpha$_1$	Increases force of contraction of heart. Vasoconstriction: increases blood pressure. Mydriasis: dilates pupils of the eyes. Glandular (salivary): decreases secretions. Bladder and prostate: capsule increases contraction and ejaculation.
Alpha$_2$	Inhibits the release of norepinephrine, dilates blood vessels, and produces hypotension; decreases gastrointestinal motility and tone
Beta$_1$	Increases heart rate and force of contraction; increases rennin secretion, which increases blood pressure
Beta$_2$	Dilates bronchioles; promotes GI and uterine relaxation; promotes increase in blood sugar through glycogenolysis in the liver; increases blood flow in the skeletal muscles

15.16   The Fight or Flight Response

The flight or flight response is produced by norepinephrine and acetylcholine neurotransmitters.

The fight response prepares the body to fight by improving vision, increasing oxygen, increasing circulation, and redirecting energy from less important body functions (digestion) to body functions needed to fight (Table 15.3).

The flight response is the opposite of fight and causes relaxation, returning the body to normal function (see Table 15.3).

15.17   Adrenergics and Adrenergic Blockers

Adrenergics are medications that stimulate alpha$_1$-receptors and beta$_2$-adrenergic receptors. Alpha$_1$-receptors are in the smooth muscles of vascular (vessels) tissues. Beta$_2$-adrenergic receptors are in the smooth muscles of lungs, arterioles of skeletal muscles, and the uterine muscle. Adrenergics also increase blood flow by stimulating the dopaminergic receptor located in the renal, mesenteric, coronary, and cerebral arteries. Dopamine is the only adrenergic that can activate this receptor.

There are three ways in which adrenergic blockers inactivate these receptors:

1. Promote reuptake of the transmitter back into the neuron.
2. Degrade transmitters by enzymes, making them unable to attach to a receptor. Enzymes are:
   a. Monoamine oxidase (MAO): MAO is inside the neuron
   b. Catechol-o-methyl-transferase (COMIT): COMIT is outside the neuron
3. Diffuse transmitters away from receptors.

TABLE 15.3 Fight and Flight Action

BODY TISSUE/ORGAN	SYMPATHETIC (FIGHT) RESPONSE	PARASYMPATHETIC RESPONSE (FLIGHT)
Eye	Dilates pupil	Constricts pupil
Lungs	Dilate bronchioles	Constrict bronchioles and increases secretions
Heart	Increases heart rate	Decreases heart rate
Blood vessels	Constricts	Dilates
Gastrointestinal	Relaxes smooth muscles	Increases peristalsis
Bladder	Relaxes bladder muscle	Constricts bladder
Uterus	Relaxes uterine muscle	
Salivary gland		Increases salivation

Sympathomimetic medications that stimulate adrenergic receptors are organized into three categories. These are:

1. Direct-acting Sympathomimetics: Directly stimulate receptors
2. Indirect-acting Sympathomimetics: Stimulate the release of norepinephrine from terminal nerve endings
3. Mixed-acting Sympathomimetics: Stimulate the adrenergic receptor sites and stimulate the release of norepinephrine from terminal nerve endings
   a. Ephedrine: Ephedrine is a mixed-acting sympathomimetic used to treat idiopathic orthostatic hypotension and hypotension resulting from spinal anesthesia. Ephedrine also stimulates $beta_2$-receptors to dilate bronchi to treat bronchial asthma.

Adrenergics such as epinephrine (adrenalin) stimulate as more than one adrenergic receptor site. Epinephrine acts on $alpha_1$-, $beta_1$-, and $beta_2$-receptor sites that influence blood pressure, pupil, heart rate, and bronchodilatation. Epinephrine and other adrenergics are nonselective and affect two or more adrenergic receptor sites.

ADRENERGICS AND ADRENERGIC BLOCKERS

Use	Treatment of acute bronchial asthma attacks, reversible bronchospasm in patients with chronic bronchitis, emphysema, and hypersensitivity reactions. Restores cardiac rhythm in cardiac arrest. Ophthalmic: Management of chronic open-angle glaucoma. Systemic: Treatment of gingival/pulpal hemorrhage; priapism. Ophthalmic: Treatment of conjunctival congestion during surgery; secondary glaucoma.	Half-life: UK	Onset: SC: 5–10 minutes IM: 5–10 minutes Inhalation: 3–5 minutes Ophthalmic: 4–8 hours	Peaks: SC: 20 minutes IM: 20 minutes Inhalation: 20 minutes Ophthalmic: 4–8 hours	Duration: SC: 1–4 hours IM:1–4 hours Inhalation: 1–3 hours Ophthalmic: 12–24 hours
Example	Epinephrine (Adrenalin) $alpha_1$, $beta_1$, $beta_2$	Route: SC, IM, IV, inhalation,		Pregnancy category: C	Pharmacokinetic: Rapidly ophthalmic metabolized in the GI tract and liver and excreted in the urine; Minimal absorption after inhalation; well absorbed after parenteral administration; Ophthalmic: May have systemic absorption from drainage into nasal pharyngeal passages. Mydriasis occurs within several minutes. Persists several hours; vasoconstriction occurs within 5 min; last less than 1 hr

How it works	• Stimulates $alpha_1$, $beta_1$, and $beta_2$ receptors, resulting in relaxation of smooth muscle of bronchial tree; peripheral vasculature; Ophthalmic: Increases outflow of aqueous humor from anterior eye chamber, dilates pupils (constricts conjunctival blood vessels)
Adult dose	• Asthma and anaphylaxis: SC; 0.1–0.5 ml of 1:1000 PRN; IV: 0.1–0.25 ml of 1:1000; Potent inotropic (increasing the force of the muscular contraction of the heart); Cardiac arrest: 1:10,000 solution IV (1 mg/ml) which may be diluted in 10 ml of saline solution; this can also be instilled in the endotracheal tube (tube inserted in patient airway into lungs during resuscitation)
Before administration	• Assess and monitor vital signs. • Check IV site frequently; infiltration of this category of drugs can result in tissue necrosis. • Assess lung sounds. • Monitor arterial blood cases. • Monitor ECG, B/P, and pulse in cardiac arrest.

Administration	• SC: Use tuberculin syringe into lateral deltoid region; massage injection site (minimizes vasoconstriction effect) • For IV infusion, give at 1–10 mcg/min (titrate to desired response)
After administration	• Report side effects. • Monitor urine output. • Offer food to avoid nausea and vomiting if patient is not NPO. • Monitor laboratory tests results and arterial blood gases as prescribed.
Contraindications	• Cardiac dysrhythmias, cerebral arteriosclerosis, pregnancy, narrow-angle glaucoma, cardiogenic shock; Use with caution in hypertension, prostatic hypertrophy, hyperthyroidism, pregnancy, diabetes mellitus
Side effects/ adverse reactions	• Anorexia, nausea, vomiting, nervousness, tremors, agitation, headaches, pallor, insomnia, syncope, dizziness • Palpitations, tachycardia, dyspnea; urinary retention can result from high dose or continuous use
Patient education	• Read labels on all OTC drugs for cold symptoms and diet pills. Many of these contain sympathetic (adrenergic, sympathomimetic) drugs and should not be taken if hypertensive or diabetic, or if the patient has cardiac dysrhythmias, coronary artery disease, or prostate hypertrophy. • These drugs pass into breast milk. • Continuous use of nasal sprays or drops that contain adrenergics may result in nasal congestion rebound (inflamed and congested nasal tissue). • Do not use bronchodilator sprays in excess.

OTHER ADRENERGICS AND ADRENERGIC BLOCKERS

Ephedrine HCl (alpha$_1$, beta$_1$, beta$_2$)	PO 25–50 mg TID/QID; SC/IM: 25–50 mg; IV: 10–25 mg PRN; maximum dose 150 mg/24 h; effective for relief of hay fever, sinusitis, and allergic rhinitis; may be used for treating mild cases of asthma; Pregnancy category: C; PB: UK; half-life 3–6 h.
Norepinephrine bitartrate (Levophed) (alpha$_1$,beta$_1$)	Potent vasoconstrictor; IV: 4 mg in 250–500 ml of D$_5$W or NSS infused initially 8–12 mcg/min; then 4 mcg/min; titrated according to blood pressure; Pregnancy category: C, D; PB: UK; half-life: UK.
Metaraminol bitartrate (Aramine) (alpha$_1$, beta$_1$)	IV/Inf: 15–100 mg in 500 mg D5W at a rate adjusted according to blood pressure; Pregnancy category: C; PB: UK; half-life UK.
Dobutamine HCl (Dobutrex) (beta$_1$)	To treat cardiac decompensation because of depressed myocardial contractility, which may result from organic heart disease, cardiac surgery. IV: 2.5–20 mcg/kg/min initially; increase dose gradually; maximum dose of 40 mcg/kg/min. Pregnancy category: C; PB:UK; half-life 2 min.
Dopamine HCl (Intropin) (alpha$_1$, beta$_1$) IV/Inf	1–5 mcg/kg/min initially; gradually increase 5–10 mcg/kg/min to a maximum of 50 mcg/kg/min; it does not decrease renal function in doses less than 5 mcg/kg/min. Pregnancy category: C; PB: UK; half-life 2 min.

15.18   Alpha-Adrenergic Blockers

Alpha-adrenergic blockers inhibit the response at the alpha-adrenergic receptor sites. There are two types of alpha-adrenergic blockers:

- Selective Alpha-adrenergic Blockers: Affect a specific alpha-adrenergic receptor site
- Nonselective Alpha-adrenergic Blockers: Affect multiple alpha-adrenergic receptor sites

Alpha-adrenergic blockers are prescribed to treat symptoms of benign prostatic hypertrophy (BPH) and to treat peripheral vascular disease. Alpha-adrenergic blockers also cause vasodilation.

Adverse effects of alpha-adrenergic blockers are:

- Orthostatic hypotension
- Dizziness
- Reflex tachycardia

15.19   Beta-Adrenergic Blockers

Beta-adrenergic blockers decrease the heart rate, decrease blood pressure, and cause bronchoconstriction. There are two types of beta-adrenergic blockers.

Selective Beta-Adrenergic Blockers

Selective blockers affect a specific beta-adrenergic receptor site. Tartrate (Lopressor) is a selective beta-adrenergic blocker that blocks beta$_1$ to decrease pulse rate and decreased blood pressure.

Nonselective Beta-Adrenergic Blockers

Nonselective blockers affect multiple beta-adrenergic receptor sites. Propranolol NCL (Inderal) is a nonselective beta-adrenergic blocker that blocks both beta$_1$ and beta$_2$ receptors, resulting in a slower heart rate, decreased cardiac output, and lower blood pressure.

Caution: Use caution when administering beta-adrenergic blockers to a patient who has COPD or asthma.

BETA-BLOCKERS					
Use	Treatment of hypertension, angina, various cardiac arrhythmias, hypertrophic subaortic stenosis, migraine headache, essential tremor, and as an adjunct to alpha-blocking agents in the treatment of pheochromocytoma. Used to reduce risk of cardiovascular mortality and reinfarction in patients who have previously suffered a myocardial infarction (MI). Treatment of adjunct anxiety, thyrotoxicosis, and mitral valve prolapse syndrome.	Half-life: 3–5 hours	Onset: PO: UK PO (long-acting): IV: immediate	Peaks: 60–90 minutes 6 hours 1 minute	Duration: PO:UK
Example	Propranolol HCl (Inderal) beta$_1$ and beta$_2$	Route: PO/IV		Pregnancy category: C	Pharmaco-kinetic: Absorbed from the GI tract; metabolized in the liver; excreted in urine. Crosses the blood–brain barrier and the placenta and is found in breast milk; PB: 93%; not removed by hemodialysis
How it works	• Blocks beta$_1$ (cardiac) and beta$_2$ (pulmonary); decreases myocardial ischemia severity by decreasing oxygen requirements; slows AV conduction; increases refractory period in AV node; exhibits antiarrhythmic activity				
Adult dose	• Hypertension: Initially 40 mg two times/day or 80 mg daily as extended-release capsule; increase at 3- to 7-day intervals. Maintenance: 120–140 mg/day as tablets or oral solution, 120–160 mg/day as extended-release capsules. Maximum: 640 mg/day • Angina: PO: Initially, 80–320 mg/day in two to four divided doses or 80 mg/day (sustained-release). Maximum: 320 mg/day; Maintenance: 160 mg/day • Cardiac arrhythmias: PO: 10–30 mg 3–4/day • Life-threatening arrhythmias: IV: 0.5–3 mg; Repeat once in 2 min. Give additional doses at intervals of at least 4 hours • Hypertropic subaortic stenosis: PO: 20–40 mg in three to four divided doses or 80–160 mg/day as extended-release capsule • Pheochromocytoma: PO: 60 mg/day in divided doses with alpha-blocker for 3 days before surgery; Maintenance (inoperable tumor): 30 mg/day with alpha-blocker				

	• Migraine headache: PO: 80 mg/day in divided doses or 80 mg once daily as extended-release capsule; increase up to 160–240 mg/day in divided doses
	• Myocardial infarction: PO: 180–240 mg/day in divided doses beginning 5–21 days after MI
	• Essential tremor: PO: Initially 40 mg 2 times/day increased up to 120–320 mg/day in divided doses
Before administration	• Assess and monitor vital signs and ECG.
	• Assess medical and drug history, report if taking phenothiazines, digoxin, calcium channel blockers, or other antihypertensives.
	• Assess urine output for baseline.
	• Assess respiratory status before administering drug.
	• Anginal: Record onset, type (sharp, dull, squeezing) radiation, location, intensity, and duration of anginal pain and precipitating factors (exertion, emotional stress).
Administration	• PO: May crush scored tablets
	• PO: Give at same time each day
	• IV: Give undiluted for IV push
	• For IV infusion, give 1 mg over 10–15 min
After administration	• Report symptoms of excessive dizziness or lightheadedness; dose may need adjustment.
	• Report complaints of stuffy nose.
	• Monitor blood glucose in diabetics; insulin dose may need to be adjusted.
	• Maintain safe environment in case of orthostatic hypotension.
	• Monitor pulse for strength/weakness, irregular rate, and bradycardia.
	• Monitor ECG for cardiac arrhythmias.
	• Assess fingers for color, numbness (Raynaud's) disease.
	• Assess for evidence of CHF (dyspnea [particularly on exertion or lying down], night cough, peripheral edema, distended neck veins).
	• Monitor I and O (increase in weight, decrease in urine output may indicate CHF).
	• Assess for rash, fatigue, or behavioral changes.
	• Therapeutic response ranges from a few days to several weeks.
	• Measure B/P near end of dosing interval (determine if BP is controlled throughout day).
Contraindications	• Congestive heart failure, secondary heart block, cardiogenic shock, bronchial asthma, bronchospasm. Use with caution in patients with renal or liver problems.
Side effects/ adverse reactions	• Bradycardia, confusion, drowsiness, fatigue, vertigo, pruritus, dry mouth, nasal stuffiness, brown discoloration of the tongue (rare)
	• Visual hallucinations, thrombocytopenia
	• Life-threatening: Laryngospasm, atrioventricular heart block, agranulocytosis
Patient education	• Do not abruptly stop a beta-blocker; rebound hypertension and tachycardia or an angina attack could result.
	• Diabetics on insulin therapy should be aware that early signs of hypoglycemia may be masked by the beta-blocker.
	• Teach patient and family how to monitor pulse and blood pressure.
	• Rise slowly from supine (lying) or sitting positions to avoid orthostatic hypotension.
	• Mood changes can occur which range from depression, nightmares, and suicidal tendencies (although rare).
	• Certain beta-blockers such as propranolol, metoprolol, and pindolol, and alpha-blockers such as prazosin, may cause impotence or a decrease in libido, which is usually dose related and should be reported to the prescriber.

OTHER BETA-BLOCKERS

Doxazosin mesylate (Cardura) alpha$_1$	Mild to moderate hypertension; PO: 1 mg/d; titrate dose up to maximum of 16 mg/d; maintenance 4–8 mg/day. Pregnancy category: C; PB: 95%; half-life 3 hours
Carvedilol (Coreg) alpha$_1$, beta$_1$, beta$_2$	Use for hypertension and mild to moderate heart failure; can be used with a thiazide diuretic; PO 6.25 mg BID; may increase to 12.5 mg BID to maximum 50 mg/d; Pregnancy category: C; PB: UK; half-life 7–10 hours
Labetalol (Normodyne) alpha$_1$, beta$_1$, beta$_2$	Mild to severe hypertension; angina pectoris; PO 100 mg BID; dose may be increased to a maximum of 2.4 g/day. IV: 20 mg OR 102 mg/kg; repeat 20–80 mg at 10-min intervals to maximum dose of 300 mg/day. Pregnancy category: C; PB: 50%; half-life 6–8 hours.

(Continued)

(Continued from previous page)

OTHER BETA-BLOCKERS

Nadolol (Corgard) beta$_1$, beta$_2$	Management of hypotension and angina pectora. Contraindicated in bronchial asthma and severe COPD. PO 40–80 mg/d; maximum 320 mg/day. Pregnancy category: C; PB: 30%; half-life 10–24 hours

SELECTIVE BETA-ADRENERGICS

Metoprolol tartrate (Lopressor)—beta$_1$	Management of hypertension, angina pectoris, postmyocardial infarction. Hypertension: PO 50–100 mg/d in one dose or two divided doses; maintenance 100–450 mg/d in divided doses. Myocardial infarction: IV: 5 mg q2 min × three doses, then PO 100 mg BID. Pregnancy category: C; PB: 12%; half-life 3–4 hours
Atenolol (Tenormin)—beta$_1$	Mild to moderate hypertension and angina pectoris. May be used in combination with antihypertensive drugs. PO 25–100 mg/d. Pregnancy category: C; PB: 6%–16%; half-life 6–7 hours Esmolol HCl (Brevibloc)—beta$_1$Supraventricular tachycardia, atrial fibrillation/flutter, and hypertension. Contraindications: heart block, bradycardia, cardiogenic shock, uncompensated CHF; IV: Loading dose 500 μ/kg/min for 1 min; then 50 mcg/kg/min for 4 min. Pregnancy category: C; PB: UK; half-life 9 minutes

15.20   Cholinergics

Cholinergics mimic acetylcholine (a parasympathetic neurotransmitter). Acetylcholine (ACH) is a neurotransmitter at the ganglions and terminal nerve endings of parasympathetic nerves.

There are two types of cholinergic receptors.

- Muscarinic receptors: Stimulate smooth muscles and slow the heart rate
- Nicotinic receptors: Affect skeletal muscles

Cholinergic medication (cholinesterase inhibitors, anticholinesterase) has either a direct- or indirect-acting effect on receptor sites. Direct and indirect effects inhibit the action of the enzyme cholinesterase (acetylcholinesterase). By inhibiting cholinesterase, more acetylcholine is available to stimulate the receptor and remains in contact with the receptor longer.

Pilocarpine is direct acting cholinergic used to treat glaucoma, reducing intraocular pressure by constricting pupils and opening the canal of Schlemm, which enable drainage of aqueous humor.

There are two types of cholinesterase inhibitors.

- Reversible inhibitors: binds to the cholinesterase enzyme for a period and then releases, enabling the cholinesterase enzyme to properly function
- Irreversible inhibitors: permanently binds to the cholinesterase enzyme

Cholinergics:

- Stimulate the bladder.
- Constrict pupils.
- Increase neuromuscular transmission.
- Provide muscle tone to the GI tract.
- Decrease heart rate.
- Decrease blood pressure.
- Increase salivary glands secretion.

EFFECTS OF CHOLINERGIC AND ANTICHOLINERGIC DRUGS

Body Tissue	Cholinergic Response	Anticholinergic Response
Cardiovascular*	Decreases heart rate, lowers blood pressure because of vasodilation, and slows conduction of atrioventricular node.	Increases heart rate with large doses. Small doses can decrease heart rate.
Gastrointestinal+	Increases the tone and motility of the smooth muscles of the stomach and intestine. Peristalsis is increased and the sphincter muscles are relaxed.	Relaxes smooth muscle tone of GI tract, decreasing GI motility and peristalsis. Decreases gastric and intestinal secretions.
Genitourinary	Contracts the muscles of the urinary bladder, increases tone of the ureters, and relaxes the bladder's sphincter muscles. Stimulates urination.	Relaxes the bladder detrusor muscle and increases constriction of the internal sphincter. Urinary retention can result.
Eye+	Increases papillary constriction, or miosis (pupil becomes smaller), and increases accommodation (flattening or thickening of eye lens for distant or near vision).	Dilates pupils of the eye (mydriasis) and paralyzes ciliary muscle (cycloplegia), causing a decrease in accommodation.
Glandular*	Increases salivation, perspiration, and tears.	Decreases salivation, sweating, and bronchial secretions.
Bronchi (lung)*	Stimulates bronchial smooth muscle contraction and increases bronchial secretions.	Dilates the bronchi and decreases bronchial secretions.
Striated muscle+	Increases neuromuscular transmission and maintains muscle strength and tone.	Decreases tremors and rigidity of muscles.
Central nervous system	Stimulates transmissions of nerve impulses to smooth and striated muscles	Drowsiness, disorientation, and hallucination can result from large doses.

* Tissue responses to large doses of cholinergic drugs.

+ Major tissue responses to normal doses of cholinergic drugs.

DIRECT-ACTING CHOLINERGIC

Use	Increase urination	Half-life: UK	Onset: 0.5–1.5 hours	Peaks: 1–2 hours	Duration: 4–6 hours
Example	Bethanechol chloride (Urecholine)	Route: PO or SC. Do not give IM or IV	Pregnancy category: C	Pharmacokinetic: Poorly absorbed from GI tract; PB: UK; Excreted in urine.	

How it works
- Acts directly at cholinergic receptor of smooth muscle of urinary bladder and GI tract. Increases tone of detrusor muscle, may initiate micturation (urination), bladder emptying. Stimulates gastric intestinal motility.

Adult dose
- PO 10–50 BID/TID/QID—maximum 120 mg/day; SC 2.5–5 mg; repeat at 15–30 minutes. intervals; PRN

Before administration
- Obtain baseline vital signs.
- Assess urine output (should be greater than 600 ml/d).
- Assess medical and drug history. Cholinergics can aggravate symptoms of peptic ulcer, urinary obstruction, or asthma.

Administration
- Do not give IM or IV. Violent cholinergic reaction (circulatory collapse; severe hypotension, bloody diarrhea, shock, cardiac arrest) will occur. Antidote: 0–0.6–1.2 mg atropine sulfate
- Give 1 hour before or 2 hour after meals. If patient complains of gastric pain, the drug may be given with meals.

(Continued)

(Continued from previous page)

DIRECT-ACTING CHOLINERGIC

After administration	• Monitor vital signs. • Monitor fluid intake and output. • Observe for side effects. • Auscultate bowel sounds. Report decreased or hyperactive sounds. • Auscultate breath sounds. Bronchial secretions may increase. • Diaphoresis (excessive perspiration) may occur; change linens as needed. • Monitor of the possibility of cholinergic crisis (overdose); symptoms include muscular weakness and increased salivation.
Contraindications	• Hyperthyroidism, peptic ulcer, latent or active bronchial asthma, mechanical GI and urinary obstruction or recent GI resection, acute inflammatory GI tract conditions, anastomosis, bladder wall instability, pronounced bradycardia, hypotension, hypertension, cardiac disease, coronary artery disease, vasomotor instability, epilepsy, Parkinsonism. *Cautions:* None significant.
Side effects/ adverse reactions	• Effects are more noticeable with SC administration. • Occasional: Belching, change in vision, blurred vision, diarrhea, frequent urinary urgency • Rare: (SC): Shortness of breath, tight chest, bronchospasm Adverse/toxic: • Overdosage produces CNS stimulation (insomnia, nervousness, orthostatic hypotension) and cholinergic stimulation (headache, increased salivation/sweating, nausea, vomiting, flushed skin, stomach pain, seizures).
Patient education	• Take drug as prescribed. • Report any side effects. • Sit up or stand up slowly to avoid dizziness.

15.21   Anticholinergics

Anticholinergics mimic acetylcholine (parasympathetic neurotransmitter). Anticholinergics inhibit acetylcholine by occupying the acetylcholine receptors blocking parasympathetic nerve enabling impulses from sympathetic nerves to take control. Anticholinergic and adrenergic drugs produce many of the same responses.

Anticholinergics are also called:

- Parasympatholytics
- Cholinergic blocking agents
- Cholinergic antagonists
- Muscarinic antagonists
- Antiparasympathetic agents
- Antimuscarinic agents
- Antispasmodics

ANTICHOLINERGIC/PARASYMPATHOLYTIC

Use	Preoperative medication to reduce salivation, increase heart rate, dilate pupils of the eye; treatment of cardiac arrhythmias, sinus bradycardia	Half-life: 2–3 hours	Onset: 0.5–1 hour	Peaks: 1–2 hours	Duration: 4 hours
Example	Atropine SO$_4$	Route: PO/IM/IV	Pregnancy category: C	Pharmacokinetic: Well absorbed; crosses the placenta; 75% excreted in urine; PB: UK.	
How it works	• Inhibits action of acetylcholine on structures innervated by postganglionic sites (smooth/cardiac muscle, SA/AV nodes, exocrine glands). Larger doses may decrease motility, secretory activity of GI system, tone of ureter and urinary bladder.				

Adult dose	• PO/Q/IM/IV: Preoperative: 0.4–0.6 mg q4h–6h 30 to 60 minutes before time of induction of anesthesia or other preanesthetic medications; Anti-arrhythmic: IV: 0.4–1 mg q1–2 hours PRN with a maximum dose of 2 mg; Antisecretory: IM: 0.2–0.6 mg 30–60 min before surgery.
Before administration	• Have the patient void before giving medication; this reduces the risk of urinary retention. • Assess vital signs. • Keep the patient NPO before surgical procedures as per agency policies. • Food decreases absorption of medication if taken PO.
Administration	• IV: Must be given rapidly (prevents paradoxical slowing of heart rate)
After administration	• Monitor for changes in BP, pulse, or temperature. • Assess skin turgor and mucous membranes to evaluate hydration status. • Monitor bowel sounds for peristalsis. • Be alert for fever (increased risk of hyperthermia). • Monitor intake and output. • Palpate bladder for urinary retention. • Assess stool frequency and consistency. • Monitor heart rate and ECG.
Contraindications	• Narrow-angle glaucoma, severe ulcerative colitis, toxic megacolon, obstructive disease of GI tract, paralytic ileus, intestinal atony, bladder neck obstruction because of prostatic hypertrophy, myasthenia gravis in those not treated with neostigmine, tachycardia secondary to cardiac insufficiency or thyrotoxicosis, cardiospasm, unstable cardiovascular status in acute hemorrhage • *Caution:* Hyperthyroidism, hepatic or renal disease, hypertension, tachyarrhythmias, CHF, coronary artery disease, gastric ulcer, esophageal reflux or hiatal hernia associated with reflux esophagitis, infants, elderly persons, systemic administration in those with COPD • *Extreme Caution:* Autonomic neuropathy, known or suspected GI infections, diarrhea, mild to moderate ulcerative colitis
Side effects/ adverse reactions	• Discontinue medication immediately if dizziness, increased pulse, or blurring of vision occurs • Frequent: Dry mouth/nose/throat (may be severe), decreased sweating, constipation, irritation at SC/IM injection site • Occasional: Swallowing difficulty, blurred vision, bloated feeling, impotence, urinary hesitancy • Rare: Allergic reaction (rash, urticaria), mental confusion/excitement (particularly children), fatigue Adverse/Toxic • Overdose may produce tachycardia, palpitations, hot/dry/flushed skin, absence of bowel sounds, increased respiratory rate, nausea, vomiting, confusion, drowsiness, slurred speech, CNS stimulation, psychosis (agitation, restlessness, rambling speech, visual hallucinations, paranoid behavior, delusions), followed by depression.
Patient education	• Take oral form 30 min before meals. • Avoid becoming overheated during exercise in hot weather (which may result in heat stroke). • Avoid hot baths and saunas. • Avoid tasks that require alertness until response to drug is established. • Sugarless gum and sips of tepid water may relieve dry mouth. • Do not take antacids or medicine for diarrhea within 1 hour of taking this medication (decreases effectiveness). • If given as a preoperative medication, explain that a warm, dry, flushing feeling may occur. • Remind the patient to stay in bed and remain NPO.

ANTICHOLINERGIC: GI

Use	Treatment of functional disturbances of GI motility (i.e., irritable bowel syndrome)	Half-life: 9–10 hours	Onset: 1 hour	Peaks: 2 hours	Duration: 6 hours
Example	Dicyclomine HCl (Bentyl, Antispas, Di-Spaz)	Route: PO/IM	Pregnancy category: B		Pharmacokinetic: Readily absorbed from GI tract. Widely distributed; metabolized in liver.
How it works	• Direct relaxant action on smooth muscle reducing tone and motility of GI tract				
Adult dose	• PO: 10–20 mg two to four times/day up to 40 mg four times/day; IM: 20 mg q4–6 hours				
Before administration	• Store capsules, tablets, syrup, parenteral form at room temperature • PO: Dilute oral solution with equal volume of water just before administration • IM: Injection should appear colorless • Void before taking medication to avoid risk of urinary retention				

(Continued)

(Continued from previous page)

ANTICHOLINERGIC: GI

Administration	• PO: May give without regard to meals (food may slightly decrease absorption) • IM: Do not administer IV or SC; inject deep into large muscle mass; do not give longer than 2 days
After administration	• Monitor daily bowel activity and stool consistency. • Assess for urinary retention. • Monitor changes in vital signs including temperature. • Assess for hydration. • Assess bowel sounds for peristalsis. • Be alert for fever.
Contraindications	• Narrow-angle glaucoma, severe ulcerative colitis, toxic megacolon, obstructive disease of GI tract, paralytic ileus, intestinal atony, bladder neck obstruction because of prostatic hypertrophy, myasthenia gravis in those not treated with neostigmine, tachycardia secondary to cardiac insufficiency or thyrotoxicosis, cardiospasm, unstable cardiovascular status in acute hemorrhage • *Caution:* Hyperthyroidism, hepatic or renal disease, hypertension, tachyarrhythmias, CHF, coronary artery disease, gastric ulcer, esophageal reflux or hiatal hernia associated with reflux esophagitis, infants, elderly persons, systemic administration in those with COPD • *Extreme Caution:* Autonomic neuropathy, known or suspected GI infections, diarrhea, mild to moderate ulcerative colitis
Side effects/ adverse reactions	• Frequent: Dry mouth (sometimes severe), constipation, decreased sweating • Occasional: Blurred vision, intolerance to light, urinary hesitancy, drowsiness (with high dosage), agitation/excitement/drowsiness noted in elderly (even with low doses). IM may produce transient lightheadedness, irritation at injection site. • Rare: Confusion, hypersensitivity reaction, increased intraocular pressure, nausea, vomiting, unusual tiredness. Adverse/toxic • Overdosage may produce temporary paralysis of ciliary muscle papillary dilation, tachycardia, palpitation, hit/dry/flushed skin, absence of bowel sounds, hyperthermia, increased respiratory rate, ECG abnormalities, nausea, vomiting, rash over face/upper trunk, CNS stimulation, psychosis (agitation, restlessness, rambling speech, visual hallucination, paranoid behavior, delusions), followed by depression
Patient education	• Avoid becoming overheated during exercise in hot weather (may result in heat stroke). • Avoid hot baths and saunas. • Avoid tasks that require alertness until a response to drug is established. • Sugarless gum and sips of tepid water may relieve dry mouth. • Do not take antacids or medicine for diarrhea within 1 hour of taking this medication (decreases effectiveness).

15.22 Antiparkinsonism-Anticholinergic Medication

Antiparkinsonism-anticholinergic medication treats pseudoparkinsonism and the early stages of Parkinson's disease. They are prescribed for pseudoparkinsonism. Pseudoparkinsonism is parkinsonism-like side effects of the antipsychotic medication phenothiazines. Antiparkinsonism-anticholinergic medication is combined with levodopa to control parkinsonism.

ANTICHOLINERGIC-ANTIPARKINSONISM DRUGS

Use	Adjunctive treatment for all forms of Parkinson's disease, including postencephalitic, arteriosclerotic, idiopathic types. Controls symptoms of drug-induced extrapyramidal symptoms.	Half-life: 5–10 hours	Onset: 1 hour SR: UK	Peaks: 2–3 hours SR: UK	Duration: 6–12 hours SR: 12–24 hours
Example	Trihexyphenidyl HCl (Artane)		Route: PO	Pregnancy category: C	Pharmacokinetic: PB: UK; Well absorbed; excreted in urine.

How it works	• Blocks central cholinergic receptors (aids in balancing cholinergic and dopaminergic activity). Decreases salivation, relaxes smooth muscle; decreases involuntary movements.
Adult dose	• Parkinsonism: PO: Initially 1–2 mg/d; increase to 6–10 mg/day in divided doses. Extrapyramidal symptoms: drug induced: PO 1 mg/d; increase to 5–15 mg/day in divided doses.
Before administration	• Do not use sustained-release capsules for initial therapy. Once stabilized, may switch, on mg-for-mg basis; giving a single daily dose after breakfast or two divided doses 12 hours apart.
Administration	• No known interaction with foods or herbals.
After administration	• Be alert to neurologic effects: headache, lethargy, mental confusion, agitation. • Assess for clinical improvement of parkinsonism: tremor of head/hands at rest, masklike facial expression, shuffling gait, muscular rigidity. • Maintain a safe environment for patient.
Contraindications	• Angle-closure glaucoma, GI obstruction, paralytic ileus, intestinal atony, severe ulcerative colitis, prostatic hypertrophy, myasthenia gravis, megacolon • *Caution:* Treated open-angle glaucoma, autonomic neuropathy, pulmonary disease, esophageal reflux, hiatal hernia, heart disease, hyperthyroidism, hypertension
Side effects/ adverse reactions	• Elderly (greater than 60) tend to develop mental confusion, disorientation, agitation, psychotic-like symptoms • Frequent: Drowsiness, dry mouth • Occasional: Blurred vision, urinary retention, constipation, dizziness, headache, muscle cramps • Rare: Skin rash, seizures, depression Adverse/Toxic • Hypersensitivity reaction (eczema, pruritus, rash, cardiac disturbances, photosensitivity) may occur. Overdose may vary from CNS depression (sedation, apnea, cardiovascular collapse, death) to severe paradoxical reaction (hallucinations, tremor, seizures).
Patient education	• Avoid tasks that require alertness until response to drug is established. • Expect dry mouth, drowsiness, and dizziness. • Avoid use of alcohol. • Sugarless gum and sips of tepid water may relieve dry mouth. • Caffeine in coffee, tea, and soft drinks may help reduce drowsiness.

ANTICHOLINERGIC-ANTIPARKINSONISM

Use	Treatment of Parkinson's disease, drug-induced extrapyramidal reactions, except tardive dyskinesia		Half life: UK	Onset: 2 hours	Peak: 4 hours	Duration: 12 hours
Example	Benztropine mesylate (Cogentin)	Route: PO/IM/IV	Pregnancy category: C	Pharmacokinetic: PB: UK		

How it works	• Selectively blocks central cholinergic receptors, assists in balancing cholinergic/dopaminergic activity. Reduces incidence, severity of akinesia, rigidity, and tremor
Adult dose	• Idiopathic parkinsonism: PO/IM: initially 0.5–1 mg/day at bedtime up to 6 mg/day • Postencephalitic parkinsonism: PO/IM: 2 mg/day as single or divided dose • Drug-induced extrapyramidal symptoms: PO/IM: 1–4 mg one to two times/day • Acute dystonic reactions: IM/IV: 1–2 mg, then 1–2 mg PO two times/day to prevent recurrence
Before administration	• Assess mental status for confusion, disorientation, agitation, psychotic-like symptoms.
Administration	• Administer as ordered.
After administration	• Be alert to neurologic effects: headache, lethargy, mental confusion, agitation. • Assess for clinical improvement of parkinsonism: tremor of head/hands at rest, masklike facial expression, shuffling gait, muscular rigidity. • Maintain a safe environment for patient.
Contraindications	• Angle closure glaucoma, GI obstruction, paralytic ileus, intestinal atony, severe ulcerative colitis, prostatic hypertrophy, myasthenia gravis, megacolon, children less than 3 years • *Caution:* Treated open-angle glaucoma, heart disease, hypertension, patients with tachycardia, arrhythmias, prostatic hypertrophy, liver/renal impairment, obstructive diseases of the GI or GU tract, urinary retention

(Continued)

(Continued from previous page)

ANTICHOLINERGIC-ANTIPARKINSONISM

Side effects/ adverse reactions	• Elderly patients (greater than 60) tend to develop mental confusion, disorientation, agitation, psychotic-like symptoms • Frequent: Drowsiness, dry mouth, blurred vision, constipation, decreased sweating/urination, GI upset, photosensitivity • Occasional: Headache, memory loss, muscle cramping, nervousness, peripheral paresthesia, orthostatic hypotension, abdominal cramping • Rare: Rash, confusion, eye pain Adverse/toxic • Overdose may vary: Severe anticholinergic effects (unsteadiness, severe drowsiness, severe dryness of mouth/nose/throat, tachycardia, shortness of breath, skin flushing); also produces severe paradoxical reaction (hallucinations, tremor, seizures, toxic psychosis)
Patient education	• Avoid tasks that require alertness until response to drug is established. • Expect dry mouth, drowsiness, and dizziness. • Avoid the use of alcohol. • Sugarless gum and sips of tepid water may relieve dry mouth. • Caffeine in coffee, tea, and soft drinks may help reduce drowsiness.

CHOLINESTERASE INHIBITOR

Use	To improve memory in mild to moderate Alzheimer's dementia. Drug enhances cholinergic function.	Half-life: 1.5–3.5 hours	Onset: 1 hour	Peaks: 4 hours	Duration: 12 hours
Example	Reminyl (galantamine)	Route: PO	Pregnancy category: B	Pharmacokinetic: Rapidly absorbed from GI tract, metabolized in the liver, and excreted in urine. PB: 18%	

How it works	• Prevents the breakdown of acetylcholine and stimulates nicotinic receptors to release more acetylcholine in the brain
Adult dose	• 4 mg, twice a day (8 mg/day) • Increase by 8 mg/day after 4 weeks to 8 mg, twice a day (16 mg/day) • After another 4 weeks, increase to 12 mg, twice a day (24 mg/day), if well tolerated. Note: If therapy is interrupted for several days or longer, must retitrate as noted.
Before administration	• Obtain the baseline cognitive, behavioral, and functional deficits of the patient. • Assess liver and renal function.
Administration	• Give with morning and evening meals.
After administration	• Monitor cognitive, behavioral, and functional status of patient. • Evaluate ECG, periodic rhythm strips in patient with underlying arrhythmias. • Monitor for symptoms of ulcer, GI bleeding.
Contraindica-tions	• Severe hepatic or renal impairment *Cautions:* • Moderately impaired renal/hepatic function • History of ulcer disease, those on concurrent NSAIDs, asthma, COPD, bladder outflow obstruction, supraventricular cardiac conduction conditions
Side effects/ adverse reactions	• Frequent: Nausea, vomiting, diarrhea, anorexia • Occasional: Abdominal pain, insomnia, depression, headache, dizziness, fatigue, rhinitis • Rare: Tremors, constipation, confusion, cough, anxiety, urinary incontinence Adverse/toxic: • Overdose can cause cholinergic crises (increased salivation, lacrimation, urination, defecation, bradycardia, hypotension, increased muscle weakness). Treatment aimed at general supportive measures, use of anticholinergics (e.g., atropine)

Patient education	• Take with morning and evening meals to reduce risk of nausea.
	• Do not reduce or stop medication.
	• Do not increase dosage without healthcare provider direction.
	• If therapy is interrupted for several days, restart at lowest dose and titrate to current dose at 4-week intervals.

CHOLINESTERASE INHIBITOR

Use	Slows the progression of Alzheimer's	Half-life:	Onset:	Peaks:	Duration:
Example	Aricept (donepezil)	Route: PO	Pregnancy category: C	Pharmacokinetic: PB: 96% Well absorbed in GI tract, metabolized in liver, and eliminated in urine and feces	

How it works	• Enhances cholinergic function by increasing the concentration of acetylcholine through inhibition of the hydrolysis of acetylcholine by the enzyme acetylcholinesterase
Adult dose	• 5–10 mg/day as a single dose. Infinitival dose is 5 mg. Do not increase to 10 mg for 4–6 weeks.
Before administration	• Same as Reminyl
Administration	• May be given without regard to meals or time of administration (morning versus evening dose), although it is suggested the dose be given in the evening just before bedtime
After administration	• Same as Reminyl
Contraindications	• History of hypersensitivity to donepezil or piperidine derivatives.
	• Use with caution, same as Reminyl
Side effects/ adverse reactions	• Same as Reminyl
Patient education	• Same as Reminyl

OTHER: COMT INHIBITOR

Use	Adjunct therapy with levodopa/carbidopa for treatment of idiopathic Parkinson's disease	Half-life: 2–3 hours	Onset: 1 hour	Peaks: 3 hours	Duration: 8 hours
Example	Tolcapone (Tasmar)	Route: PO	Pregnancy category: UK	Pharmacokinetic: PB: UK	

How it works	• Inhibits the enzyme COMT; sustaining plasma levels and thereby increasing the duration of action of levodopa, resulting in greater effect, relieving signs and symptoms of Parkinson's disease
Adult dose	• Initially, 100–200 mg three/times/day; Maximum dose of 600 mg/day
Before administration	• May combine tolcapone with both the immediate and sustained-release form of levodopa/carbidopa
	• Obtain vital signs; assess for hypotension.
Administration	• Give without regard to food.
After administration	• Serum transaminase levels should be monitored q2 weeks for the first year; q4 weeks for the next 6 months and q8 weeks thereafter.
	• Treatment should be discontinued if ALT (SGPT) exceeds the upper limit of normal or clinical signs of hepatic failure occur.
	• If hallucinations occur, they may be eliminated if levodopa dosage is reduced. Hallucinations generally are accompanied by confusion and to a lesser extend insomnia.
	• Have patient sit and rise slowly to prevent risk of postural hypotension.
	• Assist with ambulation if dizziness occurs.
	• Assess for clinical reversal of symptoms.

(Continued)

(Continued from previous page)

OTHER: COMT INHIBITOR

Contraindica-tions	• None significant • *Caution:* Severe renal impairment; severe liver impairment, those with history of hallucinations, baseline hypotension, history of orthostatic hypotension
Side effects/ adverse reactions	• Frequency of occurrence of side effects increases with dosage amount. • Frequent: Nausea; insomnia, somnolence, anorexia, diarrhea, muscle cramps, orthostatic hypotension, excessive dreaming • Occasional: Headache, vomiting, confusion, hallucinations, constipation, increased sweating, urine discoloration (bright yellow), dry eyes, abdominal pain, dizziness, flatulence • Rare: Dyspepsia, neck pain, hypotension, fatigue, chest discomfort Adverse/Toxic • Upper respiratory infection and urinary tract infection occur occasionally; too-rapid withdrawal from therapy may produce withdrawal emergent hyperpyrexia characterized by elevated temperature, muscular rigidity, altered consciousness. An increase in dyskinesia (impaired voluntary movement) or dystonia (impaired muscular tone) occurs frequently.
Patient education	• If nausea occurs, take medication with food. • Side effects of drowsiness, dizziness, and nausea diminish or stop as therapy continues. • Postural hypotension may occur more frequently during initial therapy; arise from lying and sitting position slowly. • Avoid tasks that require mental alertness until response to the drug is established. • Hallucinations may occur in the first weeks of therapy. • Inform healthcare provider if pregnancy occurs. • Urine will change color to a bright yellow.

15.23 Skeletal Muscle Relaxants

Muscle relaxants are prescribed to relieve muscular spasms (spasticity) and pain associated with traumatic injuries and chronic debilitating disorders:

- Multiple sclerosis
- Cerebrovascular accident
- Cerebral palsy
- Spinal cord injuries

Increased stimulations from the cerebral neurons or lack of inhibition in the spinal cord or at the skeletal muscles cause hyperexcitable neurons, resulting in increased muscle tone and spasticity.

Two major groups of muscle relaxants are:

- Centrally acting: Depress neuron activity in the spinal cord or brain
- Peripherally acting: Act directly on the skeletal muscles

ANXIOLYTICS, SKELETAL MUSCLE RELAXANT, ANTICONVULSANT

Use		Half-life:	Onset: PO	Peaks: PO	Duration: PO
	Short-term relief of anxiety symptoms, preanesthetic medication, relief of acute alcohol withdrawal. Adjunct for relief of acute musculoskeletal conditions, treatment of seizures. Treatment of panic disorders, tension headache and tremors.	20–70 hours	30 minutes IM 15 minutes IV 1–5 minutes	1–2 hours; IM 30–90 minutes IV 15 minutes	2–3 hours IM 30–90 minutes IV 15–60 minutes

Example	Diazepam (Valium) Schedule IV	Route: PO IM IV	Pregnancy category: D	Pharmacokinetic: Well absorbed from GI tract; widely distributed; PB: 96%; metabolized in liver; excreted in urine

How it works
- Enhances action of neurotransmitter gamma-aminobutyric acid (GABA) neurotransmission at CNS producing anxiolytic effect. Enhances presynaptic inhibition elevating seizure threshold in response to electrical/chemical stimulation. Inhibits spinal afferent pathways, producing skeletal muscle relaxation.

Adult dose
- Anxiety/muscle relaxant: PO 2–10 mg two to four times/day; IM/IV: 2–10 mg repeat in 3–4 hours; Preanesthesia: IV: 5–15 mg 5–10 min before procedure; maximum of 10 mg. Alcohol withdrawal: PO 10 mg three to four times during first 24 hours, then reduce to 5–10 mg three to four times/day as needed; IM/IV: initially 10 mg followed by 5–10 mg q3–4 h. Status epilepticus: IV 5–10 mg q10–15 min up to 30 mg/8 h

Before administration
- Assess B/P, pulse, respirations immediately before administration.
- Assess and document pain.
- Check for immobility, stiffness, and swelling.
- Review history of seizure disorder.

Administration
- PO: Give without regard to food.
- Dilute oral concentrations with water, juice, carbonated beverages; may also be mixed in semisolid food.
- Tablets may be crushed; do not crush or break capsule.

IV administration:
- Give IV push
- Administer directly into a large vein (reduces risk of thrombosis/phlebitis); if not possible, administer into tubing of a flowing IV solution as close to the vein insertion point as possible
- Do not use small veins (e.g., wrist/dorsum of hand)
- Administer IV rate not exceeding 5 mg/min
- Monitor respirations q5–15 min for 2 hours. May produce arrhythmias when used before cardioversion.

After administration
- Patient must remain recumbent for up to 3 hours after parenteral administration to reduce hypotension.
- Monitor vital signs.
- Monitor for recurrence of seizure activity.
- Assess pain and immobility.

Contraindications
- Acute narrow-angle glaucoma, acute alcohol intoxication
- *Caution:* Impaired kidney/liver function

Side effects/ adverse reactions
- Frequent: Pain with IM injection, drowsiness, fatigue, ataxia (muscular incoordination)
- Occasional: Slurred speech, orthostatic hypotension, headache, hypoactivity, constipation, nausea, blurred vision
- Rare: Paradoxical CNS hyperactivity/nervousness in children, excitement/restlessness in elderly/debilitated (generally noted during first 2 weeks of therapy, particularly noted in presence of uncontrolled pain).
Adverse/Toxic
- IV route may produce pain, swelling thrombophlebitis, carpal tunnel syndrome.
- Abrupt or too rapid withdrawal may result in pronounced restlessness, irritability, insomnia, hand tremors, abdominal/muscle cramps, sweating, vomiting, seizures.
- Abrupt withdrawal in patients with epilepsy may produce increase in frequency and/or severity of seizures.
- Overdosage results in somnolence, confusion, diminished reflexes, coma.

Patient education
- Discomfort may occur with IM injection.
- Drowsiness usually diminishes with continued therapy.
- Smoking reduces drug effectiveness.
- Do not abruptly withdraw medication after long-term therapy.
- Strict maintenance of drug therapy is essential for seizure control.
- Avoid alcohol.

CENTRALLY ACTING MUSCLE RELAXANTS

Use	• For muscle spasms caused by multiple sclerosis and spinal cord injury	Half-life: 8 hours	Onset: 30 minutes	Peaks: 3–4 hours	Duration: 4–6 hours

- For muscle spasms and other painful musculoskeletal disorders. Available in compound form with aspirin and aspirin with codeine.
- For short-term treatment of muscle spasms; not effective for relieving cerebral or spinal cord disease.
- For acute muscle spasms; drug used for treatment of tetanus.

Example	• Baclofen (Lioresal)	Route: PO/ IM /IV	Pregnancy category: C	Pharmacokinetic: Well absorbed; PB: UK; excreted in urine

- Carisoprodol (Soma)
- Cyclobenzaprine HCl (Flexeril)
- Methocarbamol (Robaxin)

How it works   Blocks interneuronal activity

Adult dose
- Initially 5 mg TID may increase dose; maintenance 10–20 mg TID/QID; maximum dose 80 mg/day
- PO 350 mg TID hs
- PO 10 mg TID may increase dose to a maximum of 60 mg/d
- PO initially 1.5 g QID; maintenance 1 g QID; IM/IV: 0.5–1 g q8h; max 3 g/d

Before administration
- Assess drug and medical history.
- Obtain baseline vital signs.
- Assess history or muscle spasms (acute versus chronic).

Administration
- Administer with food to decrease GI upset.

After administration
- Monitor vital signs.
- Monitor serum liver enzyme levels and report if liver enzyme levels elevate.
- Monitor for CNS side effects such as dizziness.
- Maintain a safe environment to avoid injury from side effects.

Contraindications
- Severe liver or renal disease

Side effects/ adverse reactions
- Nausea/vomiting
- Dizziness
- Weakness
- Insomnia

Adverse/Toxic
- Asthmatic attack
- Tachycardia
- Hypotension
- Diplopia

Patient education
- Do not stop muscle relaxants abruptly; take over 1 week to avoid rebound spasms.
- Do not drive or operate dangerous machinery when taking muscle relaxants; sedative effect can cause drowsiness.
- Avoid alcohol and CNS depressants.
- These drugs are contraindicated during pregnancy or by lactating mothers.
- Report side effects.

DEPOLARIZING MUSCLE RELAXANTS (ADJUNCT TO ANESTHESIA)

Use	Used in surgery for relaxation of skeletal muscle; also used during endoscopy and with intubated patients	Half-life: • 2 hours • UK • 1–1.5 hours • 2–18 minutes	Onset: 5 minutes	Peak: 2 hours	Duration: 6 hours

Example	• Pancuronium bromide (Pavulon)	Route: IV/IM	Pregnancy category: C Rocuronium is B	Pharmacokinetic: • PB: 10% • UK • 60%–80% • 30%

- Succinylcholine Cl (Anectine Cl)
- Vecuronium bromide (Norcuron)
- Rocuronium bromide

How it works	• Blocks the normal neuromuscular transmission
Adult dose	• IV: 0.04–0.1 mg/kg than 0.01 mg/kg every 30–60 min • IM: 2.5–4 mg/kg; max: 150 mg; IV: 0.3–1.1 mg/kg; max: 150 mg • IV: Initially 0.08–01 mg/kg/dose; maintenance 0.05–0.1 mg/kg/h as needed
Before administration	• These are not nurse-administered medications. Except in Critical Care; they cannot be administered unless the patient is intubated or has an airway. Be sure all resuscitation equipment and medications are available.
Administration	• Give IV push or IV drip to maintain muscle paralysis. • Norcuron is given after general anesthesia has been started. • Patients who are conscious and ventilated should also receive an anxiolytic drug to reduce anxiety created by the inability to move or speak. • If necessary used eye blinking as a method of communication for the patient (blink once for yes; twice for no).
After administration	• Monitor vital signs, including ECG. • Maintain patent airway.
Side effects/ adverse reactions	• Pavulon does not cause bronchospasm or hypotension.
Patient education	• If patient is conscious and intubated, explain why he or she cannot speak or move.

PERIPHERALLY ACTING MUSCLE RELAXANT

Use	PO: Relief of signs and symptoms of spasticity because of spinal cord injuries, stroke, cerebral palsy, multiple sclerosis, especially flexor spasms; concomitant pain, clonus, and muscular rigidity; IV, Parenteral: Management of fulminant hypermetabolism of skeletal muscle because of malignant hyperthermia crisis. Treatment of neuroleptic malignant syndrome, relief induced pain in patients with muscular of exercise-dystrophy, treatment of flexor spasms	Half-life: IV: 4–8 hours PO: 8.7 hours	Onset: 1 hours	Peaks: 2 hours	Duration: 6 hours
Example	Dantrolene sodium (Dantrium)	Route: PO/IV	Pregnancy category: C	Pharmacokinetic: Poorly absorbed from GI tract; PB: 95%; metabolized in liver, excreted in urine.	

How it works	• Reduces muscle contraction by interfering with release of calcium ion, dissociating excitation-contraction coupling. Reduces calcium concentration interfering with the catabolic process, which is associated with malignant hyperthermic crisis.
Adult dose	• Spasticity: PO initially 25 mg/day; increase to 25 mg two to four times/day, then by 25 mg increments up to 100 mg 204 times/day. Prevention of malignant hyperthermia; PO 4–8 mg/kg/day in three to four divided doses 1–2 days before surgery (give last dose 3–4 hours before surgery). IV Infusion: 2.5 mg/kg about 1.25 h before surgery. • Management of hyperthermia crisis: IV: Initially 1 mg/kg (minimum) rapid infusion; may repeat up to total maximum dose of 10 mg/kg. May follow with 4–8 mg/kg/day orally in four divided doses up to 3 days after crisis.
Before administration	• PO: Give without regard to food. • IV: Store at room temperature; use within 6 hours after reconstitution. • Solution is clear, colorless. Discard if cloudy, precipitate formed; Reconstitute 20 mg vial with 60 ml of sterile water for injection to provide concentration of 0.33 mg/ml. • Obtain baseline liver function tests. • Record onset, type, location of muscular spasm. • Check for immobility, stiffness, swelling.
Administration	• IV infusion; administer over 1 h

(Continued)

(Continued from previous page)

PERIPHERALLY ACTING MUSCLE RELAXANT

After administration	• Diligently monitor IV site for signs of extravasation (high pH of IV preparation may cause severe complications). • Assist with ambulation. • Monitor liver function and blood counts periodically for those on long-term therapy. • Evaluate for therapeutic response: decreased intensity of skeletal muscle spasticity and pain.
Contraindications	• PO: Active liver disease (i.e., hepatitis, cirrhosis), when spasticity is needed to maintain upright posture and balance when walking or to achieve or support increased function • Severely impaired cardiac function • Previous liver disease/dysfunction • *Caution:* Women; those greater than 35 years of age; impaired liver or pulmonary function
Side effects/ adverse reactions	Effects are generally transient • Frequent: Drowsiness, dizziness, weakness, general malaise, diarrhea (may be severe) • Occasional: Confusion, headache, insomnia, constipation, urinary frequency • Rare: Paradoxical CNS excitement/ restlessness, paresthesia, tinnitus, slurred speech, diarrhea, nocturia, impotence Adverse/Toxic • Risk of hepatotoxicity, most notably in females, those greater than 35 years of age, those taking other medications concurrently • Overt hepatitis noted most frequently between third and twelfth month of therapy • Overdosage results in vomiting, muscular hypotonia, muscle twitching, respiratory depression, seizures
Patient education	• Drowsiness usually diminishes with continued therapy. • Avoid tasks that require alertness or motor skills until response to drug is established. • Avoid alcohol or other depressants while taking medication. • Report continued weakness, fatigue, nausea, or diarrhea, skin rash, itching, bloody/black stools.

15.24   Parkinsonism Medication

Parkinsonism (Parkinson's disease) is a chronic neurologic disorder affecting balance and motion at the extrapyramidal motor tract. Five major symptoms of Parkinsonism are:

1. Rigidity: An abnormal increase in muscle tone, resulting in postural changes (shuffling gate, the chest and head thrust forward, knees and hips flexed, walks without swinging arms)
2. Bradykinesia: Slow movement.
3. Involuntary tremors: Head and neck involuntary tremors at rest
4. Pill-rolling: Pill-rolling movement of the hands
5. Masked facies: No facial expression

TABLE 15.4 MAOIs* Can Cause a Hypertensive Crisis if Taken with These Foods

FOODS	EFFECTS
Cheese (cheddar, Swiss, blue)	Sweating, tremors
Bananas, raisins	Bounding heart rate
Pickled foods	Increased blood pressure
Red wine, beer	Increased temperature
Cream, yogurts	
Chocolate, coffee	
Italian green beans	
Liver	
Yeast	
Soy sauce	

* Avoid taking barbiturates, tricyclic antidepressants, antihistamines, central nervous system depressants, and OTC cold medications with MAOIs.

Parkinsonism is treated with four medications. These are:

1. Dopaminergics: Decrease the symptoms by enabling an increase of levodopa at nerve terminals where levodopa is transformed into dopamine. Increased dopamine reduces tremors.
2. Dopamine agonists: Stimulate dopamine receptors, reducing signs and symptoms of Parkinsonism.
3. MAO-B inhibitor: Inhibit the catabolic enzymes that break down dopamine, resulting in extending the dopamine effects. MAO-B inhibitors cause a hypertensive crisis if taken with foods shown in Table 15.4.
4. Anticholinergics: (see 15.22 Antiparkinsonism-Anticholinergic Medication)

DOPAMINERGICS

Use	Antiparkinsonism	Half-life: 1–2 hours	Onset: 15 minutes	Peaks: 1–3 hours	Duration: 5–12 hours
Example	Carbidopa-Levodopa (Sinemet)	Route: PO	Pregnancy category: C	Pharmacokinetic: Carbidopa: Rapidly and completely absorbed from GI tract. Widely distributed; excreted primarily in urine. Levodopa: converted to dopamine; excreted in urine.	

How it works
- Converted to dopamine in basal ganglia. Increases dopamine concentration in brain, inhibiting hyperactive cholinergic activity, reducing tremor. Carbidopa prevents peripheral breakdown of levodopa, allowing more levodopa to be available for transport into brain.

Adult dose
- Not receiving levodopa: 25/100 mg tablets three times/day or 10/100 mg tablets three to four times/day. May increase by 1 tablet q1–2 days up to 8 tablets/day
- Sustained-release: 1 tablet two times/day no closer than 6 hours between doses; range of two to eight tablets at 4- to 8-hour intervals. May increase dose at intervals of not less than 3 days.
- Receiving only levodopa: Less than 1500 mg levodopa/day: 1 tablet (25/100 mg) three to four times/day; greater than 1500 mg levodopa/day; 1 tablet (25/250 mg) three to four times/day
- Sustained-release: 1 tablet two times/day
- Receiving carbidopa/levodopa: Provide about 10% more levodopa; may increase up to 30% more at 4- to 8-hour dosing intervals

Before administration
- Receiving only levodopa: Discontinue levodopa at least 8 hours before carbidopa/levodopa
- Have patient void before taking medication to reduce risk of urinary retention.

Administration
- Scored tablets may be crushed. Do not crush sustained-release tablets; may cut in half.
- May be given without regard to meals. However, administer with low-protein foods. High-protein diets interfere with drug transport to the CNS.

After administration
- Be alert to neurologic effects: Headache, lethargy, mental confusion, agitation.
- Monitor for evidence of dyskinesia (difficulty with movement). Assess for clinical reversal of symptoms (improvement of tremor of head/hands at rest, masklike facial expression, shuffling gait, muscular rigidity).
- Monitor VS and ECG. Orthostatic hypotension may occur during the early use of levodopa and bromocriptine.

Contraindications
- Narrow-angle glaucoma, those of MAO inhibitor therapy
- *Caution:* History of MI, bronchial asthma, emphysema, severe cardiac, pulmonary, renal, hepatic, endocrine disease; active peptic ulcer, treated open-angle glaucoma

Side effects/ adverse reactions
- Frequent: Uncontrolled body movements (including face, tongue, arms, upper body), nausea and vomiting, anorexia
- Occasional: Depression, anxiety, confusion, nervousness, difficulty urinating, irregular heartbeats, dizziness, lightheadedness, decreased appetite, blurred vision, constipation, dry mouth, flushed skin, headache, insomnia, diarrhea, unusual tiredness, darkening of urine
- Rare: Hypertension, ulcer, hemolytic anemia (tiredness/weakness)
  Adverse/Toxic
- High incidence of involuntary choreiform, dystonic, dyskinetic movements may be noted in patients on long-term therapy. Mental changes (paranoid ideation, psychotic episodes, depression) may be noted. Numerous mild to severe CNS, psychiatric disturbances may include reduced attention span, anxiety, nightmares, daytime somnolence, euphoria, fatigue, paranoia, hallucination.

(Continued)

(Continued from previous page)

DOPAMINERGICS

Patient education	• Do not abruptly discontinue the medication. Rebound parkinsonism can occur. • Urine may be discolored and will darken with exposure to air. • Perspiration also may be dark. This is a harmless side effect but clothes may be stained. • Avoid tasks that require alertness until response to drug is established. • Avoid alcoholic beverages. • Sugarless gum, sips of tepid water may relieve dry mouth. • Take with low-protein food to minimize GI symptoms. • Report uncontrolled movement of face, eyelids, mouth, tongue, extremities, mental changes, palpitations, severe or continuing nausea/vomiting, and difficulty in urinating.

DOPAMINE AGONISTS

Use	• Prevention and treatment of respiratory tract infections because of influenza virus, Parkinson's disease, drug-induced extrapyramidal reactions. Treatment of fatigue associated with multiple sclerosis, AHDH. • Treatment of hyperprolactinemia conditions (amenorrhea with or without galactorrhea, prolactin-secreting adenomas, infertility). Treatment of Parkinson's disease, acromegaly. Treatment of neuroleptic malignant syndrome, cocaine addiction, hyperprolactemia associated with pituitary adenomas. • Adjunctive treatment with levodopa/carbidopa in Parkinson's disease.	Half-life: • 11–15 hours • 15 hours • UK	Onset: Growth hormone reduction: 1–2 hours Prolactin reduction: 2 hours	Peaks: Growth hormone: 1.5–8 hours Prolactin reduction: 8 hours	Duration: Growth hormone: 4–5 hours Prolactin reduction: 24 hours
Example	• Amantadine HCl (Symmetrel) • Bromocriptine (Parlodel) • Pergolide mesylate (Permax)	Route: All PO drugs	Pregnancy category: • C • C • B	Pharmacokinetic: Rapidly absorbed in GI tract; PB: 67%; excreted in urine; Minimal absorption in GI tract; PB: 90%–96%; excreted in feces; Well absorbed from GI tract. PB: 90%; remetabolized in liver; excreted in urine.	

How it works	• Antiviral action against influenza A virus believed to prevent uncoating of virus, penetration of host cells, release of nucleic acid into host cells. • Antiparkinsonism because of increased release of dopamine. Virustatic. • Activated at postsynaptic dopamine receptors. Directly inhibits prolactin secretion, reduces elevated growth hormone concentration, suppresses galactorrhea and reinitiates the ovulatory menstrual cycle. • Inhibits prolactin secretion; directly stimulates postsynaptic dopamine receptors, assisting in reduction in tremor, improvement in akinesia (absence of movement), posture and equilibrium disorders, and rigidity of parkinsonism
Adult dose	• Viral: 200 mg/day (give as single or in two divided doses) • Parkinson's: 100 mg two times/day; may increase up to 200 mg/day in divided doses • Hyperprolactinemia: Initially, 1.25–2.5 mg/day; may increase by 2.5 mg/day at 3- to 7-day intervals; Range: 2.5–15 mg/day
Before administration	• Symmetrel: May be given without regard to food; administer nighttime dose several hours before bedtime (prevents insomnia) • Parlodel: Patient should be lying down before administering first dose; give after food intake (decreases incidence of nausea); obtain pregnancy test if given for infertility • Permax: Scored tablets may be crushed; give without regard to meals

Administration	• Administer with meals to prevent GI disturbances.
After administration	• Assist with ambulation if dizziness is noted after administration. • Assess for therapeutic response. • Monitor for constipation. • Monitor I and O. • Check for peripheral edema. • Evaluate food tolerance. • Assess skin for rash and blotching. • Assess for clinical response.
Contraindications	• None significant. *Caution:* History of seizures, orthostatic hypotension, CHF, peripheral edema, liver disease, recurrent eczematoid dermatitis, cerebrovascular disease, renal dysfunction, those receiving CNS stimulation • Pregnancy, peripheral vascular disease, severe ischemic heart disease, uncontrolled hypertension, hypersensitivity to ergot alkaloids. *Caution:* Impaired hepatic/cardiac function, hypertension, psychiatric disorders. • None significant. *Caution:* Cardiac dysrhythmias.
Side effects/ adverse reactions	• Frequent: Nausea, dizziness, poor concentration, insomnia, nervousness • Occasional: Orthostatic hypotension, anorexia, headache, livedo reticularis (reddish blue, netlike blotching of skin), blurred vision, urinary retention, dry mouth/nose • Rare: Vomiting depression, irritation/swelling of eyes, rash. Incidence of side effects is high, especially at beginning of therapy or with high dosage • Frequent: Nausea, headache, dizziness; Occasional: fatigue, lightheadedness, vomiting abdominal cramps, diarrhea, constipation, nasal congestion, drowsiness, dry mouth • Rare: Muscle cramping urinary hesitancy • Frequent: Nausea, dizziness, hallucinations, constipation, rhinitis, dystonia (impaired muscle tone), confusion, somnolence • Occasional: Postural hypotension, insomnia, dry mouth, peripheral edema, anxiety, diarrhea, dyspepsia, abdominal pain, headache, abnormal vision, anorexia, tremor, depression, rash • Rare: Urinary frequency, vivid dreams, neck pain, hypotension, vomiting Adverse/Toxic • CHF, leucopenia, neutropenia, occur rarely. Hyperexcitability, convulsions, ventricular arrhythmias may occur. • Visual or auditory hallucinations noted in Parkinsonism syndrome. Long-term, high-dose therapy may produce continuing runny nose, fainting, GI hemorrhage, peptic ulcer, severe abdominal/stomach pain. • Overdose may require supportive measures to maintain arterial B/P (monitor cardiac function, vital signs, blood gases, serum electrolytes). Activated charcoal may be more effective than emesis or lavage.
Patient education	• Continue therapy for full length of treatment. • Doses should be evenly spaced. • Do not take any other medications (prescribed, OTC, or herbal) without consulting healthcare provider. • Avoid alcoholic beverages. • Do not drive or engage in activities that require mental acuity if experiencing dizziness or blurred vision. • Get up slowly from a sitting or lying position. • Report all side effects. • Take nighttime dose several hours before bedtime to prevent insomnia. • If taking Parlodel, use other than oral forms of birth control during treatment.

MAOB INHIBITOR

Use	Adjunctive to levodopa/carbidopa in treatment of Parkinson's disease	Half-life: 16–69 hours	Onset: 1 hour	Peaks: 2.5 hours	Duration: 12 hours
Example	Selegiline HCl (Eldepryl)	Route: PO	Pregnancy category: C	Pharmacokinetic: Rapidly absorbed from GI tract; crosses blood–brain barrier; metabolized in liver and excreted in urine.	

How it works	• Irreversibly inhibits monoamine oxidase type B activity. Increases dopaminergic action, assisting in reduction in tremor, akinesia (absence of sense of movement), posture and equilibrium disorders, rigidity of parkinsonism
Adult dose	• 10 mg/d in two divided doses (5 mg at breakfast and lunch)
Before administration	• Give before meals.
Administration	• None significant
After administration	• Be alert to neurologic effects. • Monitor for evidence of dyskinesia (difficulty with movement). • Assess for clinical reversal of symptoms.
Contraindications	• None significant • *Caution:* History of peptic ulcer disease, dementia, psychosis, tardive dyskinesia, profound tremor, cardiac dysrhythmias
Side effects/ adverse reactions	• Frequent: Nausea, dizziness, lightheadedness, faintness, abdominal discomfort • Occasional: Confusion, hallucinations, dry mouth, vivid dreams, dyskinesia (impairment of voluntary movement). • Rare: Headache, generalized aches, anxiety, diarrhea, insomnia Adverse/Toxic • Overdose may vary from CNS depression (sedation, apnea, cardiovascular collapse, death) to severe paradoxical reason (hallucinations, tremor, seizures); impaired motor coordination (loss of balance of, blepharospasm [blinking]; facial grimace, feeling of heavy leg/stiff neck, involuntary movements), hallucinations, confusion, depression, nightmares, delusions, overstimulation, sleep disturbance, anger occurs in some patients.
Patient education	• Rise slowly from sitting or lying position (tolerance will develop during therapy). • Avoid tasks that require alertness until response to drug is established. • Dry mouth, drowsiness, dizziness may be expected side effects. • Avoid alcoholic beverages during therapy. • Coffee/tea and other caffeinated beverages may help reduce drowsiness.

15.25 Myasthenia Gravis

Myasthenia gravis is a disease in which nerve impulses do not reach the nerves in muscle endings (myoneural junction); it is caused by inadequate secretion or loss of acetylcholine resulting from action of acetylcholinesterase, an enzyme that destroys acetylcholine at the myoneural junction.

Myasthenia gravis signs and symptoms are:

- Fatigue
- Weak respiratory muscles, leading to respiratory paralysis and respiratory arrest
- Weak facial muscles

- Weak extremities
- Ptosis (drooping eyelids)
- Difficulty in chewing

Myasthenia gravis is treated with acetylcholinesterase (AChE inhibitors):

- Ambenonium (Mytelase)
- Edrophonium Cl (Tensilon)
- Neostigmine bromide (Prostigmin)
- Pyridostigmine bromide (Mestinon)

15.26   Multiple Sclerosis

Multiple sclerosis (MS) is an autoimmune disease that results in the absence of myelin sheath around some nerve fiber, enabling impediment of transmission of nerve impulses. Multiple sclerosis is relapsing-remitting as patients might experience no symptoms and other times experience debilitating symptoms.

Multiple sclerosis is treated symptomatically using:

- Corticosteroids: Treat periods of exacerbations known as attacks, relapses and flare-ups
- Interferon-ß: Interferon-ß–1B (Betaseron.) and interferon-ß–1a (Avonex) reduce the frequency and severity of relapses
- Copaxone (glatiramer acetate injection): Reduces new brain lesions and the frequency of relapses

15.27   Alzheimer's Disease

Alzheimer's disease (dementia) affects the ability to carry out daily activities, caused by impairment of portions of the brain that control thought, memory and language. The cause of Alzheimer's disease is unknown.

Medications that provide relief to patients in the early and middle stages of Alzheimer's disease are:

- Tacrine (Cognex), donepezil (Aricept), rivastigmine (Exelon), and galantamine (Reminyl): Temporarily limit the progression of some symptoms
- Memantine (Namenda): Treats moderate to severe cases
- Tranquilizers, mood elevators, sedatives: Control behavior (sleeplessness, agitation, wandering, anxiety, and depression)

15.28   Muscle Spasms

Muscle spasms are caused by hyperexcitable neurons stimulated by cerebral neurons or from lack of inhibition of the stimulus in the spinal cord or at the skeletal muscles. Muscle spasms are treated with muscle relaxants. There are two groups of muscle relaxants.

Centrally Acting Muscle Relaxants

Centrally acting muscle relaxants depress neuron activity in the spinal cord or in the brain and are used to treat acute spasms from muscle trauma. Centrally acting muscle relaxants decrease pain, increase range of motion, and have a sedative effect. These are not taken concurrently with central nervous system depressants (barbiturates, narcotics, alcohol). Commonly used centrally acting muscle relaxants are:

- Carisoprodol (Soma) (for muscle trauma)
- Cyclobenzaprine (Flexeril) (for muscle trauma)
- Methocarbamol (Robaxin) (for muscle trauma)
- Diazepam (Valium) (for chronic neurologic disorders and muscle trauma)
- Baclofen (Lioresal) (for chronic neurologic disorders and muscle trauma)

Peripherally Acting Muscle Relaxants

Peripherally acting muscle relaxants are primarily use for chronic neurologic disorders because they depress neuron activity at the skeletal muscles and have a minimal effect on the central nervous system. Commonly prescribed peripherally acting muscle relaxants is:

- Dantrolene sodium (Dantrium)

15.29   Epilepsy

Epilepsy is when abnormal electric discharges from the cerebral neurons result in a loss or disturbance of consciousness and convulsion (seizure).
   Seizures are defined as:

- Tonic-clonic (grand mal): Occurs in three phases:
  - Feels a sense of strong déjà vu, lightheadedness and/or dizziness, unusual, altered vision and hearing
  - Tonic: Falls unconscious, muscles tense up, extremities are pulled toward or rigidly pushed away from the body
  - Clonic: Muscles contract and relax, causing convulsions
- Absence (petit mal): Person stares with or without jerking eye movements
- Psychomotor: Clouding consciousness and amnesia affecting multiple sensory, motor, and/or psychic components

Epilepsy is treated by using anticonvulsant medication. These include:

- Hydantoins (phenytoin, mephenytoin, ethotoin): Treat tonic-clonic and psychomotor seizures
- Barbiturates (Phenobarbital, mephobarbital, primidone): Treat grand mal and acute episodes or status epilepticus, meningitis, toxic rations, and eclampsia
- Succinimides (ethosuximide): Treat absence seizures
- Oxazolidine (trimethadione): Treats absence seizures
- Benzodiazepines (diazepam, clonazepam): Treat absence seizures
- Carbamazepine: Treats tonic-clonic and psychomotor seizures
- Valproate (valproic acid): Treats absence and tonic-clonic seizures

Functions of anticonvulsant medication:

- Suppresses sodium influx by binding to the sodium channel, prolonging the sodium channel's inactivation, and preventing neurons from firing
- Suppresses calcium influx, preventing stimulation of the T-calcium channel
- Increases the action of the GABA, inhibiting neurotransmitters and resulting in suppression seizure activity.

BARBITURATES

Use	Management of generalized tonic-clonic (grand mal) seizures, partial seizures, control of acute convulsive episodes (status epilepticus, eclampsia, febrile seizures). Relieves anxiety, provides preop sedation. Prophylaxis/treatment of hyperbilirubinemia	Half-life: 50–140 hours	Onset: PO 20–60 minutes IM 10–15 minutes IV 5 minutes	Peaks: PO, IM, IV 30 minutes	Duration: PO, IM 4–6 hours IV 4–6 hours
Example	Phenobarbital (Luminal) Schedule IV	Route: PO/IM/IV	Pregnancy category: D	Pharmacokinetic: Well-absorbed after PO, parenteral administration. PB: 35%–50%; Rapidly, widely distributed; metabolized in liver; excreted in urine	

How it works
- Decreases motor activity to electrical/chemical stimulation; producing anticonvulsant effect. CNS depressant effect produces all levels from mild sedation, hypnosis to deep coma.

Adult dose
- Status epilepticus: IV; 15–18 mg/kg; max: 30 mg/kg.
- Maintenance: 1–3 mg/kg/d; 100–300 mg/d
- Therapeutic serum range 15–40 mcg/ml

Before administration
- Assess vital signs immediately before administration.
- Hypnotic: Raise side rails to provide environment conducive to sleep (back rub, quiet environment, low lighting).
- Seizures: Review history of seizure disorder (length, presence of auras, LOC).
- Initiate seizure precautions as per agency policy.

Administration
- Give PO without regard to meals.
- Tablets may be crushed.
- Elixir may be mixed with water, milk, or fruit juice.
- IM do not inject more than 5 ml in any one IM injection site (produces tissue irritation).
- Inject IM. Keep into gluteus maximus or lateral aspect of thigh.
- IV may give undiluted or may dilute with NaCl, D5W, lactated Ringer's

After administration
- Assess elderly, debilitated, and children for evidence of paradoxical reaction—particularly during early therapy.
- Evaluate for therapeutic response.
- Monitor for therapeutic serum levels (10–30 mcg/ml; toxic level is greater than 40 mcg/ml).

Contraindications
- History of porphyria, bronchopneumonia
- *Extreme Caution:* Nephritis, renal insufficiency
  Caution: Uncontrolled pain (may produce paradoxical reaction), impaired liver function)

Side effects/ adverse reactions
- Occasional: Somnolence
- Rare: Confusion, paradoxical CNS hyperactivity/nervousness in children, excitement/restlessness in elderly (generally noted during first 2 weeks of therapy, particularly noted in presence of uncontrolled pain)
  Adverse/side
- Abrupt withdrawal after prolonged therapy may produce effects ranging from markedly increased dreaming, nightmares and/or insomnia, tremor, sweating, and vomiting to hallucinations, delirium, seizures, and status epilepticus.
- Skin eruptions appear as hypersensitivity reaction.
- Blood dyscrasias, liver disease, and hypocalcemia occur rarely.
- Overdosage produces cold, clammy skin, hypothermia, severe CNS depression, cyanosis, rapid pulse, Cheyne-Stokes respirations. Toxicity may result in severe renal impairment.

Patient education
- Drowsiness may gradually decrease/disappear with continued use.
- Do not abruptly withdraw medication following long-term use (may precipitate seizures).
- Avoid tasks that require alertness and motor skills until response to drug is established.
- Tolerance/dependence may occur with prolonged use of high doses.
- Strict maintenance of drug therapy is essential for seizure control.

BENZODIAZEPINES (ANXIOLYTICS)

Use	For petit mal, myoclonus akinetic seizures and treatment of panic disorder. Adjunct treatment of seizures, treatment of simple/complex partial seizures, tonic-clonic seizures.	Half-life: 18–50 hours	Onset: 1 hour	Peaks: 4 hours	Duration: 24 hours
Example	Clonazepam (Klonopin)	Route: PO	Pregnancy category: C	Pharmacokinetic: Well-absorbed from GI tract, PB: 85%; metabolized in liver, excreted in urine.	

How it works	• Elevates seizure threshold in response to electrical/chemical stimulation by enhancing presynaptic inhibition in CNS, suppressing seizure activity.
Adult dose	• 1.5 mg daily. Dosage may be increased in 0.5–1 mg increments at 3 day intervals until seizures are controlled. Do not exceed maintenance dose of 20 mg daily. Panic disorder: Initially 0.25 mg two times/day. Increase up to target dose of 1 mg/day after 3 days.
Before administration	• Give without regard to meals. • Tablets may be crushed.
Administration	• Review history of seizure disorder. • Implement safety measures.
After administration	• Observe frequently for recurrence of seizure activity. • When replacement by another anticonvulsant is necessary; decrease clonazepam gradually as therapy begins with low replacement dose. • On long-term therapy liver/renal function tests, CBC should be performed periodically. • Assist with ambulation if drowsiness and ataxia occur. • Evaluate for therapeutic response.
Contraindications	• Significant liver disease, narrow-angle glaucoma • *Caution:* Impaired kidney/liver function, chronic respiratory disease
Side effects/ adverse reactions	• Frequent: Mild transient drowsiness, ataxia, behavioral disturbances (especially in children) manifested as aggression, irritability, agitation • Occasional: Rash, ankle/facial edema, nocturia, dysuria, change in appetite/weight, dry mouth, sore gums, nausea, blurred vision • Rare: Paradoxical reaction (hyperactivity/nervousness in children, excitement/restlessness in elderly; particularly noted in presence of uncontrolled pain) Adverse/Toxic • Abrupt withdrawal may result in pronounced restlessness, irritability, insomnia, hand tremors, abdominal/muscle cramps, sweating, vomiting, and status epilepticus. • Overdosage results in somnolence, confusion, diminished reflexes, and coma.
Patient education	• Drowsiness may gradually decrease/disappear with continued use. • Do not abruptly withdraw medication after long-term use (may precipitate seizures). • Avoid tasks that require alertness and motor skills until response to drug is established. • Strict maintenance of drug therapy is essential for seizure control. • Avoid alcohol.

15.30 Antipsychotics

Psychosis is characterized by:

• Difficulty processing information
• Difficulty reaching a conclusion
• Delusions
• Hallucinations

- Incoherence
- Catatonia
- Aggressive and/or violent behavior

Psychosis is caused by a dopamine (neurotransmitter) imbalance in the brain. Antipsychotic medications (dopamine antagonists) block the D_2 dopamine receptors, reducing the psychotic symptoms. Some antipsychotic medications block the chemoreceptor trigger zone and vomiting (emetic) center, producing an antiemetic effect. Blocking dopamine causes the side effects of Parkinsonism (see 15.24 Parkinsonism Medication). Psychosis is treated with antipsychotic medications. Categories of antipsychotic are:

- Typical: Typical antipsychotic medications are subdivided:
  - Blocks norepinephrine, causing sedative and hypotensive effects. Prescribed early in the treatment for psychosis
  - Nonphenothiazines: Blocks the dopamine receptor sites and causes similar effects as phenothiazines
- Atypical: Prescribed if the patient does not respond to typical antipsychotic medication

15.31 Phenothiazines

There are three groups of phenothiazines and each have different side effects (Table 15.5). These are:

1. Aliphatic: Decreases blood pressure, strong sedate effect, and moderate extrapyramidal symptoms
2. Piperazine: Produces low sedative effect, strong antiemetic effect, and increases extrapyramidal symptoms
3. Piperidine: Decreases blood pressure, minimum extrapyramidal symptoms, and minimum antiemetic effect

TABLE 15.5 The Effects of Categories of Phenothiazines

GROUP	SEDATION	HYPOTENSION	EPS	ANTIEMETIC
Aliphatic (chlorpromazine	+++	+++	++	++
and triflupromazine)				+++
Piperazine	++	+	+++	+++
Piperidine	+++	+++	+	−
Nonphenothiazines				
Haloperidol	+	+	+++	++
Loxapine	++	++	+++	−
Molindone	+/++	+	+++	−
Thiothixene	+	+	+++	−
Atypical antipsychotics				
Risperidone	+	+	+/0	−

−, No effect; + mild effect; ++ moderate effect; +++ severe effect.

PHENOTHIAZINE (ALIPHATIC)

Use	Management of psychotic disorders, manic phase of manic-depressive illness, severe nausea or vomiting, preop sedation, severe behavioral disturbances in children. Relief of intractable hiccups, acute intermittent porphyria. Treatment of choreiform movement of Huntington's disease.	Half-life: 8–30 hours	Onset: PO 30–60 minutes PO: SR: 30–60 minutes PR: 1–2 hours IM 15–20 minutes IV 5–10 minutes	Peaks: PO: 2–4 hours PO: SR: 2–4 hours PR: 3 hours IM: 30 minutes IV: 10 minutes	Duration: PO: 4–6 hours PO SR: 10–12 hours; PR: 3–4 hours IM 4–8 hours IV UK
Example	Chlorpromazine (Thorazine)	Route: PO/ PO-SR/PR/ IM/IV	Pregnancy category: C	Pharmacokinetic: Absorption varies; PB: 95%; metabolized in liver; excreted in urine.	

How it works
- Blocks dopamine neurotransmission at postsynaptic dopamine receptor sites. Possesses strong anticholinergic sedative, antiemetic effects, moderate extrapyramidal effects, slights antihistamine action. Reduces psychosis, relieves nausea and vomiting, controls intractable hiccups and porphyria.

Adult dose
- Psychosis: IM/IV initially 25 mg, may repeat in 1–4 hours. May gradually increase to 400 mg q4–6 h; maximum 300–800 mg/day. PO: 30–800 mg/day in 1–4 divided doses.
- Nausea and vomiting: IM/IV 25–50 mg q4–6 h; PO 10–25 mg q4–6 h; Rectal: 50–100 mg q6–8 h
- Hiccups: PO 25–50 mg three times/day. May give IM/IV.

Before administration
- Obtain baseline vital signs.
- Obtain medical and drug history.
- Assess mental status, cardiac, eye, and respiratory disorders before start of therapy.
- Assess for dehydration if using as antiemetic.

Administration
- Avoid skin contact with liquid concentrates to prevent contacting dermatitis.
- Liquids must be protected from light and should be diluted with fruit juice.
- Administer oral doses with food or milk to decrease gastric irritation.
- Remain with patient while taking oral medications to avoid them hiding the drug.
- Administer IM deep into muscle because drug is irritating to fatty tissue. Do not inject into subcutaneous tissue.
- Do not mix in same syringe as heparin, pentobarbital, cimetidine, or dimenhydrinate.
- Chill suppository in refrigerator for 30 min before removing foil wrapper.

After administration
- Monitor blood pressure for hypotension.
- Assess for extrapyramidal symptoms.
- Monitor WBC, differential count for blood dyscrasias.
- Monitor for fine tongue movement (may be early sign of tardive dyskinesia).
- Place on suicide precautions if necessary.
- Monitor for symptoms of neuroleptic malignant syndrome (NMS): increased fever, pulse, and blood pressure, muscle rigidity, increased creatine phosphokinase, and WBC count; altered mental status, acute renal failure, varying levels of consciousness; pallor; diaphoresis, tachycardia, and dysrhythmias.
- Monitor urine output. Urinary retention may occur.
- Monitor serum glucose level.
- Assess for therapeutic response. Blood serum level 50–300 mcg/ml; toxic greater than 750.

Contraindications
- Severe CNS depression, comatose states, severe cardiovascular disease, bone marrow depression, and subcortical brain damage
- *Caution:* Impaired respiratory/hepatic/renal/cardiac function, alcohol withdrawal, history of seizures, urinary retention, glaucoma, prostatic hypertrophy, and hypocalcemia (increases susceptibility to dystonias)

Side effects/ adverse reactions
- Frequent: Drowsiness, blurred vision, hypotension, defective color vision, difficulty in night vision, dizziness, decreased sweating, constipation, dry mouth, nasal congestion
- Occasional: Difficulty urinating, increased skin sensitivity to sun, skin rash, decreased sexual ability, swelling or pain in breasts, weight gain, nausea, vomiting, stomach pain, tremors

Adverse/Toxic
- Extrapyramidal symptoms appear dose related (particularly high dose): divided into three categories: akathisia, parkinsonian symptoms, and acute dystonias. Acute dystonias symptoms are torticollis (neck muscle spasm), opisthotonos (rigidity of back muscles), and oculogyric crisis (rolling back of eyes). Dystonic reaction may also produce profuse sweating, pallor. Tardive dyskinesia occurs rarely and may be irreversible.
- Abrupt withdrawal after long-term therapy may precipitate nausea, vomiting, gastritis, dizziness, and tremors.
- Blood dyscrasias: Particularly agranulocytosis; mild leucopenia may occur. May lower seizure threshold.

Patient education	<ul><li>Take drug exactly as ordered.</li><li>May take up to 6 weeks or longer to achieve full clinical effect.</li><li>Do not consume alcohol or other CNS depressants such as narcotics.</li><li>Do not abruptly discontinue the drug.</li><li>Read labels on OTC and herbal preparations. Some are contraindicated when taking antipsychotics.</li><li>Advise healthcare provider if you smoke. The dose may need to be adjusted as smoking increases metabolism of some antipsychotics.</li><li>Maintain good oral hygiene by frequent brushing and flossing.</li><li>Effects of antipsychotics on the fetus are unknown; discuss family planning with healthcare provider.</li><li>Drug passes into breast milk which could cause drowsiness and unusual muscle movement in a baby.</li><li>Maintain routine follow-up appointments with healthcare provider.</li><li>Obtain laboratory tests as scheduled.</li><li>Be alert to symptoms of malaise, fever, and sore throat which may be an indication of agranulocytosis, a serious blood dyscrasia. Report this promptly to healthcare provider.</li><li>Wear an identification bracelet indicating medication taken.</li><li>Tolerance to sedative effect develops over a period of days or weeks.</li><li>Avoid potentially dangerous situations such as driving until drug dose has been stabilized.</li><li>Be aware of EPS and report them immediately to provider.</li><li>Avoid direct sunlight or use a sun block and protective clothing. Sunbathing can cause a skin rash.</li><li>Avoid arising from a lying or sitting position quickly as orthostatic hypotension can occur.</li><li>Urine may be pink or red-brown; this is harmless.</li><li>Changes may occur related to sexual functioning and menstruation. Women may experience irregular periods or amenorrhea. Men might experience impotence and gynecomastia (enlargement of breast tissue).</li><li>Lozenges or hard candy may help mouth dryness. If dry mouth persists for more than 2 weeks, advise provider.</li><li>Avoid extremes in temperatures and increased exercise.</li></ul>

NONPHENOTHIAZINE

Use	Management of psychotic disorders, control of tics, vocal utterances in Tourette's syndrome. Used in management of severe behavioral problems in children, short-term treatment of hyperactivity in children; treatment of infantile autism, Huntington's chorea, nausea/vomiting associated with cancer therapy.	Half-life: PO 12–37 hours IM 17–25 hours IV 10–19 hours	Onset: PO: Erratic IM: 15–30 minutes IM: Decanoate UK	Peaks: PO 2–6 hours IM: 30–45 minutes IM: Decanoate 6–7 days	Duration: PO: 24–72 hours IM: 4–8 hours IM: Decanoate 3–4 weeks
Example	Haloperidol (Haldol)		Route: PO/IM/IV	Pregnancy category: C	Pharmacokinetic: PB: 80%–90%; readily absorbed from GI tract; extensively metabolized in liver, excreted in urine; not removed by hemodialysis
How it works	<ul><li>Competitively blocks postsynaptic dopamine receptors, interrupts impulse movement, and increases turnover of brain dopamine, producing a tranquilizing effect. Strong extrapyramidal, antiemetic effects, weak anticholinergic, sedative effects</li></ul>				

Adult dose	• PO: 0.5–5 mg two to three times/day. Maximum 100 mg/day • IM (lactate): 2–5 mg q4–8 h as needed • IM (decanoate): 10–15 times stabilized oral dose given at 3–4 wk intervals • IV: Only lactate is given IV; IV push at rate of 5 mg/min.; infuse piggy back over 30 min; up to 25 mg/h has been used titrated to patient response
Before administration	• Obtain baseline vital signs. • Obtain medical and drug history. • Assess mental status, cardiac, eye, and respiratory disorders before start of therapy.
Administration	• PO: Give without regard to meals. • PO: Scored tablets may be crushed. • Prepare Decanoate IM injection with 21-gauge needle; do not exceed maximum volume of 3 ml per IM site; inject slowly, deep IM into upper outer of gluteus maximus • IV may given undiluted; flush with at least 2 ml 0.9% NaCl before and after administration; may add to 30–50 ml most solutions (D5W preferred)
After administration	• IM: Patient must remain recumbent for 30–60 min in head-low position with legs raised to minimize hypotensive effect. • Monitor blood pressure for hypotension. • Assess for extrapyramidal symptoms. • Monitor WBC and differential count for blood dyscrasias. • Monitor for fine tongue movement (may be an early sign of tardive dyskinesia). • Place on suicide precautions if necessary.
Contraindications	• Coma, alcohol ingestion, Parkinson's disease, thyrotoxicosis • *Caution:* Impaired respiratory/hepatic/cardiovascular function, alcohol withdrawal, history of seizures, urinary retention, glaucoma, prostatic hypertrophy, elderly persons
Side effects/ adverse reactions	• Frequent: Blurred vision, constipation, orthostatic hypotension, dry mouth, swelling or soreness of female breasts, peripheral edema • Occasional: Allergic reaction, difficulty urinating, decreased thirst, dizziness, decreased sexual ability, drowsiness, nausea, vomiting, photosensitivity, lethargy 　Adverse/Toxic • Extrapyramidal symptoms appear to be dose related and may be noted in first few days of therapy. Marked drowsiness and lethargy, excessive salivation, fixed stare may be mild to severe in intensity. Less frequently seen are severe akathisia and acute dystonias. Tardive dyskinesia may occur with long-term therapy and is more common in female geriatric patients. This may be irreversible. Abrupt withdrawal after long-term therapy may provoke signs of transient dyskinesia. • Toxic blood serum level greater than 1 mcg/ml
Patient education	• Take drug exactly as ordered. • May take up to 6 weeks or longer to achieve full clinical effect. • Do not consume alcohol or other CNS depressants such as narcotics. • Do not abruptly discontinue the drug. • Read labels on OTC and herbal preparations. Some are contraindicated when taking antipsychotics. • Advise healthcare provider if you smoke. The dose may need to be adjusted as smoking increases metabolism of some antipsychotics. • Maintain good oral hygiene by frequent brushing and flossing. • Effects of antipsychotics on the fetus are unknown; discuss family planning with healthc are provider. • Drug passes into breast milk which could cause drowsiness and unusual muscle movement in a baby. • Maintain routine follow-up appointments with healthcare provider. • Obtain laboratory tests as scheduled. • Wear an ID bracelet indicating medication taken. • Tolerance to sedative effect develops over a period of days or weeks. • Avoid potentially dangerous situations such as driving until drug dose has been stabilized. • Be aware of EPS and report them immediately to provider. • Avoid direct sunlight or use a sun block and protective clothing. Sun bathing can cause a skin rash. • Avoid arising from a lying or sitting position quickly as orthostatic hypotension can occur.

15.32　Anxiolytics

Anxiolytics treat anxiety and insomnia by providing a sedative-hypnotic effect, few side effects, and no risk of the overdose that is common to traditional sedative medications. Anxiolytics are prescribed when the patient is unable to perform activities of daily life.

There are two types of anxiety:

- Primary anxiety: Caused by a situation and not a medical condition or use of medication. Anxiolytics are prescribed for primary anxiety.
- Secondary anxiety: Caused by a medical condition or use of medication. Anxiolytics are not prescribed for secondary anxiety. The cause of the anxiety is treated.

The major group of anxiolytics is Benzodiazepines. Benzodiazepines treat severe prolonged anxiety, convulsions, hypertension, and preoperative medication. Benzodiazepines include:

- Chlordiazepoxide (Librium)
- Diazepam (Valium)
- Clorazepate dipotassium (Tranxene)
- Oxazepam (Serax)
- Lorazepam (Ativan)
- Alprazolam (Xanax)
- Lorazepam (Ativan)

15.33　Antidepressants

Depression is characterized by mood changes and loss of interest in normal activities that might result in insomnia, fatigue, a feeling of despair and an inability to concentrate. It can also lead to suicidal thoughts. Depression is caused by insufficient monoamine neurotransmitter (norepinephrine and serotonin), genetic predisposition, or environmental factors.

Three types of depression are:

1. *Reactive (exogenous)*: Caused by an event resulting in rapid onset that last for months; treated with benzodiazepine
2. *Major (unipolar)*: Caused by insufficient monoamine neurotransmitter (norepinephrine and serotonin), genetic predisposition, or environmental factors resulting in the patient unable to perform activities of daily life; treated with benzodiazepine.
3. *Bipolar Affective (manic-depressive)*: Results in mood swings from manic to depressive; treated with lithium.

Antidepressants have side effects (Table 15.6) that might mask suicidal tendencies.

Antidepressants are organized into three groups:

1. Tricyclics: Prescribed to treat major depression. More effective than SSRs. These include:
   a. Clomipramine HCl (Anafranil)
   b. Desipramine HCK (Norpramin, Pertofrane)
   c. Doxepin HCl (Sinequan)
   d. Imipramine HCl (Tofranil)

    e. Nortriptyline HCl (Aventyl)

    f. Protriptyline HCl (Vivactil)

    g. Trimipramine maleate (Surmontil)

2. Second-generation antidepressants: Have fewer side effects than tricyclic and do not cause hypotension, sedation, anticholinergic effects, or cardiotoxicity. Types of second-generation antidepressants are:

    a. Serotonin reuptake inhibitors (SSRI): fluoxetine HCl (Prozac), paroxetine HCl (Paxil), sertraline HCl (Zoloft), fluvoxamine (Luvox)

    b. Atypical: amoxapine (Asendin), bupropion HCl (Wellbutrin), maprotiline HCl (Ludiomil), nefazodone HCl (Serzone), trazodone HCl (Desyrel)

3. Monoamine oxidase inhibitors (MAOI): Neurotransmitters norepinephrine, dopamine, epinephrine, and serotonin are inactive by the enzyme monoamine oxidase. MAOI inhibits monoamine oxidase, resulting in a rise in the levels of these neurotransmitters. MAOI are isocarboxazid (Marplan), phenelzine sulfate (Nardil), and tranylcypromine sulfate (Parnate).

TRICYCLIC ANTIDEPRESSANT

Use	Treatment of various forms of depression, exhibited as persistent, prominent dysphoria (occurring nearly every day for at least 2 weeks) manifested by four of eight symptoms: appetite change, sleep pattern change, increased fatigue, impaired concentration, feelings of guilt or worthlessness, loss of interest in usually activities, psychomotor agitation or retardation, suicidal tendencies. Relieves neuropathic pain (e.g., diabetic neuropathy, postherpetic neuralgia, treatment of bulimia nervosa)	Half-life: 10–50 hours	Onset: 1–3 weeks	Peaks: 2–6 weeks	Duration: UK
Example	Amitriptyline HCl (Elavil)	Route: PO/IM	Pregnancy category: D	Pharmacokinetic: Rapid, well absorbed from GI tract. PB: 90%. Metabolized in liver, excreted in urine; minimal removal by hemodialysis	

How it works
- Blocks reuptake of neurotransmitters (norepinephrine, serotonin) at presynaptic membranes, increasing synaptic concentration at post-synaptic receptor sites, resulting in antidepressant effect; has strong anticholinergic activity

Adult dose
- PO: Initially 25 mg two to four times/day, adjust as needed; maximum: Outpatient 150 mg; inpatient 300 mg
- IM: 20–30 mg four times/day

Before administration
- Assess baseline vitals and weight for future comparisons.
- Check liver and renal function by assessing urine output (greater than 600 ml/d) BUN and creatinine and liver enzyme levels.
- Obtain a history of episodes of depression; assess mental status and suicidal tendencies.
- Obtain medical and drug history.
- Assess for tardive dyskinesia and neuroleptic malignant syndrome (NMS).

Administration
- PO: Give with food or milk if GI distress occurs.
- Give IM only if oral administration is not feasible. Give deep IM slowly.

After administration
- Monitor vital signs.
- Monitor mood, appearance, behavior, speech, level of interest, and activity.

- Monitor therapeutic drug levels (120–250 ng/ml) toxic greater than 500 ng/ml.
- Maintain safe environment; use suicide precautions if necessary.
- Monitor renal/liver function laboratory values.
- Check weight two to three times/week.
- If patient is on anticonvulsant, observe for seizures; dose may need to be increased.

Contraindications	• Acute recovery period following MI, within 14 days of MAOI ingestion • *Caution:* Prostatic hypertrophy, history of urinary retention or obstruction, glaucoma, diabetes mellitus, history of seizures, hyperthyroidism, cardiac/hepatic/renal disease, schizophrenia, increased intraocular pressure, hiatal hernia
Side effects/ adverse reactions	• Frequent: Dizziness, drowsiness, dry mouth, orthostatic hypotension, headache, increased appetite/weight changes, nausea, unusual tiredness, unpleasant taste • Occasional: Blurred vision, confusion, constipation, hallucinations, delayed micturition, eye pain, arrhythmias, fine muscle tremors, Parkinsonian syndrome, nervousness, diarrhea, increased sweating, heartburn, insomnia • Rare: Hypersensitivity, alopecia, tinnitus, breast enlargement Adverse/Toxic • High dosage may produce confusion, seizures, severe drowsiness, fast/slow/irregular heartbeat, fever, hallucinations, agitation, shortness of breath, vomiting, unusual tiredness/weakness. Abrupt withdrawal from prolonged therapy may produce headache, malaise, nausea, vomiting, vivid dreams. Rarely, blood dyscrasias and cholestatic jaundice noted.
Patient education	• Take medication as ordered. Compliance is important. • Full effectiveness may not be evident until 1 to 2 weeks. • Keep all medical appointments. • Avoid alcohol or any other CNS depressants. • Do not drive or be involved in potentially dangerous mechanical activity until response to drug is established. • Do not abruptly stop taking drug; gradually withdraw under medical supervision. • Use birth control because of possible teratogenic effects on fetus. • Take with food if GI distress occurs. • Take at bedtime to avoid sedative effect. • Monitor side effects and report to healthcare provider if persistent. • Sensitivity to sun may occur. • Change position slowly to avoid postural hypotension; tolerance to this should occur early in therapy.

TABLE 15.6 Side Effects of Antidepressants

CATEGORY	ANTICHOL-INERGIC EFFECT	SEDATION	HYPOTEN-SION	GI DISTRESS	CARDIO-TOXICITY	SEIZURES	INSOMNIA/ AGITATION
Tricyclic Antidepressants							
Amitriptyline (Elavil)	++++	++++	+++	−	++++	+++	−
Clomipramine (Anafranil)	++++	++++	++	−	++++	++	−
Desipramine (Norpramin)	+	++	++	−	++	++	+
Doxepin (Sinequan)	+++	++++	++	−	++	++	−
Imipramine (Tofranil)	+++	+++	+++	+	++++	++	+
Nortriptyline (Aventyl)	+	+++	+	−	+++	++	−
Protriptyline (Vivactil)	+++	+	++	−	+++	++	+
Trimipramine (Surmontil)	+++	++++	+++	−	++++	++	−
Selective Serotonin Reuptake Inhibitors							
Fluoxetine (Prozac)	−	+	−	+++	−	0/+	++
Fluvoxamine (Luvox)	−	++	−	+++	−	−	++

(Continued)

(Continued from previous page)

CATEGORY	ANTICHOL-INERGIC EFFECT	SEDATION	HYPOTEN-SION	GI DISTRESS	CARDIO-TOXICITY	SEIZURES	INSOMNIA/AGITATION
Paroxetine (Paxil)	−	+	−	+++	−	−	++
Sertraline (Zoloft)	−	+	−	+++	−	−	++
Atypical (Heterocyclic) Antide pressants							
Amoxapine (Asendin)	+++	++	+	−	+	+++	++
Bupropion (Wellbutrin)	++	−	0/+	+	+	++++	++
Nefazodone (Serzone)	+	++	+	+	0/+	−	−
Trazodone (Desyrel)	−	+++	++	+	+	+	−
Maprotiline (Ludiomil)	+++	+++	+	−	++	++	−
Monoamine Oxidase Inhibitors	+	+	++	+	−	−	++

Solved Problems

Central Nervous System

15.1   What are amphetamines?

Amphetamines stimulate the cerebral cortex of the brain. Amphetamines are also taken to decrease weight and increase energy, enabling the quick performance of work without rest.

15.2   What are anorexiants?

Anorexiants inhibit appetite by stimulating the cerebral cortex and the hypothalamus. Anorexiants can produce psychological dependence. A patient can build a tolerance to the therapeutic effect of anorexiants. Discontinuing anorexiants abruptly may result in withdrawal symptoms.

15.3   How do analeptics work?

Analeptics stimulate the release of neurotransmitters, norepinephrine, and dopamine from the brain and from the peripheral nerve terminals of the sympathetic nervous system, resulting in euphoria and increased alertness. Patients can experience sleeplessness, restlessness, tremors, irritability, and cardiovascular problems (increased heart rate, palpitations, dysrhythmias, and hypertension).

15.4   What are sedative-hypnotics?

Central nervous system depressants are medications that suppress the transmission of information throughout the central nervous system.

15.5   What are CNS depressants?

Sedative-hypnotics, the mildest form of central nervous system depressant, are given in low doses to diminish physical and mental responses without affecting consciousness. Short-acting sedative-hypnotics are prescribed to help the patient fall asleep, allowing the patient to awaken early without a lingering after effect. Intermediate-acting sedative-hypnotics are used for sustaining sleep and cause residual drowsiness after waking.

15.6   What are nonpharmacological methods that promote sleep?

- Arise at the same hour in the morning.
- No daytime naps.
- No heavy meals or strenuous exercise before bed.

- Relax before bed (warm bath, read, listen to music, drink warm milk).
- No loud noises.
- Do not watch disturbing television before bed.
- Do not drinking a lot of fluids before bed.

15.7   What are barbiturates?

Barbiturates are a type of sedative-hypnotic used to induce sleep and as an anesthetic. In high doses barbiturates control epileptic seizures. Barbiturates are Class II controlled substances prescribed for no more than 2 weeks because of adverse side effect such as CNS depression in elderly persons.

Anesthesia

15.8   What are general anesthetic agents?

General anesthetic agents depress the central nervous system, causing a loss of consciousness and a relief of pain.

15.9   When is a patient given a sedative-hypnotic for surgery?

A sedative-hypnotic is administered the night before surgery to assist with sleep. An hour before the surgery, premedications are administered to sedate and decrease anxiety.

15.10   What are the four stages of anesthesia?

The four stages of anesthesia are analgesia, excitement, surgical anesthesia, and medullary paralysis.

15.11   What stage of anesthesia is not reached by the patient?

The stage of anesthesia not reached by the patient is medullary paralysis. The respiratory center (medulla oblongata) becomes paralyzed. Breathing and vital functions cease. Death occurs. However, the anesthetist adjusts the general anesthetic to prevent the patient from reaching this stage.

15.12   What is spinal anesthesia?

Spinal anesthesia is a local anesthetic injected into the spinal column to produce a regional neural block.

15.13   What are side effects of spinal anesthesia?

Headaches and hypotension are common side effects of spinal anesthesia because of changes in cerebrospinal fluid pressure caused by the injection.

15.14   How are side effects of spinal anesthesia minimized?

Side effects are reduced by reaming in the supine position and increasing fluids.

Autonomic Nervous System

15.15   How do cholinergic medications work?

Cholinergic (parasympathomimetics) medications mimic acetylcholine. They initiate a response and inhibit the effect of acetylcholine.

15.16   What are adrenergics?

Adrenergics are medications that stimulate alpha$_1$-receptors and beta$_2$-adrenergic receptors. Alpha$_1$-receptors are in the smooth muscles of vascular (vessel) tissues. Beta$_2$-adrenergic receptors are in smooth muscles of lungs, arterioles of skeletal muscles, and the uterine muscle. Adrenergics also increase blood flow by stimulating the dopaminergic receptor located in the renal, mesenteric, coronary, and cerebral arteries to dilate. Dopamine is the only adrenergic that can activate this receptor.

15.17 How do adrenergic blockers inactive receptors?

Adrenergic blockers inactive receptors by promoting the reuptake of the transmitter back to the neuron and degrading transmitters by enzymes, making the transmitters unable to attach to a receptor. Adrenergic blockers also diffuse transmitters away from receptors.

15.18 What are mixed-acting sympathomimetics?

Mixed-acting sympathomimetics simulate the adrenergic receptor sites and stimulate the release of norepinephrine from terminal nerve endings

15.19 What are anticholinergics?

Anticholinergics mimics acetylcholine (parasympathetic neurotransmitter). Anticholinergics inhibit acetylcholine by occupying the acetylcholine receptors, blocking parasympathetic nerve enabling impulses from sympathetic nerves to take control.

Parkinsonism

15.20 What are dopaminergics?

Dopaminergics decrease symptoms by enabling an increase of levodopa at nerve terminals where levodopa is transformed into dopamine. Increased dopamine reduces tremors.

15.21 What are dopamine agonists?

Dopamine agonists stimulate dopamine receptors, reducing the signs and symptoms of parkinsonism.

15.22 What are MAOB inhibitors?

MAOB inhibitors inhibit the catabolic enzymes that break down dopamine, resulting in extending the dopamine effects.

Muscle Spasms

15.23 What are centrally acting muscle relaxants?

Centrally acting muscle relaxants depress neuron activity in the spinal cord or in the brain and are used to treat acute spasms from muscle trauma. Centrally acting muscle relaxants decrease pain, increase range of motion, and have a sedative effect.

15.24 What are peripherally acting muscle relaxants?

Peripherally acting muscle relaxants are primarily used for chronic neurologic disorders because they depress neuron activity at the skeletal muscles and have a minimal effect on the central nervous system.

Antipsychotics

15.25 What medication is used to treat severe, prolonged anxiety?

The medication used to treat severe, prolonged anxiety is benzodiazepines.

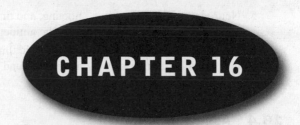

CHAPTER 16

Narcotic Agonists

16.1   Pain

There are two components of pain:

- Physical: Occurs when nerve endings are stimulated. An impulse is sent to the brain and a pain response is transmitted.
- Psychological: An emotional response based on the pain threshold. The pain threshold is the level of nerve ending stimulation that causes the feeling of unbearable pain.

16.2   The Gate Control Theory

The gate control theory describes pain transmission. The gate mechanism that alters the transmission of painful sensations from peripheral nerve fiber to the thalamus and cortex of the brain is located in the dorsal horn of the spinal cord. The thalamus and cortex of the brain are where the body recognizes painful sensations as pain.

Transmission of painful sensations flows through the gate mechanism. Large-diameter, low-threshold afferent fibers close the gate. Large-diameter fibers are stimulated when the patient feels slower-acting painful stimuli. The gate is then closed, preventing transmission of the painful stimuli. Small-diameter, high-threshold afferent fibers open the gate. The brain also closes the gate by descending control inhibition.

16.3   Defining Pain

Pain is whatever the patient says it is and is described as intensity, duration, frequency, and type of pain. There are six ways to classify pain. These are:

1. Acute Pain: A sudden uncomfortable sensation that subsides with treatment; treated with nonsteroidal anti-inflammatory drugs (NSAIDs) or opioid analgesics
2. Chronic Pain: Recurring pain for 6 months or more; treated with combinations of NSAIDs, opioid analgesics, antianxiety, and medications to reduce swelling
3. Visceral Pain: Dull and aching pain resulting from stimulation of nerve endings in smooth muscle or sympathetically innervated organs; is difficult to locate; treated with opioid analgesics
4. Somatic Pain: Aching, throbbing pain of skeletal muscles, fascia, ligaments, vessels, and joints; treated with NSAIDs

5. Neuropathic Pain: Burning, shooting, and tingling pain resulting from injury to a peripheral nerve; treated with anticonvulsants, tricyclic antidepressants, and opioid analgesics

6. Psychogenic Pain: Caused by psychiatric illness or psychosocial stimuli (anxiety, depression, and fear); treated temporarily by medication and requires psychotherapy to relieve the pain

16.4 Assessing Pain

A pain scale is used to assess the intensity of pain by asking a patient to report pain based on the pain scale. There are three commonly used pain scales:

- Zero to 10: Zero is free from pain and 10 is severe pain.
- Face Rating Scale: Cartoon faces show various expression of pain. A smile face is free from pain and a grimacing face is severe pain.
- Color Scale. The color scale ranges from blue to red. Blue is freedom from pain. Red is severe pain.

Pain is also assessed by:

- Onset
- Duration
- Frequency
- What started the pain
- What relieves the pain

16.5 Pain Management Treatment Plans

A pain management treatment plan describes pharmacological and nonpharmacological treatments for managing chronic pain. The patient is asked to track pain using a pain diary. A pain diary is kept by patients who are in chronic pain to help develop a pain management treatment plan. The patient enters into the diary:

- Time the pain starts
- What starts the pain
- Description of the pain
- What relieves the pain
- How you responded to the pain

16.6 Nonpharmacological Management of Pain

Nonpharmacological management of pain includes:

- Massage
- Imagery
- Music
- Distraction
- Humor
- Acupuncture
- Hypnosis
- Herbal therapies
- Therapeutic touch

- Transcutaneous electro-nerve stimulation
- Surgical interventions

16.7 Pharmacologic Management of Pain

Pain is managed pharmacologically by administering nonnarcotic analgesics, NSAIDs, narcotic analgesics, and salicylates.

Nonnarcotic analgesics treat mild to moderate pain such as headaches, menstrual pain (dysmenorrheal), inflammatory pain, muscular aches, and abrasions. Nonnarcotic analgesics include acetaminophen and NSAIDs (see chapter 12). Nonnarcotic analgesics are not addictive and available over the counter.

NON-NARCOTIC ANALGESICS

Use	Relief of mild to moderate pain, fever	Half-life: 1–4 hours	Onset: 15–30 minutes	Peaks: 1–1.5 hours	Duration: 4–6 hours
Example	Acetaminophen Fixed combinations: With barbital, a sedative-hypnotic; with caffeine, a stimulant (Fioricet); with codeine, a narcotic analgesic (Tylenol with Codeine); with hydrocodone, a narcotic analgesic (Vicodin); with oxycodone, a narcotic analgesic (Percocet); with propoxyphene, an analgesic (Darvocet); with tramadol, an analgesic (Ultracet).	Route: PO/rectal	Pregnancy category: B	Pharmacokinetic: Rapidly, completely absorbed from the gastrointestinal (GI) tract, rectal absorption variable. Widely distributed to most body tissues. Metabolized in liver; excreted in urine. Removed by hemodialysis. PB: 20%–50%; crosses the placenta and is found in breast milk.	

How it works	• Exact mechanism unknown, but appears to inhibit prostaglandin synthesis in central nervous system (CNS) and, to a lesser extent by blocking pain impulse through peripheral action, resulting in analgesia. Acts centrally on hypothalamic heat-regulating center, producing peripheral vasodilation (skin erythema, sweating, heat loss), resulting in antipyresis.
Adult dose	• By mouth (PO). 325–650 mg q4–6 h or 1 g three to four times/day; maximum 4 g/day • Rectal: 650 mg q4–6 h; maximum six doses 24/h
Before administration	• Assess for analgesia, assess onset, type, location, and duration of pain • Fixed combination: Obtain vital signs. If respirations are less than 12/min, withhold medication • Assess temperature if given for antipyresis 10–30 mcg/ml; toxic serum level: greater than 200 mcg/ml
Administration	• Give without regard to meals. • Tablets may be crushed. • Rectal: Moisten suppository with cold water before inserting well up into rectum.
After administration	• Assess for clinical improvement of pain. • Assess for reduced body temperature. • Therapeutic blood serum level
Contraindications	• Hypersensitivity to acetaminophen • *Caution:* Impaired hepatic function or anemia
Side effects/ adverse reactions	• Well tolerated • Rare: Hypersensitivity reaction Adverse/Toxic: • Early signs of acetaminophen toxicity: anorexia, nausea, diaphoresis, generalized weakness within first 12–24 h. Later signs of toxicity; vomiting, right upper quadrant tenderness, elevated liver function tests within 48–72 hours after ingestion. Antidote: Acetylcysteine (N-acetylcysteine) Mucomyst.

Patient education	• If used for more than 3 days for fever consult health care provider • Severe/recurrent pain or high/continuous fever may indicate serious illness • Not drug of choice for acute injuries because it has no anti-inflammatory properties

16.8 Narcotic Analgesics

Narcotic analgesics (narcotic agonists) such as opioids act on the central nervous system to treat moderate and severe pain, suppress respiration and coughing by acting on the respiratory and cough centers in the medulla of the brain stem. All narcotic analgesics relieve pain. All except meperidine (Demerol) are also antitussive (cough suppression) and antidiarrheal.

NARCOTIC AGONIST-OPIATE ANALGESIC

Use	Relief of severe, acute, chronic pain, preop sedation, anesthesia supplement, analgesia during labor. Drug of choice for pain due to myocardial infarction, dyspnea from pulmonary edema not resulting from chemical respiratory irritant.	Half-life: 2.5–3 h	Onset: PO: variable PO SR: SC/IM: 5–30 minutes IV: rapid Rectal: 20–60 min Epidural: 15–60 min Intrathecal: 15–60 min	Peaks: PO: 1–2 hours PO SR: 1–2 h SC: 50–90 minutes IM: 0.5–1 h IV: 20 minutes Rectal/ Epidural/ Intrathecal	Duration: PO: 4–5 hours; PO SR: 8–12 h IM: 3–7 h IV: 4–5 hours Rectal: 4–5 h Epidural 16–24 h Intrathecal 16–24 h
Example	Morphine sulfate (Astramorph, Duramorph) Schedule II	Route: PO/SC/ IM/IV Rectal/ Epidural/ Intrathecal	Pregnancy category: B	Pharmacokinetic: variably absorbed from GI tract; readily absorbed after SC and IM administration; PB: 20%–35%; widely distributed, metabolized in liver; excreted in urine; removed by hemodialysis	

How it works	• Binds with opioid receptors within CNS, altering processes affecting pain perception, emotional response to pain. Decreases intestinal motility by local and central actions.
Adult dose	• Pain: PO 10–30 mg q4h as needed; SR: 15–30 mg q8–12 h PRN • IV/IM/SC: 2.5–20 mg/dose q2–6h; IV continuous infusion: 0.8–10 mg/h • Range: up to 80 m/h • Epidural: Initially, 5 mg; may give 1–2 mg in 1 h if no relief; maximum 20 mg/24h • Intrathecal: 1/10 epidural dose; 0.2–1 mg/dose • PCA: Loading dose 5–0 mg; intermittent bolus 0.5–3 mg; Lockout interval: 5–12 min; Continuous infusion: 1–10 mg/hr (4-h limit): 20–30 mg
Before administration	• Obtain medical and drug history. • Assess vital signs. • Assess pain using a pain scale; assess onset, type, location, and duration of pain. • Assess urinary output. Morphine can cause urinary retention. • Administer before pain reaches its peak to maximize the effectiveness of the drug. • Patient should be in recumbent position before administering by parenteral route. • If patient will receive opioids on a regular base, obtain orders for stool softeners before beginning therapy. • Have naloxone (Narcan) available as an antidote if opioid overdose occurs. • Provide a safe environment.
Administration	• Give by IM injection if repeated dose is necessary (repeated SC may produce local tissue irritation, induration). May also be given by slow IV injection or IV infusion.

- PO mix liquid form with fruit juice to improve taste. Do not crush or break extended-release capsule.
- SC/IM administer slowly, rotating injection sites; patients with circulatory impairment experience higher risk of overdosage because of delayed absorption of repeated administration.
- Always administer very slowly over 4–5 minutes. Rapid IV increases risk of severe adverse reaction.
- If suppository is too soft, chill for 30 min in refrigerator or run cold water over foil wrapper; moisten with cold water before inserting well up into rectum.
- If respirations are less than 12, drug may need to be withheld; notify healthcare provider.

After administration	• Monitor vital signs 5–10 minutes after IV administration; 15–30 minutes after SC or IM. Be alert for decreased respirations and hypotension.
	• Check for adequate urine output. Palpate bladder if output is decreased to determine if retention has occurred.
	• Monitor stools. Avoid constipation.
	• Initiate deep breathing and coughing exercises.
	• Assess pain regularly. Notify provider if relief is not adequate (4 or less on a scale of 0–10).
	• Check for pupil changes and reaction. Pinpoint pupils can indicate opioid overdose.
Contraindications	• Postoperative biliary tract surgery; surgical anastomosis
	• Extreme caution: CNS depression, anoxia, hypercapnia, respiratory depression, seizures, acute alcoholism, shock, untreated myxedema, respiratory dysfunction
	• *Caution:* Toxic psychoses, increased intracranial pressure, impaired hepatic function, acute abdominal conditions, hypothyroidism, prostatic hypertrophy, Addison's disease, urethral stricture, COPD
Side effects/ adverse reactions	*Note:* Effects dependent on dosage amount, route of administration. Ambulatory patients (those not in severe pain) may experience dizziness, nausea, vomiting, and hypotension more frequently than those in supine position or who have severe pain.
	• Frequent: Sedation, decreased B/P, increased sweating, flushed face, constipation, dizziness, drowsiness, nausea, vomiting
	• Occasional: Allergic reaction (rash, itching,) difficulty breathing, confusion, pounding heartbeat, tremors, decreased urination, stomach cramps, vision changes, dry mouth, headache, decreased appetite, pain/burning at injection site
	• Rare: Paralytic ileus
	Adverse/Toxic
	• Overdosage results in respiratory depression, skeletal muscle flaccidity, cold clammy skin, cyanosis, extreme somnolence progressing to convulsions, stupor, coma. Tolerance to analgesic effect, physical dependence may occur with repeated use. Prolonged duration of action, cumulative effect may occur in those with impaired hepatic and renal function.
Patient education	• Do not take alcohol or CNS depressants with narcotic analgesics. Respiratory depression can occur.
	• Avoid constipating foods such as eggs and cheese.
	• Take stool softeners as ordered.
	• Try nonpharmacological measures to relieve pain as an adjunct to drug; i.e., imagery, relaxation techniques, music, and humor
	• Report dizziness or difficulty in breathing.
	• Do not drive or operate machinery while taking opioids. Do not make major decisions.
	• Opioids are addicting. Tolerance and dependence may occur with prolonged use of high doses.
	• Instruct patient/family to use a pain scale and a pain diary if necessary.
	• Maintain a safe environment while taking opioids.

OPIOID AGONIST

Use	Relief of mild to moderately severe pain	Half-life: 2–3 hours	Onset: 10–15 minutes	Peaks: 30–60 minutes	Duration: 3–6 hours
Example	Oxycodone (OxyContin); Schedule II Fixed combinations: With acetaminophen; a	Route: PO	Pregnancy category: B	Pharmacokinetic: Moderately absorbed	

(Continued)

(Continued from previous page)

OPIOID AGONIST

	nonnarcotic analgesic (Percocet); with aspirin (Percodan)	from GI tract. PB: 38%–45%; widely distributed; metabolized in liver; excreted in urine; unknown if removed by hemodialysis

How it works	• Binds with opioid receptors within CNS, altering processes affecting pain, perception, and emotional response to pain
Adult dose	• Initially 10 mg q12 h; may increase q1–2 days by 25%–50%. Usual 40 mg/day; cancer pain 100 mg/day
Before administration	• Obtain medical and drug history. • Assess vital signs. • Assess pain using a pain scale; assess onset, type, location, and duration of pain. • Administer before pain reaches its peak to maximize the effectiveness of the drug. • If patient will receive opioids on a regular basis, obtain orders for stool softeners before beginning therapy. • Provide a safe environment.
Administration	• May give without regard to meals. • Tablets may be crushed. • Controlled-release: Swallow whole. Do not crush, break, or chew.
After administration	• Assess vital signs. • Assess for pain relief (4 or less on 0–10 scale).
Contraindications	• None significant • *Extreme Caution:* CNS depression, anoxia, hypercapnia, respiratory depression, seizures, acute alcoholism, shock, untreated myxedema, respiratory dysfunction • *Caution:* Increased intracranial pressure, impaired hepatic function, acute abdominal conditions, hypothyroidism, prostatic hypertrophy, Addison's disease, urethral stricture, COPD
Side effects/ adverse reactions	*Note:* Effects are dose dependent; ambulatory patients and those not in severe pain may experience dizziness, nausea, vomiting, and hypotension more frequently than those in supine position or having severe pain. • Frequent: Drowsiness, dizziness, hypotension, anorexia • Occasional: Confusion, diaphoresis, facial flushing, urinary retention, constipation, dry mouth, nausea, vomiting, headache • Rare: Allergic reaction, depression, paradoxical CNS hyperactivity/nervousness in children, excitement/restlessness in elderly/debilitated patients Adverse/Toxic • Overdose results in respiratory depression; skeletal muscle flaccidity; cold, clammy skin; cyanosis; extreme somnolence progressing to convulsions, stupor, coma. Hepatotoxicity may occur with overdosage of acetaminophen component. Tolerance to analgesic effect with physical dependence may occur with repeated use.
Patient education	• Do not take alcohol or CNS depressants with narcotic analgesics. Respiratory depression can occur. • Avoid constipating foods such as eggs and cheese. • Take stool softeners as ordered. • Try nonpharmacological measures to relieve pain as an adjunct to drug such as imagery, relaxation techniques, music, and humor. • Report dizziness or difficulty in breathing. • Do not drive or operate machinery while taking opioids; do not make major decisions. • Opioids are addicting. Tolerance and dependence may occur with prolonged use of high doses.

- Instruct patient/family to use a pain scale and a pain diary if necessary.
- Maintain a safe environment while taking opioids.

OTHER NARCOTIC ANALGESICS OF THE OPIUM AND SYNTHETIC GROUP

Drug	Purpose
Codeine (sulfate, phosphate), CSS II	For mile to moderate pain
Hydromorphone HCl (Dilaudid) CSS II	For severe pain
Levorphanol tartrate (Levo-Dromoran) CSS II	For moderate to severe pain
Meperidine (Demerol) Synthetic narcotic CSS II	For moderate pain
Fentanyl (Duragesic, Sublimaze) CSS II	Short-acting potent—used with short-term surgery; patches for controlling chronic pain
Sufentanil (Duragesic, Sublimaze) CSS II	Short-acting potent—used as part of balanced anesthesia
Methadone (Dolophine)	Similar to morphine, but longer duration of action; used in drug abuse programs

16.9 Narcotic Agonist-Antagonists

Narcotic agonist-antagonists are medications that have both agonist and antagonist effects on the opioid receptors, making them less potent and have a lower dependency potential than opioids. Withdrawal symptoms from narcotic agonist-antagonists are not as severe as with narcotic agonists (narcotic analgesics).

Commonly prescribed narcotic agonist-antagonists are:

- Pentazocine (Talwin)
- Butorphanol tartrate (Stadol)
- Diprenorphine (Buprenex)
- Nalbuphine hydrochloride (Nubain)

16.10 Narcotic Antagonists

Narcotic antagonists are antidotes for narcotic analgesics and have a higher affinity to the opiate receptor site than the narcotic analgesic, resulting in blocking the narcotic analgesic from binding to the opiate receptor site. Narcotic antagonists are prescribed to reverse an overdose of narcotic analgesics. Reverse narcotic analgesics cause respiratory and CNS depression.

Naloxone (Narcan) is a narcotic agonist and is prescribed to reverse the effects of narcotic analgesics. Naloxone (Narcan) is also used to determine if a patient's unconsciousness is caused by an overdose of narcotic analgesics. If the patient regains consciousness after administering Naloxone (Narcan) IV, then it can be assumed that the patient's unconsciousness is caused by an overdose of narcotic analgesics

NARCOTIC AGONIST-ANTAGONISTS

Use	Management of pain (including postop pain). Nasal: Migraine headache pain. Parenteral: Preop, preanesthetic medication, supplement balanced anesthesia, relief of pain during labor.	Half-life: 2.5–4 hours	Onset: IM 10–30 minutes IV less than 1 minute Nasal 15 minutes	Peaks: IM 30–60 minutes IV 30 minutes Nasal 1–2 hours	Duration: IM 3–4 hours IV 2–4 hours Nasal 4–5 hours

(Continued)

(Continued from previous page)

NARCOTIC AGONIST-ANTAGONISTS

Example	Butorphanol tartrate (Buprenex)	Route: IM/IV/nasal	Pregnancy category: B	Pharmacokinetic: Rapidly absorbed from IM injection; PB: 60%; extensively metabolized in liver; excreted in urine.

How it works
- Binds at opiate receptor sites in CNS. Reduces intensity of pain stimuli incoming from sensory nerve endings, altering pain perception and emotional response to pain

Adult dose
- Analgesia: IM: 1–4 mg q3–4 h as needed; IV 0.5–2 mg q3–4 h as needed; nasal 1 mg (one spray in one nostril); may repeat in 60–90 min. May repeat two-dose sequence q3–4 h as needed. Alternatively, 2 mg (one spray each nostril if pt remains recumbent) may repeat in 3–4 h

Before administration
- Obtain medical and drug history.
- Assess vital signs.
- Assess pain using a pain scale; assess onset, type, location, and duration of pain.
- Assess urinary output. Morphine can cause urinary retention.
- Administer before pain reaches its peak to maximize the effectiveness of the drug.
- Patient should be in recumbent position before administering by parenteral route.
- If patient will receive opioids on a regular basis, obtain orders for stool softeners before beginning therapy.
- Have naloxone (Narcan) available as an antidote if opioid overdose occurs.
- Provide a safe environment.

Administration
- If respirations less than 12/min withhold medication and notify healthcare provider
- May given undiluted. Administer over 3–5 minutes.
- Intranasal: Instruct patient to blow nose to clear nasal passages as much as possible; tilt head slightly forward and insert spray tip into nostril, pointing toward nasal passages, away from nasal septum. Spray into nostril while holding other nostril closed and concurrently inspire through nose to permit medication as high into nasal passages as possible.

After administration
- Monitor vital signs 5–10 minutes after IV administration. Be alert for decreased respirations and hypotension.
- Check for adequate urine output. Palpate bladder if output is decreased to determine if retention has occurred.
- Monitor stools. Avoid constipation.
- Initiate deep breathing and coughing exercises.
- Assess pain regularly. Notify provider if relief is not adequate (4 or less on a scale of 0–10).
- Check for pupil changes and reaction. Pinpoint pupils can indicate opioid overdose.

Contraindications
- CNS disease that affects respirations, pulmonary disease, preexisting respiratory depression, physical dependence on other opioid analgesics
- *Caution:* Impaired hepatic/renal function, elderly persons, debilitated, head injury, hypertension, before biliary tract surgery (produces spasm of sphincter of Oddi), MI with nausea and vomiting

Side effects/ adverse reactions
- Frequent: Parenteral: drowsiness, dizziness. Nasal: nasal congestion, insomnia
- Occasional: Parenteral confusion, sweating/clammy skin, lethargy, headache, nausea, vomiting, dry mouth. Nasal: vasodilation, constipation, unpleasant taste, dyspnea, epistaxis, nasal irritation, upper respiratory infection, tinnitus
- Rare: Parenteral: Hypotension, pruritus, blurred vision, sensation of heat, CNS stimulation, insomnia. Nasal: hypertension, tremor, ear pain, paresthesia, depression, sinusitis

Adverse/Toxic
- Abrupt withdrawal after prolonged use may produce symptoms of narcotic withdrawal (abdominal cramping, rhinorrhea, lacrimation, anxiety, increased temperature, piloerection [goose bumps]).
- Overdosage results in severe respiratory depression, skeletal muscle flaccidity, cyanosis, extreme somnolence progressing to convulsions, stupor, coma.
- Tolerance to analgesic effect and physical dependence may occur with chronic use. If taking MAO inhibitors may produce a severe, fatal reaction.

Patient education
- Do not take alcohol or CNS depressants with narcotic analgesics. Respiratory depression can occur.
- Avoid constipating foods such as eggs and cheese.
- Take stool softeners as ordered.
- Try nonpharmacological measures to relieve pain as an adjunct to drug such as imagery, relaxation techniques, music, and humor.
- Report dizziness or difficulty in breathing.
- Do not drive or operate machinery while taking opioids; do not make major decisions.
- Opioids are addicting; tolerance and dependence may occur with prolonged use of high doses.
- Instruct patient/family to use a pain scale and a pain diary if necessary.
- Maintain a safe environment while taking opioids.

Solved Problems

Pain

16.1 What are the two components of pain?

The two components of pain are physical and psychological.

16.2 What is the psychological component of pain?

The psychological component is an emotional response based on the pain threshold. The pain threshold is the level of nerve ending stimulation that causes the feeling of unbearable pain.

16.3 What is the gate control theory?

The gate control theory describes pain transmission. The gate mechanism that alters the transmission of painful sensations from peripheral nerve fiber to the thalamus and cortex of the brain is located in the dorsal horn of the spinal cord. The thalamus and cortex of the brain is where painful sensations are recognized as pain.

16.4 What are the six ways to classify pain?

The six ways to classify pain are acute, chronic, visceral, somatic, neuropathic, and psychogenic.

16.5 What is somatic pain?

Somatic pain is the aching, throbbing pain of skeletal muscles, fascia, ligaments, vessels, and joints.

16.6 What is psychogenic pain?

Psychogenic pain is caused by psychiatric illness or psychosocial stimuli (anxiety, depression, and fear).

16.7 What is visceral pain?

Visceral pain is dull and aching pain resulting from stimulation of nerve endings in smooth muscle or sympathetically innervated organs. Visceral pain is difficult locate.

16.8 How is psychogenic pain treated?

Psychogenic pain is treated temporarily by medication and requires psychotherapy to relieve the pain.

16.9 How is chronic pain treated?

Chronic pain is treated with combinations of NSAIDs, opioid analgesics, antianxiety, and medications to reduce swelling.

16.10 Name three types of pain scales.

Three types of pain scales are 0–10, face rating scale, and color scale.

16.11 What is a pain management treatment plan?

A pain management treatment plan describes pharmacological and nonpharmacological treatments for managing chronic pain.

16.12　What is a pain diary?

A pain diary is kept by patients who are in chronic pain to help develop a pain management treatment plan. The patient enters into the daily time pain starts, what starts the pain, description of the pain, what relieves the pain, and how the patient responded to the pain.

16.13　Name three nonpharmacological ways to manage pain.

Three nonpharmacological ways to manage pain are massage, imagery, and music.

Pharmacological Pain Management

16.14　What is pharmacological pain management?

Pain is managed pharmacologically by administering nonnarcotic analgesics, NSAIDs, narcotic analgesics, and salicylates.

16.15　What are nonnarcotic analgesics used to treat?

Nonnarcotic analgesics are used to treat mild to moderate pain such as headaches, menstrual pain (dysmenorrhea), inflammatory pain, muscular aches, and abrasions.

16.16　Name a common type of nonnarcotic analgesic.

A common type of nonnarcotic analgesic is NSAIDs.

16.17　Name an advantage of a nonnarcotic analgesic.

An advantage of a nonnarcotic analgesic is that it is not addictive.

16.18　What are narcotic analgesics?

Narcotic analgesics (narcotic agonists) act on the central nervous system to treat moderate and severe pain, suppress respiration and coughing by acting on the respiratory and cough centers in the medulla of the brainstem.

16.19　Name an example of a narcotic analgesic.

An example of a narcotic analgesic is an opioid.

16.20　What are narcotic agonist-antagonists?

Narcotic agonist-antagonists are medications that have both agonist and antagonist effects on the opioid receptors.

16.21　What are the advantages of prescribing narcotic agonist-antagonists?

Narcotic agonist-antagonists are less potent and have a lower dependency potential than opioids. Withdrawal symptoms from narcotic agonist-antagonists are not as severe as with narcotic agonists (narcotic analgesics).

16.22　What are narcotic antagonists?

Narcotic antagonists are antidotes for narcotic analgesics.

16.23　How do narcotic antagonists work?

Narcotic antagonists have higher affinity to the opiate receptor site than the narcotic analgesic, resulting in blocking the narcotic analgesic from binding to the opiate receptor site.

16.24　Why are narcotic antagonists prescribed?

Narcotic antagonists are prescribed to reverse an overdose of narcotic analgesics. Reverse narcotic analgesics cause respiratory and CNS depression.

16.25　Name a narcotic antagonist.

Naloxone (Narcan) is a narcotic antagonist.

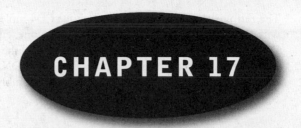

CHAPTER 17

Immunologic Agents

17.1 The Immune System

The immune system uses self-tolerance to neutralize, destroy, and eliminate any non-self proteins and cells, including microorganisms. Non-self proteins and cells include self-cells (the body's own cells) that have become infected or debilitated (cancer cells). The immune system recognizes self-cells by unique proteins on the surface of self-cells. Foreign cells have different proteins called *antigens* that stimulate the immune response by the immune system. Immune system cells originate and mature in bone marrow and release into the blood, where immune system cells search for non–self-cells.

Immunity requires three processes:

1. *Inflammation*: (see chapter 12)

2. *Antibody-Mediated Immunity (Humoral Immunity)*: This is the production of antibodies by B lymphocytes to neutralize and destroy an antigen. Antibodies are created in response to sufficient exposure to the antigen through an invasion by the antigen or a vaccination. A vaccination contains small amounts of the antigen sufficient to trigger the immune system to create antibodies.

3. *Cell-Mediated Immunity (cellular immunity) (CMI)*: This uses T-leukocytes (natural killer cells, NK cells) to attack non-self cells. This includes cells infected by a microorganism and mutated cells that are abnormal and potentially harmful, which is the mechanism for preventing cancer after being exposed to a carcinogen.

17.2 Human Immunodeficiency Virus and the Immune System

The retrovirus destroys the immune system, resulting in human immunodeficiency virus (HIV). An HIV patient develops acquired immunodeficiency syndrome (AIDS) when the retrovirus becomes active and results in opportunistic infection and malignant neoplasm.

The retrovirus disables and kills CD4+ T cells. CD4+ T cells trigger other cells in the immune system to attack invading organisms. With a reduced amount of CD4+ T cells, the immune system has a reduced capability to fight infection. A healthy person has between 800 and 1200 CD4+ T cells per cubic millimeter (mm^3) of blood. An HIV-positive patient has 200 CD4+ T cells mm^3.

The retrovirus uses three enzymes to genetically encode, replicate, and assemble a new retrovirus within a host cell. The retrovirus can replicate only inside cells. These enzymes are:

- Reverse transcriptase
- Integrase
- Protease

The retrovirus enters the cell through the CD4 molecule on the cell surface. Once inside, the virus is uncoated with the help of the reverse transcriptase enzyme, enabling the virus' single-stranded RNA to be converted into DNA. The viral DNA migrates to the nucleus of the cell, where it is spliced into the host DNA with the help of the integrase enzyme. Once combined, the HIV DNA is called the provirus and is duplicated each time the cell divides. The protease enzyme assists in the assembly of a new form of the viral particles.

17.3   Human Immunodeficiency Virus Therapies

Two common treatments for HIV are:

- *Highly Active Antiretroviral Therapy (HAART)*: HAART slows or inhibits reverse transcriptase and protease enzymes by using several antiretroviral agents. HAART decreases the viral load. The viral load measures the amount of virus in the body. A decreased viral load causes an increase in CD4+ T cells and results in the immune system being able to identify, neutralize, and destroy non–self-cells. HAART therapy must be adhered to because the virus can become resistant to the antiretroviral agents. The patient must also adhere to nutritional therapy and avoid infections.

- *Antiretroviral Therapy*: Antiretroviral therapy is given when there is less than 500 CD4+ T cells mm³ or plasma HIV RNA levels are greater than 10,000 copies/mL (B-DNA assay) or 20,000 copies/mL (R-PCR assay). Therapy should be considered for all HIV-infected patients who have detectable HIV RNA in plasma. There are risks and benefits regarding antiretroviral therapy:

    ○ Benefits:
      ▪ Controls viral replication and mutation
      ▪ Prevents progression of immunodeficiency
      ▪ Reconstructs the normal immune system
      ▪ Delays AIDS
      ▪ Decreases the risk of resistant virus
      ▪ Decreases the risk of drug toxicity
    ○ Risks:
      ▪ Adverse effects of medication reduce quality of life
      ▪ Inconvenient medication regimen
      ▪ Transmission of drug-resistant virus
      ▪ Limitation of future antiretroviral agents (due to viral resistance)
      ▪ Unknown long-term toxicity of antiretroviral drugs
      ▪ Unknown duration of effectiveness of current antiretroviral therapies

17.4   Human Immunodeficiency Virus Medication

There are four classes of HIV medication. These are:

1. Nonnucleoside Reverse Transcriptase Inhibitors (NNRTIs): These bind to reverse transcriptase, disabling the reverse transcriptase. NNRTI medications are:
    a. Delavirdine (DLV; Rescriptor)
    b. Efavirenz (EFV; Sustiva)
    c. Nevirapine (NVP; Viramune)
2. Nucleoside Reverse Transcriptase Inhibitors (NRTIs): These are faulty versions of reverse transcriptase. The retrovirus uses NRTI instead of normal reverse transcriptase, resulting in a failed attempt of reproduction. NRTI medications are:

   a. Abacavir (ABC, Ziagen)

   b. Abacavir

   c. Lamivudine (Epzicom)

   d. Abacavir

   e. Lamivudine

   f. Zidovudine (Trizivir)

   g. Didanosine (Videx, ddI, Videx EC)

   h. Emtricitabine (Emtriva, FTC, Coviracil)

   i. Emtricitabine

   j. Tenofovir DF (Truvada)

   k. Lamivudine (3TC, Epivir)

   l. Lamivudine

   m. Zidovudine (Combivir)

   n. Stavudine (d4T, Zerit)

   o. Tenofovir DF (TDF, Viread)

   p. Zalcitabine (ddC, Hivid)

   q. Zidovudine (AZT, AZV, Retrovir)

3. Protease Inhibitors (PIs): These disable protease and therefore disrupt replication of the retrovirus. PI medications are:

   a. Amprenavir (Agenerase, APV)

   b. Atazanavir (Reyataz, ATV)

   c. Fosamprenavir (Lexiva, FPV)

   d. Indinavir (Crixivan, IDV)

   e. Lopinavir

   f. Ritonavir (Kaletra, LPV/r)

   g. Nelfinavir (Viracept, NFV)

   h. Ritonavir (Norvir, RTV)

   i. Saquinavir (Fortovase, SQV, Invirase)

4. Fusion Inhibitors: These prevent the retrovirus entry into cells. A commonly prescribed fusion inhibitor is Enfuvirtide (Fuzeon, T–20).

NONNUCLEOSIDE REVERSE TRANSCRIPTASE INHIBITOR (NNRTI) ANTIRETROVIRAL

Use	Treatment of HIV infection in combination with other antivirals	Half-life: 2–11 hours	Onset: UK	Peaks: UK	Duration: UK
Example	Delavirdine mesylate (Rescriptor)	Route: PO	Pregnancy category: C	Pharmacokinetic: Rapidly absorbed following PO administration; primarily distributed in blood plasma; PB 98%; metabolized in liver; eliminated in feces and urine.	

How it works	• Inhibits catalytic reaction of HIV reverse transcriptase that is independent of nucleoside binding, interrupting HIV replication, slowing progression of HIB infection.
Adult dose	• 400 mg three times/day
Before administration	• Obtain baseline laboratory testing, especially liver function tests, before beginning therapy. • Offer emotional support.

Administration	• May disperse in water before consumption
	• May give with or without food
	• Patients with achlorhydria should take with orange juice or cranberry juice.

After administration	• Assess skin for rash.
	• Question if nausea is noted.
	• Determine pattern of bowel activity and stool consistency.
	• Assess eating pattern.
	• Monitor for weight loss.
	• Monitor lab values carefully, particularly liver function.

Contraindications	• None significant
	• *Caution:* Liver impairment

Side effects/adverse reactions	• Frequent: Rash, pruritus
	• Occasional: Headache, nausea, diarrhea, fatigue, anorexia
	Adverse/Toxic
	• None significant

Patient education	• Do not take any medications, including OTC drugs, without consulting your healthcare provider.
	• Small frequent meals may offset anorexia and nausea.
	• Delavirdine is not a cure for HIV infection, nor does it reduce risk of transmission to others.

NUCLEOSIDE REVERSE TRANSCRIPTASE INHIBITOR (NRTI) ANTIRETROVIRAL

Use	IV: Management of select adult patients with symptomatic HIV infection (AIDS, advanced HIV disease). PO: Management of patients with HIV infection having evidence of impaired immunity. HIV-infected children (older than 3 mo) who have HIV-related symptoms or asymptomatic with abnormal lab values showing significant HIV-related immunosuppression. Prevents maternal–fetal HIV transmission. Prophylaxis in occupational exposure at risk of acquiring HIV.	Half-life: 0.8–1.2 hours	Onset: NA	Peaks: 30–90 minutes	Duration: UK
Example	Zidovudine (ZDV, AZT, Retrovir)	Route: PO/IV	Pregnancy category: C	Pharmacokinetic: Rapidly, completely absorbed from GI tract. PB 25%–38%; metabolized in liver; widely distributed; crosses blood–brain barrier, cerebrospinal fluid; primarily excreted in urine; minimal removal by hemodialysis.	

How it works	• Interferes with viral RNA-dependent DNA polymerase, an enzyme necessary for viral HIV replication, slowing HIV replication, reducing progression of HIV infection.
Adult dose	• HIV: IV: 1–2 mg/kg/dose q4h. PO: 200 mg q8h or 300 mg q12 h

Before administration	• Obtain specimens for viral diagnostic tests before starting therapy (therapy may begin before results are received).
	• Check hematology reports for accurate baseline.
	• Provide emotional support.
	• Keep capsules in cool, dry place. Protect from light.
	• After dilution, IV solution is stable for 24 hours at room temperature, 48 hours if refrigerated.
	• Use within 8 hours if stored at room temperature; 24 hours if refrigerated.
Administration	• Must dilute before administration.
	• Remove calculated dose from vial and add to D5W to provide a concentration no greater than 4 mg/mL.
	• IV: Infuse over 1 hour.
	• Do not mix with any other medications.
After administration	• Avoid drugs that are nephrotoxic, cytotoxic, or myelosuppressive—may increase risk of toxicity.
	• Monitor hematology reports for anemia and granulocytopenia; check for bleeding.
	• Assess for headache and dizziness.
	• Determine pattern of bowel activity.
	• Evaluate skin for acne or rash.
	• Be alert to development of opportunistic infections (e.g., fever, chills, cough, myalgia).
	• Monitor I&O, renal, and liver function tests.
	• Check for insomnia.
Contraindications	• Life-threatening allergies to zidovudine or components of preparation
	• *Cautions:* Bone marrow compromise, renal and hepatic dysfunction, decreased hepatic blood flow
Side effects/adverse reactions	• Common: Nausea, headache
	• Frequent: GI pain, asthenia (loss of strength, energy), rash, fever
	• Occasional: Diarrhea, anorexia, malaise, myalgia, somnolence
	• Rare: Dizziness, paresthesia, vomiting, insomnia, dyspnea, altered taste
	Adverse/Toxic
	• Anemia (occurs most commonly after 4–6 weeks of therapy) and granulocytopenia, particularly significant in those with pretherapy low baselines, occur rarely.
	• Nausea, vomiting, neurotoxicity (ataxia, fatigue, lethargy, nystagmus), seizures
Patient education	• Continue therapy for full length of treatment.
	• Doses should be evenly spaced around the clock.
	• Zidovudine does not cure AIDS or HIV disease but acts reduce symptomatology and slow progress of disease.
	• Do not take any medications without healthcare provider approval. Even acetaminophen/aspirin may have serious consequences.
	• Bleeding from gums, nose, or rectum may occur and should be reported immediately.
	• Blood counts are essential because of bleeding potential.
	• Dental work should be done before therapy or after blood counts return to normal (often weeks after therapy has stopped).

PROTEASE INHIBITORS ANTIRETROVIRAL

Use				
Used in combination with nucleoside analogues for treatment of advanced HIV infection in selected patients.	Half-life: 13 hours	Onset: NA	Peaks: NA	Duration: NA

Example	Saquinavir (Fortovase, Invirase)	Route: PO	Pregnancy category: B	Pharmacokinetic: Poorly absorbed following oral administration (high-caloric/high fat meal increases absorption); PB: 99%; metabolized in liver; eliminated in feces; unknown if removed by hemodialysis

How it works
- Inhibits HIV protease, rendering the enzyme incapable of processing the polyprotein precursor to generate functional proteins in HIV-infected cells, slowing HIV replication, reducing progression of HIV infection.

Adult dose
- Fortovase: 1200 mg three times/day; Saquinavir: three 200 mg capsules given three times daily within 2 hours after a full meal; do not give less than 600 mg/day (does not produce antiviral activity). Recommended daily doses of ddC or AZT: ddC 0.75 mg three times daily; AZT 200 mg three times daily.

Before administration
- Obtain baseline laboratory testing, especially liver function tests, before beginning saquinavir therapy and at periodic intervals during therapy.
- Offer emotional support.
- Obtain medication history.

Administration
- Give within 2 hours after a full meal (if taken without food in stomach, may result in no antiviral activity).

After administration
- Closely monitor for evidence of GI discomfort.
- Monitor stool frequency and consistency (watery, loose, soft).
- Inspect mouth for signs of mucosal ulceration.
- Monitor clinical chemistry tests for marked laboratory abnormalities.
- If serious or severe toxicities occur, interrupt therapy, contact healthcare provider.

Contraindications
- Clinically significant hypersensitivity to drug
- *Caution:* Impaired hepatic function

Side effects/adverse reactions
- Occasional: Diarrhea, abdominal discomfort or pain, nausea, photosensitivity, buccal mucosa ulceration
- Rare: Confusion, ataxia, weakness, headache, rash

Adverse/Toxic
- None significant

Patient education
- Continue therapy for full length of treatment.
- Doses should be evenly spaced.
- Saquinavir is not a cure for HIV infection, nor does it reduce risk of transmission to others.
- Patients may continue to acquire illnesses associated with advanced HIV infection.
- Take within 2 hours after a full meal.
- Avoid coadministration with grapefruit products.

FUSION INHIBITORS

Use	There is no cure for HIV, but enfuvirtide is one of a number of anti-HIV medicines that lower the amount of virus in the body (viral load) and slow the progression of the disease from HIV to AIDS. Enfuvirtide must be used in conjunction with other anti-HIV	Half-life: UK	Onset: UK	Peaks: UK	Duration: UK

drugs that attack the HIV virus
in different ways. It is added to
existing treatment in people
who are failing an antiretroviral
regimen because their virus has
become resistant, and is not
responding to the existing
treatment.

Example	Enfuvirtide	Route: IM	Pregnancy category: C	Pharmacokinetic: Metabolized in liver and excreted in feces.

How it works	• Enfuvirtide works by stopping the HIV virus from invading CD4 cells. It does this by binding to a protein on the outside of the virus that helps the virus attach to the CD4 cells. With enfuvirtide bound to this protein, the virus is prevented from fusing with the CD4 cell membrane. This stops it injecting its genetic material into the cell. The virus can only replicate and increase in numbers once its genetic material is inside CD4 cells, so enfuvirtide stops the virus from replicating. This mechanism of action is different from all the other currently available anti-HIV drugs, which only work once the virus has infected the CD4 cells. This means that enfuvirtide is active against strains of HIV that have become resistant to other anti-HIV medicines.
Adult dose	• 300 mg BID
Before administration	• Do not shake to reconstitute or cause the solution to foam. It may take up to 45 minutes for medication to dissolve. • After reconstituted give drug immediately or refrigerate. May be kept for 24 hours after reconstitution; however, it must be brought to room temperature before injected. Any unused medication in the vial must be discarded. It cannot be used for next dose. • Obtain baseline laboratory tests, including liver function. • Obtain medication history and history of HIV/AIDS disease and therapies.
Administration	• Rotate injection sites.
After administration	• Monitor for side effects.
Contraindications	• Use with caution in individuals with liver disease and acute renal dysfunction.
Side effects/adverse reactions	• Headache • Abdominal pain • Constipation • Difficulty in sleeping (insomnia) • Depression • Muscle cramps • Sweating • Cold or flulike symptoms • Back pain • Disorder of the peripheral nerves, causing weakness and numbness (peripheral neuropathy) • Dizziness • Inflammation of the lining of the eye, causing pain and redness (conjunctivitis) • Dry skin • Alteration in taste • Swollen glands (lymph nodes) • Loss of appetite • Weakness or loss of strength (asthenia) • Cough • Anxiety • Yeast infection of the mouth and throat (oral thrush) • Inflammation of the hair follicles (folliculitis)

- Inflammation of the sinuses (sinusitis)
- Pain in the muscles and joints
- Pneumonia
- Herpes simplex infections such as cold sores
- Injection site reactions such as pain, discomfort, redness, itching, hardening of skin, nodules and cysts, blood spots under the skin

Patient education

- Take medications as ordered to maintain adequate blood levels or the medication may not be effective.
- If the blood levels drop, the virus will be given more chance to replicate and develop resistance to the drugs. Skipping even a few doses increases the risk of treatment failure, so you should try to ensure that you take all your doses at the correct time, and that you visit your doctor for repeat prescriptions before you run out.
- Taking this medication does not cure HIV or AIDS. It does not decrease the chance of spreading it to another individual. Use condoms if you are sexually active.

  This medicine can occasionally cause an allergic reaction characterized by symptoms, including rash, fever, nausea and vomiting, chills, stiff muscles, low blood pressure, and difficulty breathing. Stop using this medicine and consult your doctor immediately if you experience these symptoms while using this medicine. If your doctor considers you to have experienced an allergic reaction, treatment with this medicine should not be restarted.
- A healthcare professional will explain to you how to administer this medicine. Make sure you follow their instructions carefully. Once you have added the water for injections to the vial you should gently tap the vial with your fingertip until the powder begins to dissolve. After the powder begins to dissolve you can leave it to completely dissolve, which may take up to 45 minutes. You can gently roll the vial between your hands to speed this up, but never shake the vial or turn it upside down to mix, as this will cause excessive foaming.
- Once reconstituted, the solution should be injected immediately, as directed by your doctor. If the reconstituted solution cannot be injected immediately, it must be kept refrigerated until use and used within 24 hours. Reconstituted solution that has been refrigerated should be brought to room temperature before injection. The contents of each vial are suitable for one injection only—any remaining solution should be discarded.
- Each injection should be given at a different site to the previous injection, and where there is no current injection site reaction.
- Do not breastfeed while taking this medication.

17.5 Human Immunodeficiency Virus Therapy and Pregnancy

A pregnant HIV patient is at risk of transmitting the retrovirus to the fetus. This risk is reduced by:

- Administering 100 mg of ZDV five times daily starting at the 14 week of gestation
- Administering ZDV IV in a 10-hour loading dose of 2 mg per kg of body weight, followed by a continuous infusion of 1 mg per kg of body weight per hour at beginning of labor and until delivery
- Administering to the newborn ZDV at 2 mg/kg/per PO beginning 8 to 12 hours after birth and every 6 hours for the first 6 weeks of age

17.6 Postexposure Prophylaxis

Healthcare workers exposed to the retrovirus are administered postexposure prophylaxis according to the Public Health Service Statement on the Management of Occupational Exposures to HIV and Recommendations (Table 17–1).

TABLE 17–1 Basic and Expanded Postexposure Prophylaxis Regimens

REGIMEN CATEGORY	APPLICATION	DRUG REGIMEN
Basic	Occupational HIV exposures for which there is a recognized transmission risk.	4 week (28 d) of both zidovudine 600 mg every day in divided doses (i.e., 300 mg twice a day, 200 mg three times a day, or 100 mg every 4 h) and lamivudine 150 mg twice a day
Expanded	Occupational HIV exposures that pose an increased risk for transmission (e.g., larger volume of blood and/or higher virus titer in blood)	Basic regimen plus either indinavir 800 mg every 8 hours or nelfinavir 750 mg three times a day

17.7　Types of Immunity

There are two ways antibodies are created.

Active Natural Immunity

Active natural immunity occurs when antibodies are created when exposed to the pathogen. Active immunity is slow. The immune system is slow to react to the first exposure but quick to respond to subsequent exposure because antibodies are already created. Exposure is from either infection or a vaccine, which contains a small amount of the pathogen.

Passive Immunity

Passive immunity occurs when antibodies from another source are administered to the patient. Antibodies are prescribed when a patient needs immediate protection that lasts a few months, giving time for a vaccine to develop active natural immunity.

- Passive Natural Immunity: This occurs when antibodies cross the placenta and to the fetus to protect the newborn.
- Passive Acquired Immunity: Antibodies from a human or animal source are administered to the patient.

17.8　Vaccines

There are five kinds of vaccines. These are:

1. Inactivated (dead) microorganism (whole or part)
2. Live weakened microorganisms
3. Toxoids, which are inactivated toxins produced by microorganisms
4. Conjugates, in which the disease-causing microorganism is coated with toxoid from an unrelated microorganism
5. Recombinant subunit vaccine, in which a pathogen's DNA is inserted into a cell or organism, which then produces massive quantities of the pathogen that are used in place of the whole pathogen.

A vaccine booster is administered to maintain immunity. A blood test determines detectable levels of specific antibodies in the bloodstream. The patient is immune to a pathogen if sufficient quantity of the corresponding antibody is detected in the patient's blood.

17.9 Administering Vaccinations

Before administering a vaccination:

- Obtain immunization history.
- Determine if the patient is immune deficient.
- Determine if the patient is pregnant. Do not administer the vaccine to a pregnant patient.
- Determine if the patient has a history of receiving immunosuppressants.
- Determine if the patient has a history of blood transfusions.
- Determine if the patient has received immune globulin.
- Determine if the patient has allergies.
- Determine if anyone in the patient's household is not vaccinated or is immunodeficient.
- Assess for symptoms of moderate to severe acute illness, with or without fever.
- Adhere to storage requirements for the vaccine to ensure its potency.
- Keep epinephrine available in the case of anaphylactic reaction.

Administering a vaccination:

- Administer vaccine within stated time limit after preparation.
- Use different injection site if multiple vaccinations are given on the same day.
- Do not mix vaccines in the same syringe.

After administering a vaccination:

- Observe for signs and symptoms of adverse reactions.
- Document that a vaccine information statement (VIS), available from the Centers for Disease Control and Prevention (CDC) for each vaccine administered, is provided to the patient and his or her family.
- Document the date of vaccination, route and site, vaccine type, manufacturer, lot number, and expiration date, as well as the name, address, and title of individual administering vaccine.
- Provide the patient with a record of immunizations.

17.10 Patient Education

The patient should be told the following facts about vaccinations:

- Explain the risk of contracting vaccine-preventable diseases.
- Female patients of childbearing age should avoid becoming pregnant within a month of the vaccination.
- Provide the patient with a current VIS available from the CDC for each vaccine administered.
- Remind the patient to bring the VIS record to all visits.
- Provide the patient with the date for the next vaccination.
- Discuss common side effects of a vaccine.
- Tell the patient to contact the healthcare provider if there are signs of an adverse reaction.

17.11 Immunosuppressant Medication

Immunosuppressant medications suppress the body's ability to reject non–self-cells. These medications are prescribed to patients who have organ transplants.

Commonly prescribed immunosuppressant medications are:

- Azathioprine (Imuran)
- Cyclosporine (Sandimmune)
- Muromonab-DC3 (Orthoclone OKT3)
- Mycophenolate mofetil (Cell Cept, and tacrolimus FK506, Prograf)

Immunosuppressant medications cause:

- Nausea
- Vomiting
- Risk of tumor growth
- Leukopenia
- Thrombocytopenia

Solved Problems

Immune System

17.1 What is self-tolerance?

Self-tolerance is the immune system's ability to neutralize, destroy, and eliminate any non-self proteins and cells in the body.

17.2 What is a non-self protein?

A non-self protein is a marker on a cell that is different from proteins found on self-cells, enabling the immune system to differentiate between a self-cell and a non-self cell.

17.3 Does the immune system neutralize and destroy only non-self cells?

No. The immune system also destroys self-cells that have become infected or debilitated.

17.4 What is antibody-mediated immunity?

Antibody-mediated immunity is the production of antibodies by B lymphocytes to neutralize and destroy an antigen. Antibodies are created in response to sufficient exposure to the antigen through an invasion by the antigen or by a vaccination. A vaccination contains small amounts of the antigen sufficient to trigger the immune system to create antibodies.

17.5 What is cell-mediated immunity?

Cell-mediated immunity (cellular immunity) uses T-leukocytes (natural killer cells, NK cells) to attack non-self cells. This includes cells infected by a microorganism and mutated cells that are abnormal and potentially harmful, which is the mechanism for preventing cancer after being exposed to a carcinogen.

Human Immunodeficiency Virus

17.6 What action does the retrovirus have on the body?

The retrovirus disables and kills CD4+ T cells. CD4+ T cells trigger other cells in the immune system to attack invading organisms. With a sufficient amount of CD4+ T cells, the immune system has a reduced capability to fight infection.

17.7 What are the three enzymes used by the retrovirus?

The three enzymes used by the retrovirus are reverse transcriptase, integrase, and protease.

17.8   What happens once the retrovirus is inside the cell?

Once inside, the virus is uncoated with the help of the reverse transcriptase enzyme, enabling the virus' single-stranded RNA to be converted into DNA. The viral DNA migrates to the nucleus of the cell, where it is spliced into the host DNA with the help of the integrase enzyme. Once combined, the HIV DNA is called the provirus and is duplicated each time the cell divides. The protease enzyme assists in the assembly of a new form of viral particles.

17.9   What is highly active antiretroviral therapy?

Highly active antiretroviral therapy (HAART) slows or inhibits reverse transcriptase and protease enzymes by using several antiretroviral agents. HAART decreases the viral load. The viral load measures the amount of virus in the body. A decreased viral load causes an increase in CDE4+ T cells, resulting in the immune system's ability to identify, neutralize, and destroy non-self-cells. HAART therapy must be adhered to because the virus can become resistant to the antiretroviral agents. The patient must also adhere to nutritional therapy and avoid infections.

17.10   When is antiretroviral therapy administered?

Antiretroviral therapy is given when less than 500 CD4+ T cells mm^3 or plasma HIV RNA levels are greater than 10,000 copies/mL (B-DNA assay) or 20,000 copies/mL (R-PCR assay).

17.11   What are the risks of antiretroviral therapy?

- Adverse effects of medication, which reduce quality of life
- Inconvenient medication regimen
- Transmission of drug-resistant virus
- Limitation of future antiretroviral agents (due to viral resistance)
- Unknown long-term toxicity of antiretroviral drugs
- Unknown duration of effectiveness of current antiretroviral therapies

17.12   How do nonnucleoside reverse transcriptase inhibitors work?

NNRTIs bind to reverse transcriptase, disabling the reverse transcriptase.

17.13   How do NRTIs work?

NRTI are faulty versions of reverse transcriptase. The retrovirus uses NRTI instead of normal reverse transcriptase, resulting in a failed attempt of reproduction.

17.14   Name three NRTI medications.

Three NRTI medications are Abacavir (Ziagen, ABC), Abacavir, and Lamivudine (Epzicom).

17.15   How do protease inhibitors work?

Protease inhibitors disable protease and therefore disrupt replication of the retrovirus.

17.16   How do fusion inhibitors work?

Fusion inhibitors prevent the retrovirus entry into cells.

17.17   What is the treatment for a pregnant HIV patient?

- Administer 100 mg of ZDV five times daily starting at the 14 week of gestation.
- Administer ZDV IV in a 10 hour loading dose of 2 mg per kg of body weight, followed by a continuous infusion of 1 mg per kg of body weight per hour at beginning of labor and until delivery.
- Administer to the newborn ZDV at 2 mg/kg/per PO beginning 8 to 12 hours after birth and every 6 hours for the first 6 weeks of life.

Vaccines

17.18 What is an inactivated vaccine?

An inactivated vaccine contains whole or part of a dead microorganism.

17.19 What is a toxoids vaccine?

A toxoids vaccine is a vaccine that contains inactivated toxins produced by a microorganism.

17.20 What is a conjugates vaccine?

A conjugates vaccine is a vaccine in which the disease-causing microorganism is coated with toxoid from an unrelated microorganism.

17.21 What is a booster vaccine?

A booster vaccine is a vaccine designed to maintain immunity.

17.22 How is it determined if a patient has been vaccinated?

A blood test determines detectable levels of specific antibodies in the bloodstream. The patient is immune to a pathogen if sufficient quantity of the corresponding antibody is detected in the patient's blood.

17.23 Name three facts about administering a vaccine.

- Administer the vaccine within stated time limit after preparation.
- Use different injection sites if multiple vaccinations are given on the same day.
- Do not mix vaccines in the same syringe.

17.24 Why keep epinephrine on hand when administering a vaccination?

Keep epinephrine available in case of anaphylactic reaction to a vaccination.

Immunosuppressants

17.25 Why is immunosuppressant medication administered?

Immunosuppressant medications suppress the body's ability to reject non-self-cells. These medications are prescribed to patients who have organ transplants.

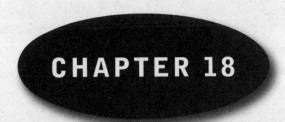

CHAPTER 18

The Gastrointestinal System

18.1 The Gastrointestinal System

The gastrointestinal (GI) system consists of alimentary canal (digestive tract):

- Oral cavity (mouth, tongue, and pharynx)
- Esophagus
- Stomach
- Small intestine (duodenum, jejunum, and ileum)
- Large intestine (cecum, colon, and rectum)
- Anus

The GI system also has accessory organs and glands:

- Salivary glands
- Pancreas
- Gallbladder
- Liver

18.2 The Esophagus

Food is broken into small pieces by chewing. Amylase in saliva digests starches. Food is swallowed and moves down the esophagus to the stomach in an involuntary movement called *peristalsis*. The esophagus is lined with mucous membranes that secrete mucus. The esophagus has two sphincters. These are:

- Superior (Hyperpharyngeal) Sphincter: Allows food to enter the esophagus
- Lower Sphincter: Prevents gastric juices from entering the esophagus (gastric reflux)

18.3 The Stomach

The stomach holds 2000 ml of content and takes about 2 to 3 hours to empty. The stomach has two sphincters:

- Cardiac Sphincter: At the opening of stomach
- Pyloric Sphincter: At the end of stomach leading to the duodenum

Mucosal folds in the stomach contain glands that secrete gastric juices used to digest food. Digestion is the breaking down of food into its chemical elements.

There are four types of cells in the stomach. These are:

1. Chief Cells: Secrete proenzyme pepsinogen (pepsin)
2. Parietal Cells: Secrete hydrochloric acid (HCl)
3. Gastrin-Producing Cells: Secrete gastrin, a hormone that regulates the release of enzymes during digestion
4. Mucus-Producing Cells: Release mucus, which protects the stomach lining from gastric juices

18.4   The Intestines

The duodenum is the shortest part of the small intestine, where most chemical digestion occurs. The duodenum releases secretin, a hormone, which suppresses gastric acid. Cholecystokinin, a hormone, is released by the duodenum that simulates flow of bile from the gallbladder into the duodenum. Bile (produced by the liver), trypsin, chymotrypsin, lipase, and amylase (all produced by the pancreas) digest carbohydrates, protein, and fat in preparation for absorption in the small intestine. The duodenum connects the stomach to the jejunum. The jejunum is the second division of the small intestine and connects the duodenum to the ileum. The ileum is the end of the small intestine.

The ileum is connected to the cecum (beginning of the large intestine) by the ileocecal valve. The cecum connects to the colon (ascending, transverse, descending, sigmoid), and then to the rectum and anus. The large intestine absorbs water and secretes mucus as undigested material moves through peristaltic contractions to the rectum where undigested material is eliminated through defecation.

18.5   Vomiting and Nausea

Nausea is a queasy sensation that sometimes precedes vomiting. Vomiting (emesis) is the expulsion of gastric contents of the stomach through the esophagus and out the oral cavity. Vomiting is the result of stimulating the chemoreceptor trigger zone (CTZ) vomiting center in the cerebral cortex. These are neurotransmitters that stimulate this center:

- Dopamine: Impulses from medication, toxins, and the vestibular center in the ear are transmitted by dopamine to the CTZ, resulting in a vomiting response.
- Acetylcholine: Impulses from odor, smell, taste, and gastric mucosal irritation are transmitted by acetylcholine to the CTZ, resulting in a vomiting response.

When stimulated, the chemoreceptor trigger zone sends impulses to motor neurons to contract the diaphragm, anterior abdominal muscles, and stomach. This contraction results in the closing of the glottis as the abdominal wall moves upward, forcing the stomach contents up the esophagus.

Hint: Vomiting can occur without being preceded by nausea.

18.6   Causes of Vomiting

Common reasons for vomiting are:

- Motion sickness
- Viral and bacterial infections
- Food intolerance
- Surgery

- Pregnancy
- Pain
- Shock
- Medication
- Radiation
- Middle ear disturbances

18.7   Nonpharmacological Treatment of Vomiting

Nonpharmacological ways to treat vomiting are:

- Identify the cause first.
- Drink weak tea.
- Drink flattened carbonated beverages.
- Eat gelatin.
- Drink Gatorade (Pedialyte for children).
- Eat crackers.
- Eat dry toast.

Hint: Vomiting and nausea during the first trimester of pregnancy should be treated nonpharmacologically. Antiemetics can harm the fetus.

18.8   Pharmacological Treatment of Vomiting

Pharmacological ways to treat vomiting are:

- Administer IV fluids if the patient is dehydrated, caused by a fluid imbalance due to severe vomiting.
- Administer antiemetics.

Over-the-Counter Antiemetics

Commonly used to prevent motion sickness. Take 30 minutes before vomiting might occur (i.e., before traveling). There is no therapeutic effect once vomiting occurs, and no therapeutic effect with severe vomiting. These medications are:

- Antihistamine Antiemetics (inhibits stimulation of the middle ear):
  - Dimenhydrinate (Dramamine)
  - Meclizine hydrochloride (Antivert)
  - Diphenhydramine hydrochloride (Benadryl)
- Bismuth Subsalicylate (Pepto-Bismol): Acts directly on the gastric mucosa, do not give to children due to risk for Reyes syndrome
- Phosphorated Carbohydrate Solution (Emetrol): Changes the gastric pH, decreases stomach contractions, high in sugar; not for diabetics

18.9   Prescription Antiemetics

Prescription antiemetics act as antagonists to dopamine, histamine, serotonin, and acetylcholine. Prescription antiemetics are classified as:

- Antihistamines: Decrease nausea and vomiting associated with motion sickness and postsurgery. These include:
  - Vistaril
  - Atarax
  - Phenergan.
- Anticholinergics: Prevent nausea and vomiting associated with vertigo, motion sickness, and vestibular system disease. These include:
  - Scopolamine
- Dopamine Antagonists: Block dopamine receptors in the CTZ, preventing nausea and vomiting. Side effects are extrapyramidal symptoms and hypotension. These include:
  - Phenothiazines (largest group of antiemetics)
  - Butyrophenones (haloperidol (Haldol) and droperidol (Inapsine))
  - Metoclopramide (Reglan) (blocks dopamine and serotonin receptors in the CTZ)
  - Chlorpromazine (Thorazine) (also prescribed as tranquilizers)
  - Prochlorperazine edisylate (Compazine) (also prescribed as tranquilizers)
- Benzodiazepines: Indirectly control nausea and vomiting. These include:
  - Lorazepam (Ativan)
- Serotonin Antagonists: Block the serotonin receptors in the CTZ and the afferent vagal nerve terminals in the upper GI tract. Two commonly prescribed serotonin antagonists are:
  - Ondansetron (Zofran) (for chemotherapy-induced emesis and postsurgery, no extrapyramidal symptoms)
  - Granisetron (Kytril) (for chemotherapy-induced emesis, no extrapyramidal symptoms)
- Glucocorticoids (Corticosteroids): Administered IV to reduce side effects. These include:
  - Dexamethasone (Decadron)
  - Methylprednisolone (Solu-Medrol)
- Cannabinoids: As the active ingredient in marijuana, Cannabinoids act on the cerebral cortex and are prescribed for cancer patients who do not respond to other antiemetics. Cannabinoids are contraindicated for patients who have glaucoma and psychiatric disorders. These include:
  - Dronabinol
  - Nabilone

ANTICHOLINERGIC

Use	Prevention and treatment of nausea, vomiting, vertigo due to motion sickness. Treatment of vertigo associated with diseases affecting vestibular system.	Half-life: 6 hours	Onset: 30–60 minutes	Peaks: 10 hours	Duration: 12–24 hours
Example	Meclizine (Antivert)	Route: PO	Pregnancy category: B	Pharmacokinetic: Well absorbed from GI tract; widely distributed; metabolized in liver	
How it works	• Reduces labyrinth excitability, diminishes vestibular stimulation of labyrinth, affecting chemoreceptor trigger zone (CTZ), reducing nausea, vomiting, vertigo. Anticholinergic activity.				
Adult dose	• Motion sickness: PO: 25–50 mg 1 hour before travel				
Before administration	• Assess medical and drug history. • Assess vital signs.				
Administration	• Give without regard to meals. • Scored tablets may be crushed; do not break or crush capsule form.				
After administration	• Monitor B/P especially in elderly (increased risk for hypotension).				

- Monitor children closely for paradoxical response.
- Monitor serum electrolytes in those with severe vomiting.
- Assess skin turgor, mucous membranes to evaluate hydration status.

Contraindications	• None significant
	• *Cautions:* Narrow-angle glaucoma, prostatic hypertrophy, pyloroduodenal or bladder neck obstruction, asthma, chronic obstructive pulmonary disease (COPD), increased intraocular pressure, cardiovascular disease, hyperthyroidism, hypertension, seizure disorders
Side effects/adverse reactions	• *Note:* Elderly persons (greater than 60 years) tend to develop sedation, dizziness, hypotension, mental confusion, disorientation, agitation, psychotic-like symptoms
	• Frequent: Drowsiness
	• Occasional: Blurred vision, dry mouth, nose or throat
	Adverse/Toxic
	• Children may experience dominant paradoxical reaction (restlessness, insomnia, euphoria, nervousness, tremors). Overdosage in children may result in hallucinations, convulsions, death.
	• Hypersensitivity reaction (eczema, pruritus, rash, cardiac disturbances, photosensitivity) may occur.
	• Overdose may vary from central nervous system (CNS) depression (sedation, apnea, cardiovascular collapse, death) to severe paradoxical reaction (hallucinations, tremor, seizures).
Patient education	• Tolerance to sedative effect may occur.
	• Avoid tasks that require alertness or motor skills until a response to the drug is established.
	• Dry mouth, drowsiness, and dizziness may be expected responses of the drug.
	• Avoid alcoholic beverages during therapy.
	• Sugarless gum and sips of tepid water may relieve dry mouth.
	• Coffee or tea may help reduce drowsiness.

SELECTIVE RECEPTOR ANTAGONIST

Use	Prevention, treatment of nausea and vomiting due to cancer chemotherapy, including high-dose cisplatin. Prevention of postoperative nausea, vomiting. Prevention of radiation-induced nausea, vomiting. Treatment of postoperative nausea/vomiting.	Half-life: 4 hours	Onset: 30 minutes	Peaks: 1–2 hours	Duration: 12–24 hours
Example	Ondansetron (Zofran)	Route: PO/IM/IV	Pregnancy category: B	Pharmacokinetic: Readily absorbed from GI tract; PB: 70%–76%; metabolized in liver; excreted in urine. Unknown if removed by hemodialysis.	

How it works	• Action may be central (CTZ) or peripheral (vagus nerve terminal), preventing nausea/vomiting associated with cancer chemotherapy.
Adult dose	• Nausea, Vomiting: Chemotherapy:
	Note: All oral doses given 30 minutes before chemotherapy and repeated at 8-hour intervals
	PO: 24 mg once a day or 8 mg three times/day; IV: three doses 0.15 mg/kg. First dose given 30 minutes before chemotherapy; then 4 and 8 hours after first dose of ondansetron.
	• Nausea, Vomiting: Post op
	○ IM/IV: 4 mg undiluted over 2–5 min
	• Nausea, Vomiting: Radiation
	○ PO: 8 mg three times/day

Before administration	• Assess for dehydration if excessive vomiting occurs. • Provide emotional support. • Assess medical and drug history (reduced dose for hepatic impairment). • Assess bowel and nutritional status. • Assess electrolytes. • Assess baseline vital signs.
Administration	• PO: Give without regard to food. • IM: Inject into large muscle mass. • IV: Give IV push over 2–5 minutes; infuse over 15 minutes.
After administration	• Monitor patient in environment for safety. • Assess bowel sounds for peristalsis. • Assess mental status. • Monitor daily bowel activity and stool consistency and record time of evacuation. • Monitor for dehydration. • Monitor patient comfort.
Contraindications	• None significant
Side effects/ adverse reactions	• Frequent: Anxiety, dizziness, drowsiness, headache, fatigue, constipation, diarrhea, hypoxia, urinary retention • Occasional: Abdominal pain, xerostomia (diminished saliva secretion), fever, feeling of cold, redness/pain at injection site, paresthesia, weakness • Rare: Hypersensitivity reaction (rash, itching), blurred vision Adverse/Toxic • Overdose may produce combination of CNS stimulation and depressant effects
Patient education	• Relief from nausea/vomiting generally occurs shortly after drug administration. • Avoid alcohol or barbiturates. • Report persistent vomiting.

ANTIHISTAMINE

Use	Provides symptomatic relief of allergic symptoms; sedative/ antiemetic in surgery/labor; decreases postop nausea/ vomiting; adjunct to analgesics in control of pain; management of motion sickness.	Half-life: UK minutes IM: 20 minutes Rectal: 20 minutes IV: 3–5 minutes	Onset: PO: 20	Peaks: 1–4 hours	Duration: PO/IM Rectal/IV: 2–8 hours
Example	Promethazine hydrochloride (Phenergan)	Route: PO/IM/ Rectal/IV	Pregnancy category: C	Pharmacokinetic: Well absorbed from GI tract, after IM administration: Widely distributed; metabolized in liver; excreted in urine; PB:60%–90%	
How it works	• Antihistamine: Inhibits histamine at histamine receptor sites, preventing most allergic effects (e.g., urticaria, pruritus). • Antiemetic: Diminishes vestibular stimulation, depresses labyrinthine function, acts on chemoreceptor trigger zone (CTZ), producing antiemetic effect • Sedative-hypnotic: Decreases stimulation to brain stem reticular formation producing CNS depression				
Adult dose	• Allergic Symptoms: PO: 25 mg at bedtime of 12.5 mg four times/day; Rectal/IM/IV: 25 mg; may repeat in 2 hours • Motion Sickness: PO: 25 mg 30–60 minutes before departure; may repeat in 8–12 hours, then every morning on arising and before evening meal				

- Antiemetic: PO/IM/IV/Rectal: 12.5–25 mg q4–6 h as needed
- Preop and postop sedation; adjunct to analgesics: IM/IV: 25–50 mg

Before administration	• Assess BP and pulse for bradycardia/tachycardia if patient is given parenteral form. • If used as an antiemetic assess for dehydration (poor skin turgor, dry mucous membranes, longitudinal furrows in tongue). • Obtain baseline blood work to include electrolyte levels. • Assess medical and drug history. • If used for preop sedation, have patient void before administering medication and raise side rails to provide a safe environment.
Administration	• PO: Give without regard to meals. • Scored tablets may be crushed. • IM: *Note:* Significant tissue necrosis may occur if given SC. Inadvertent intraarterial injection may produce severe arteriospasm, resulting in severe circulation impairment. Inject deep IM. • IV: May be given undiluted or dilute with 0.9% NaCl. Final dilution should not exceed 25 mg/ml. • Administer at 25 mg/min rate through IV infusion tube. A too rapid rate of infusion may cause resulting transient fall in B/P, producing orthostatic hypotension, reflex tachycardia; if patient complains of pain at IV site, stop injection immediately (possibility of intra-arterial needle placement/perivascular extravasation). • Rectal: Refrigerate suppository; moisten with cold water before inserting well into rectum.
After administration	• Monitor vital signs. • Monitor serum electrolytes in patients with severe vomiting. • Assist with ambulation if drowsiness, lightheadedness occurs. • Maintain a safe environment.
Contraindications	• Comatose, those receiving large doses of other CNS depressants, acutely ill/dehydrated children, acute asthmatic attack, vomiting of unknown etiology in children, Reye's syndrome, those receiving MAO inhibitors. • *Extreme Caution:* History of sleep apnea, young children, family history of sudden infant death syndrome (SIDS), those difficult to arouse from sleep • *Cautions:* Narrow-angle glaucoma, peptic ulcer, prostatic hypertrophy, pyloroduodenal/ bladder neck obstruction, asthma, COPD, increased intraocular pressure, cardiovascular disease, hyperthyroidism, hypertension, seizure disorders
Side effects/ adverse reactions	• High Incidence: Drowsiness, disorientation. Hypotension, confusion, syncope more likely in elderly persons • Frequent: Dry mouth, urinary retention, thickening of bronchial secretions • Occasional: Epigastric distress, flushing, visual disturbances, hearing disturbances, wheezing, paresthesia, sweating, chills • Rare: Dizziness, urticaria, photosensitivity, nightmares. Fixed-combination form with pseudoephedrine may produce mild CNS stimulation Adverse/Toxic • Paradoxical Reaction (particularly in children) manifested as excitation, nervousness, tremors, hyperactive reflexes, convulsions. CNS depression has occurred in infants and young children (respiratory depression, sleep apnea, SIDS). Long-term therapy may produce extrapyramidal symptoms noted as dystonia (abnormal movements), pronounced motor restlessness (most frequently occurs in children), and parkinsonian symptoms (esp. noted in elderly). Blood dyscrasias, particularly agranulocytosis, have occurred.
Patient education	• Drowsiness and dry mouth may be an expected response to drug. Sugarless gum and sips of tepid water may relieve dry mouth. Coffee or tea may help reduce drowsiness. • Report visual disturbances. • Avoid tasks that require alertness and motor skills until response to drug is established. • Avoid alcohol and other CNS depressants.

18.10   Emetics

Emetics induce vomiting through nonpharmacological or pharmacological methods to expel noncaustic toxin. Nonpharmacological emetic is produced by placing a finger or object (toothbrush) in the back of the throat stimulating the gag reflex.

Pharmacological method is by administering an emetic. The mostly commonly use emetic is Ipecac syrup. Ipecac stimulates the CTZ in the medulla and acts directly on the gastric mucosa. However, Ipecac is somewhat controversial. Administer Ipecac with at least 8 ounces of water or juice. Do not use milk or carbonated beverages. Administer Ipecac again if vomiting does not occur in 20 minutes. If vomiting still does not occur, then administer activated charcoal.

Activated charcoal absorbs toxin and is excreted in feces. Activated charcoal is available in tablets, capsules, or suspension, and is the primary treatment for ingestion of caustic toxins, which would injure the esophagus if regurgitated.

18.11   Antidiarrhea Medications

Diarrhea is frequent liquid stools in one or more bowel movement that is a symptom of an underlying cause such as microorganism, foods, malabsorption syndrome, or inflammatory bowel disease. Medication is administered to treat the underlying cause. For example, diarrhea caused by *Escherichia coli* is treated with fluoroquinolone, an antibiotic.

Diarrhea can cause dehydration and electrolyte imbalance because intestinal fluids are rich in water, sodium, potassium, and bicarbonate. To rehydrate and restore electrolyte imbalance, patients are administered Gatorade, Pedialyte, Ricelyte, and electrolytes given IV. Antidiarrheal medication decreases the hypermotility (increased peristalsis) that stimulates frequent bowel movements and should be administered for less than 2 days and not if the patient experiences a fever. There are four classifications of antidiarrheal medication. These are:

1. Opiates: Opiates decrease intestinal motility for 2 hours. Side effects of opiates are constipation and CNS depression when combined with tranquilizers, alcohol, and sedatives. Commonly prescribed opiates are:
    a. Tincture of opium
    b. Paregoric (camphorated opium tincture)
    c. Codeine

2. Opiate-Related Agents: Opiate-related agents are synthetic compounds similar to opiates. Side effects are nausea, vomiting, drowsiness, abdominal distention, Tachycardia, paralytic ileus, urinary retention, decreased secretions, and physical dependence. Two common opiate-related agents are:
    a. Diphenoxylate (Lomotil): Causes greater CNS depression than loperamide and has a shorter therapeutic effect
    b. Loperamide (Imodium): Causes less CNS depression than diphenoxylate and has a longer therapeutic effect

3. Adsorbents: Adsorbents coat the GI tract, adsorbing the bacteria or toxins that cause diarrhea. Commonly used adsorbents are:
    a. Kaopectate (kaolin and pectin)
    b. Pepto-Bismol (adsorbs bacterial toxins)
    c. Colestipol
    d. Cholestyramine (Questran)

4. Antidiarrheal Combinations: Antidiarrheal combinations are
    a. Colistin sulfate
    b. Furazolidone
    c. Loperamide (Imodium)

    d. Lactobacillus

    e. Octreotide acetate

    f. Lomotil (diphenoxylate HCl with atropine sulfate)

    g. Parepectolin (paregoric, kaolin, pectin, alcohol)

ANTIDIARRHEALS

Use	Adjunctive treatment of acute chronic diarrhea	Half-life: 2.5 hours	Onset: 45–60 minutes	Peaks: 2 hours	Duration: 3–4 hours
Example	Diphenoxylate with atropine (Lomotil) Schedule V	Route: PO	Pregnancy category: C	Pharmacokinetic: Well absorbed from GI tract; metabolized in liver; eliminated in feces	

How it works	• Acts locally and centrally to reduce intestinal motility
Adult dose	• Antidiarrheal: PO: Initially, 15–20 mg/day in three to four divided doses; then 5–15 mg/day in two to three divided doses.
Before administration	• Check baseline hydration status (skin turgor, mucous membranes, urinary status). • Obtain electrolytes if diarrhea has been moderate to severe for more than 2 days.
Administration	• Give without regard to meals. If GI irritation occurs, give with food or meals • Use liquid for children younger than 12 years
After administration	• Encourage adequate fluid intake. • Assess bowel sounds for peristalsis. • Monitor daily bowel activity; stool consistency (watery loose, soft, semisolid, solid) and record times of evacuation. • Assess for abdominal disturbances. • Discontinue medication if abdominal distention occurs. • Monitor intake and output. • Provide safe environment.
Contraindications	• Obstructive jaundice, diarrhea associated with pseudomembranous enterocolitis because of broad-spectrum antibiotics or with organisms that invade intestinal mucosa (*E. coli, Shigella, Salmonella*), acute ulcerative colitis (may produce toxic megacolon) • *Cautions:* Advanced hepatorenal disease, abnormal liver function
Side effects/ adverse reactions	• Frequent: Drowsiness, lightheadedness, dizziness, nausea • Occasional: Headache, dry mouth • Rare: Flushing, tachycardia, urinary retention, constipation, paradoxical reaction (restlessness, agitation), blurred vision Adverse/Toxic • Dehydration may predispose to toxicity. Paralytic ileus, toxic megacolon (constipation, decreased appetite, stomach pain with nausea/vomiting) occurs rarely. Severe anticholinergic effects (severe drowsiness, hypotonic reflexes, hyperthermia) may result in severe respiratory depression, coma.
Patient education	• Avoid tasks that require alertness, motor skills until response to drug is established. • Do not ingest alcohol or barbiturates. • Report fever, palpitations, or abdominal distention or if diarrhea persists.

18.12   Constipation

Constipation is the accumulation of hard fecal material in the large intestine. Constipation is treated first with nonpharmacological methods, and then with pharmacological methods if necessary.

    Nonpharmacological methods develop routine bowel habits that vary with patients, but typically range from three bowel movements per day to three per week. Nonpharmacological methods are increased dietary fiber, fluids, and exercise. Pharmacological methods are to administer laxatives and cathartics. Laxatives result in soft stools. Cathartics, called purgative, result in soft to watery stools and cramping . Laxatives and cathartics should not be administered if the cause of constipation is:

- Intestinal obstruction
- Severe abdominal pain
- Appendicitis
- Ulcerative colitis
- Diverticulitis

There are four types of laxatives:

1. *Osmotic (saline)*: Osmotic laxatives (hyperosmolar) pull water into the colon and increase water in the feces to increase bulk, stimulating peristalsis. Saline cathartics cause a semiformed to watery stool depending on the dose and are contraindicated for congestive heart failure. Monitor serum electrolytes because osmotic laxatives contain electrolytes. Monitor renal function to assure excess electrolytes can be excreted. Side effects include hypermagnesemia (drowsiness, weakness, paralysis, complete heart block, hypotension, flushing, and respiratory depression), flatulence, diarrhea, abdominal cramps, nausea, and vomiting. Commonly used osmotic laxatives are:

   a. GoLYTELY: Prepares bowel for diagnostic and surgical procedures

   b. Polyethylene Glycol (PEG) with Electrolytes: Prepares bowel for diagnostic and surgical procedures.

   c. Lactulose: Draws water into the intestines and promotes water and electrolyte retention. Decreases the serum ammonia level and is useful in liver diseases such as cirrhosis. Contraindicated for diabetics. Contains glucose and fructose.

   d. Glycerin: Increases water in the feces stimulating peristalsis and defecation.

   e. Magnesium Hydroxide (Milk of Magnesia): Magnesia draws salt from blood into the intestines, causing increased fluid into the intestines.

2. *Stimulant*: Stimulant laxatives increase peristalsis by irritating sensory nerve endings in the intestinal mucosa, causing defecation within 12 hours. Commonly used stimulant laxatives are:

   a. Phenolphthalein (Ex-Lax, Feen-A-Mint, Correctol): Commonly abused.

   b. Bisacodyl (Dulcolax): Commonly abused. Used for barium enema before diagnostic tests. Turns urine reddish-brown. Can cause fluid and electrolyte imbalance and mild cramping.

   c. Cascara Sagrada, Senna (Senokot)

   d. Castor oil (purgative): Acts on small bowel to produce watery stools within 6 hours. Do not take at bedtime. Used for bowel preparation and not for constipation. Do not use in early pregnancy. Can stimulate uterine contractions and cause spontaneous abortion. Can damage nerves, resulting in loss of intestinal muscle tone.

3. *Bulk-Forming*: Bulk-forming laxatives have natural fiber that absorbs water into the intestine, increasing fecal bulk and peristalsis, which results in large soft stools between 8 hours and 3 days. This type of laxative does not cause dependency. It can be used with diverticulosis, irritable bowel syndrome, and ileostomy and colostomy. Commonly used bulk-forming laxatives are:

   a. Powdered bulk-forming laxatives: Mix with water or juice, stir, and drink immediately followed by drinking a full glass of water. The laxative can cause intestinal obstruction if insufficient fluid is consumed.

   b. Calcium polycarbophil (FiberCon): Not for patients with hypercalcemia.

   c. Methylcellulose (Citrucel)

   d. Fiber granules (Perdiem)

   e. Psyllium hydrophilic mucilloid (Metamucil): Must be mixed with water.

4. *Emollients (Surfactants)*: Emollients are stool softeners that lower surface tension and accumulate water in the intestine and stool, resulting in decreased straining during defecation. Do not administer

to patients with inflammatory disorders of the gastrointestinal (GI) tract, undiagnosed severe pain that could be caused by an inflammation of the intestines (diverticulitis, appendicitis), pregnancy, spastic colon, or bowel obstruction. Commonly used emollients are:

a. Docusate calcium (Surfak)

b. Docusate potassium (Dialose)

c. Docusate sodium (Colace)

d. Docusate sodium with casanthranol (Peri-Colace)

e. Mineral oil: Absorbs essential fat-soluble vitamins A, D, E, and K. Do not administer to children, elderly persons, or patients with debilitating conditions because mineral oil can be aspirated and result in lipid pneumonia. Side effects include nausea, vomiting, diarrhea, and abdominal cramping.

Caution: Chronic use of laxatives can cause dependency.

GI STIMULANT-LAXATIVE

Use	Facilitates defecation in those with diminished colonic motor response; for evacuation of colon for rectal, bowel examination, elective colon surgery	Half-life: UK	Onset: PO: 6–12 h Rectal: 15–60 min	Peaks: NA	Duration: NA
Example	Bisacodyl (Dulcolax)	Route: PO/Rectal	Pregnancy category: C	Pharmacokinetic: Minimal absorption following PO, rectal administration. Absorbed drug excreted in urine; remainder eliminated in feces.	

How it works
Increases peristalsis by direct effect on colonic smooth musculature (stimulates intramural nerve plexu). Promotes fluid and ion accumulation in colon to increase laxative effect.

Adult dose
- PO: 5–15 mg as needed
- Rectal: 10 mg to induce bowel movement
- Elderly people: PO: initially, 5 mg/day. Rectal; 5–10 mg/day

Before administration
- Obtain complete drug and medical history especially history of chronic constipation and long-term use of laxatives.

Administration
- PO: Give on an empty stomach (faster action).
- Offer six to eight glasses of water per day (which aids in stool softening).
- Administer tablets whole; do not chew or crush.
- Avoid giving within 1 hour of antacids, milk, or other oral medications.
- Rectal: If suppository is too soft, chill for 30 min in refrigerator or run cold water over foil wrapper.
- Moisten suppository with cold water before inserting well up into rectum.

After administration
- Encourage adequate fluid intake.
- Assess bowel sounds for peristalsis.
- Monitor daily bowel activity and stool consistency (watery, loose, soft, semisolid, solid) and record time of evacuation.
- Assess for abdominal distention.
- Monitor serum electrolytes in those exposed to prolonged, frequent, or excessive use of medication.

Contraindications
- Abdominal pain, nausea, vomiting, appendicitis, intestinal obstruction, undiagnosed rectal bleeding
- *Cautions:* None significant

Side effects/ adverse reactions
- Frequent: Some degree of abdominal discomfort, nausea, mild cramps, griping, faintness
- Occasional: Rectal administration may produce burning of rectal mucosa, mild proctitis.

Adverse/Toxic
- Long-term use may result in laxative dependence, chronic constipation, or loss of normal bowel function. Chronic use or overdosage may result in electrolyte disturbances (hypokalemia,

hypocalcemia, metabolic acidosis, or alkalosis), persistent diarrhea, malabsorption, or weight loss. Electrolyte disturbance may produce vomiting or muscle weakness.

Patient education	• Institute measures to promote defecation: Increase fluid intake, exercise, eat a high-fiber diet.
	• Do not take antacids, milk, or other medication within 1 hour of taking medication (decreased effectiveness).
	• Report unrelieved constipation, rectal bleeding, muscle pain or cramps, dizziness, weakness.

GI OSMOTIC: LAXATIVE/ANTACID, ANTICONVULSANT, ELECTROLYTE

Use	Treatment/prevention of hypomagnesemia. Treatment of hypertension, torsade de pointes, encephalopathy, seizures associated with acute nephritis, constipation, hyperacidity	Half-life: UK	Onset: Route dependent	Peaks: Route dependent	Duration: Route dependent
Example	Magnesium chloride Magnesium citrate (citrate of Magnesia) Magnesium hydroxide (MOM) Magnesium oxide (Mag-ox) Magnesium protein complex (Mg-PLUS) Magnesium sulfate (Epsom salt, magnesium sulfate injection)	Route: PO/IM/IV	Pregnancy category: C	Pharmacokinetic: Antacid, laxative: minimal absorption through intestine. Absorbed dose primarily excreted in urine; Systemic: Widely distributed; primarily excreted in urine.	

How it works	• Antacid: Acts in stomach to neutralize gastric acid, increase pH
	• Laxative: Osmotic effect primarily in small intestine. Draws water into intestinal lumen, produces distention, promotes peristalsis, bowel evacuation
	• Systemic (dietary supplement, replacement): Found primarily in intracellular fluids. Essential for enzyme activity, nerve conduction, and muscle contraction.
	• Anticonvulsant: Blocks neuromuscular transmission, amount of acetylcholine released at motor end plate, producing seizure control

Adult dose	Hypomagnesemia (magnesium sulfate):
	• IM/IV: 1 g q6h for four doses
	• PO: 3 g q6h for four doses
	Hypertension, seizures (magnesium sulfate)
	• IM/IV: 1 g q6h for four doses as needed
	Torsade de pointes (magnesium sulfate)
	• UVL 25–50 mg/kg/dose; maximum 2 g
	Laxative
	• Magnesium citrate: PO: 150–300 ml
	• Magnesium hydroxide: PO: 30–60 ml/day
	Antacid
	• Magnesium hydroxide: Note: Up to four times/day; PO: (tablet): 622–1244 mg/dose; (liquid concentrate: 2.5–7.5 ml/dose; (liquid): 5–15 ml/dose

Before administration	• Assess if the patient is sensitive to magnesium.
	• Antacid: Assess GI pain (duration, location, time of occurrence, relief with food, or caused by food or alcohol, constant or sporadic, worsened when lying down or bending over).
	• Laxative: Assess color, amount, and consistency of stool. Assess bowel habits (usual pattern) and bowel sound for peristalsis.
	• Assess patient for any abdominal pain, weight loss, nausea, vomiting, or history of recent abdominal surgery.
	• Systemic: Assess renal function and magnesium level.

| Administration | • PO (antacid): Shake suspension well before use. Chewable tablets should be chewed thoroughly before swallowing and follow with full glass of water. |

- PO (laxative): Drink full glass of liquid (8 oz) with each dose (prevents dehydration). The flavor may be improved by following with fruit juice or citrus carbonate beverage. Refrigerate citrate of magnesia (to retain potency and palatability).
- IM: Use 250 mg/ml (25%) or 500 mg/ml (50%) magnesium sulfate concentration.
- IV: Store at room temperature; must dilute (do not exceed 20 mg/ml concentration). Do not exceed magnesium sulfate concentration 200 mg/ml (20%). Do not exceed IV infusion rate of 150 mg/min.

After administration	• Antacid: Assess for relief of gastric distress. Monitor renal function (especially if dosing is long term or frequent). • Laxative: Monitor stools for diarrhea or constipation. Maintain adequate fluid intake. • Systemic: Monitor renal function, magnesium levels, EKG for cardiac function. Test patellar reflex or knee jerk reflexes before giving repeat parenteral doses (used as indication of CNS depression; suppressed reflex may be sign of impending respiratory arrest). Patellar reflex must be present, respiratory rate greater than 16/min before each parenteral dose. Provide seizure precautions.
Contraindications	• Antacids: Severe renal impairment; appendicitis or symptoms of appendicitis, ileostomy, intestinal obstruction. • Laxatives: Appendicitis, undiagnosed rectal bleeding, congestive heart failure, intestinal obstruction, hypersensitivity, colostomy, ileostomy. • Systemic: Heart block, myocardial damage, renal failure. • *Cautions:* Safety in children less than 6 years is not known. Antacids: Undiagnosed gastrointestinal or rectal bleeding, ulcerative colitis, colostomy, diverticulitis, chronic diarrhea. Laxative: Diabetes mellitus or patients on low-salt diet (some products contain sugar and sodium). Systemic: Severe renal impairment.
Side effects/ adverse reactions	• Frequent: Antacid: Chalky taste, diarrhea, laxative effect. • Occasional: Antacid: Nausea, vomiting, stomach cramps. Antacid, laxative. Prolonged use of large dose with renal impairment may cause increased magnesium (dizziness, irregular heartbeat, mental changes, tiredness, weakness). Laxative: cramping, diarrhea, increased thirst, gas. Systemic: Reduced respiratory rate, decreased reflexes, flushing, hypotension, decreased heart rate. • Adverse/Toxic: Antacid, laxative: None significant. Systemic: May produce prolonged PR interval, widening of QRS intervals; may cause loss of deep tendon reflexes, heart block, respiratory paralysis, and cardiac arrest. Antidote: 10–20 ml 10% calcium gluconate (5–10 mEq of calcium)
Patient education	**Antacid** • Give at least 2 hours apart from other medications. • Do not take for more than 2 weeks unless directed by physician. • For peptic ulcer take 1 and 3 hours after meals and at bedtime for 4–6 weeks. • Chew tablets thoroughly, followed by a glass of water. • Shake suspensions well. • Repeat dosing/large doses may have laxative effect. **Laxative** • Drink a full glass (8 oz) of liquid to aid stool softening. • Use only short term. • Do not use if abdominal pain, vomiting, or nausea are present. **Systemic** • Inform healthcare provider of any signs of hypermagnesemia (confusion, irregular heartbeat, cramping, unusual tiredness or weakness, lightheadedness, or dizziness).

18.13 Peptic Ulcers

A peptic ulcer is erosion of the mucosal lining of esophagus, stomach, or duodenum caused by hypersecretion of hydrochloric acid and pepsin. This hypersecretion is commonly the result of infection of *Helicobacter pylori* that is resolved in 2 weeks with treatment of antibiotics.

There are three types of peptic ulcers:

- Esophageal ulcer: A peptic ulcer located in the esophagus is called an *esophageal ulcer,* caused by gastroesophageal reflux disease from the stomach, which is a result of incompetent cardiac sphincter. Incompetent cardiac sphincter is caused by malfunctioning of the esophageal sphincter brought about by smoking and obesity.
- Gastric ulcer: A peptic ulcer located in the stomach is called a *gastric ulcer,* caused by the breakdown of the gastric mucosal barrier, typically by *Helicobacter pylori* bacteria. Gastric ulcer results in burning pain 30 minutes to an hour and a half after eating.
- Duodenal ulcer: A peptic ulcer located in the duodenal is called a *duodenal ulcer,* and is caused by hypersecretion of acid from the stomach because of insufficient buffers to neutralize the acid, incompetent pyloric sphincter, or hypermotility of the stomach. Duodenal ulcer results in burning pain 2 to 3 hours after eating.

There are eight groups of antiulcer medications. These are:

1. *Tranquilizers*: Tranquilizers reduce vagal stimulation and decrease anxiety. These medications are:
   a. Librax
   b. Chlordiazepoxide (Librium)
   c. Anticholinergic clidinium (Quarzan)
2. *Anticholinergics (antimuscarinics, parasympatholytics)*: Anticholinergics decrease GI motility and secretion, inhibit acetylcholine, and block histamine and hydrochloric acid, thereby reducing pain. Anticholinergics are prescribed for duodenal ulcers because they delay gastric emptying; however, this can stimulate gastric secretions and aggravate the ulceration. Take before meals to decrease acid secretion. Do not take with antacids because antacids slow absorption of anticholinergics. Side effects are dry mouth, decreased secretions, tachycardia, urinary retention, and constipation.
3. *Antacids*: Antacids neutralize hydrochloric acid and reducing pepsin activity. Two types of antacids are:
   a. Systemic effect: Antacid is absorbed.
      i. Sodium bicarbonate: This is seldom used to treat peptic ulcer because of adverse effects (hypernatremia, water retention)
      ii. Calcium carbonate: This is the most effective neutralizing acid. It can result in acid rebound, hypercalcemia, and milk-alkali syndrome. (Calcium carbonate intensifies when taken with milk products.)
   b. Nonsystemic effect: Antacid is not absorbed.
      i. Aluminum hydroxide
      ii. Aluminum carbonate
      iii. Magnesium hydroxide (greater neutralizing than aluminum hydroxide, can be constipating with long-term use)
      iv. Magnesium carbonate
      v. Magnesium trisilicate
      vi. Magnesium phosphate
4. *Histamine$_2$ blockers*: Histamine$_2$ blockers block the H$_2$ receptors of the parietal cells in the stomach, reducing gastric acid secretion and concentration. Side effects are headaches, dizziness, constipation, pruritus, skin rash, gynecomastia, decreased libido, and impotence.
5. *Proton pump inhibitors*: Proton pump inhibitors block the final step of acid production and inhibit gastric acid secretion greater than the H$_2$ blockers. Monitor liver enzymes if patient has liver function problems. Examples are:
   a. Omeprazole (Prilosec)
   b. Lansoprazole (Prevacid)
6. *Pepsin inhibitors*: Pepsin inhibitors combine with protein to form a viscous, nonabsorbable cover for the ulcers. One example of a pepsin inhibitor is:
   a. Sucralfate (Carafate)

7. *Prostaglandin analogue*: Prostaglandin analogue decreases pepsin secretion, suppresses gastric acid secretion, and increases cytoprotective mucus in the GI tract. Prescribe to patients who have gastric distress from taking nonsteroidal anti-inflammatory drugs (NSAIDs). Do not administer to women of childbearing years or who are pregnant. One example of a prostaglandin analogue is:

   a. Misoprostol

8. *Gastrointestinal stimulants*: Gastrointestinal stimulants enhance the release of acetylcholine at the mesenteric plexus and increase gastric emptying time, preventing acid reflux. Do not administer to patients who have cardiac dysrhythmias, especially ventricular tachycardia, ventricular flutter, fibrillation, ischemic heart disease, congestive heart failure, uncorrected electrolyte disorders (hypokalemia, hypomagnesemia), and renal or respiratory failure. Perform an ECG before and after therapy. One example of a gastrointestinal stimulant is:

   a. Cisapride (Propulsid)

PROTON PUMP INHIBITOR (PPIS)

Use	Short-term treatment; 4–8 weeks of erosive esophagitis (diagnosed by endoscopy); symptomatic gastroesophageal reflux disease (GERD) poorly responsive to other treatment. Long-term treatment of pathologic hypersecretory conditions; treatment of active duodenal ulcer. Maintenance healing of erosive esophagitis. Treatment of *H. pylori*–associated duodenal ulcer (with amoxicillin, clarithromycin), active benign gastric ulcers. Prevention/treatment of NSAID-induced ulcers.	Half-life: 0.5–1 hour	Onset: NA	Peaks: NA	Duration: 24 hours
Example	Omeprazole (Prilosec)	Route: PO	Pregnancy category: C		Pharmacokinetic: Rapidly absorbed from GI tract; PB: 99%; primarily distributed into gastric parietal cells; metabolized in liver; excreted in urine; unknown if removed via hemodialysis.

How it works
- Converted to active metabolites that irreversibly bind to and inhibit H+/K+ ATPase (an enzyme on surface of gastric parietal cells). Inhibits hydrogen ion transport into gastric lumen, increasing pH, and reducing gastric acid production.

Adult dose
- Erosive esophagitis, poorly responsive GERD, active duodenal ulcer, prevention/treatment of NSAID-induced ulcers: PO 20 mg/day
- Maintenance healing of erosive esophagitis: PO: 20 mg/day
- Pathologic hypersecretory conditions: PO: Initially 60 mg/day up to 120 mg three times/day
- *H. pylori* duodenal ulcer: PO: 40 mg/day for 4–8 weeks
- Active benign gastric ulcer: PO: 0.6–0.7 mg/kg/day

Before administration
- Assess patient's pain, including the type, duration, severity, frequency, and location.
- Assess GI complaints.
- Assess mental status.

- Assess fluid and electrolytes imbalances, including intake and output.
- Assess gastric pH (greater than 5 is desired), blood urea nitrogen (BUN), and creatinine.
- Assess drug history; report probable drug–drug interactions.

Administration	• Give before meals. • Do not crush or chew capsule. Swallow whole.
After administration	• Evaluate for therapeutic response (i.e., relief of GI symptoms). • Assess for GI discomfort, nausea, and diarrhea.
Contraindications	• None significant • *Cautions:* None significant
Side effects/ adverse reactions	• Frequent: Headache • Occasional: Diarrhea, abdominal pain, nausea • Rare: Dizziness, asthenia (loss of strength), vomiting, constipation, upper respiratory infection, back pain, rash, cough Adverse/Toxic • None significant
Patient education	• Report headache. • Swallow capsules whole. • Do not chew or crush. • Take before eating.

ANTIULCERS: HISTAMINE₂ BLOCKER

Use	Short-term treatment of active duodenal ulcer. Prevention of duodenal ulcer recurrence. Treatment of active benign gastric ulcer, pathological GI hypersecretory conditions. Short-term treatment of gastroesophageal reflux disease, including erosive esophagitis. Over-the-counter (OTC) formulation for relief of heartburn, acid indigestion, and sour stomach. Prophylaxis versus aspiration pneumonitis. Autism.	Half-life: 2.5–3.5 hours	Onset: 15 minutes	Peaks: 1–3 hours	Duration: 8–12 hours
Example	Famotidine (Pepcid)	Route: PO/IV	Pregnancy category: B	Pharmacokinetic: Rapidly, incompletely absorbed from GI tract. PB: 15%–20%; metabolized in liver; excreted in urine; not removed by hemodialysis	

How it works	• Inhibits histamine action at H₂ receptors of parietal cells, inhibiting gastric acid secretion (fasting, nocturnal, or when stimulated by food, caffeine, insulin)
Adult dose	• Acute therapy duodenal ulcer: PO 40 mg at bedtime or 20 mg q12 h; Maintenance: 20 mg at bedtime • Acute therapy; benign gastric ulcer: PO: 40 mg at bedtime • Gastroesophageal reflux disease: PO: 20 mg two times/day up to 6 wk; 20–40 mg two times/day up to 12 weeks in patients with esophagitis (including erosions, ulcerations); maximum 80 mg/day • Pathological hypersecretory conditions: PO: Initially, 20 mg q6h up to 160 mg q6h • Acid indigestion, heartburn, sour stomach: PO: 10 mg 15–60 min before eating; Maximum: two tablets/day • Usual parenteral dose: IV: 20 mg q12h; Maximum: 40 mg/day

Before administration
- Assess patient's pain, including the type, duration, severity, frequency, and location.
- Assess GI complaints.
- Assess mental status.
- Assess fluid and electrolyte imbalances, including intake and output.
- Assess gastric pH (greater than 5 is desired), BUN and creatinine.
- Assess drug history; report probably drug–drug interactions.

Administration
- Administer just before meals to decrease food-induced acid secretion or at bedtime.
- Be alert that reduced doses of drug are needed by elderly persons, who have less gastric acid. Prevent metabolic acidosis.
- Store tablets and suspension at room temperature.
- Give without regard to meals or antacids; best given after meals or at bedtime
- Shake suspension well before use.
- Pepcid RPD dissolves under tongue; does not require water for dosing.
- Administer drug IV in 20 to 100 mL of IV solution; IV push give over at least 2 minutes; infuse piggyback over 15–30 minutes.

After administration
- Monitor daily bowel activity and stool consistency.
- Monitor for diarrhea/constipation, headache.
- Monitor for effectiveness, i.e., pain free.

Contraindications
- None significant
- *Cautions:* Impaired renal/hepatic function

Side effects/ adverse reactions
- Occasional: Headache
- Rare: Constipation, diarrhea, dizziness

Adverse/Toxic
- None significant

Patient education
- May take without regard to meals or antacids.
- Report headache, pain, coughing, or vomiting of blood.
- Take drug as prescribed for effectiveness.
- Avoid tasks that require alertness and motor skills until drug response is established.
- Avoid foods and liquids that cause gastric irritation (individualized for each patient).

Solved Problems

The Gastrointestinal System

18.1 What is the pyloric sphincter?

The pyloric sphincter is a circular muscle at the end of the stomach leading to the duodenum that controls emptying of the stomach contents.

18.2 What is the cardiac sphincter?

The cardiac sphincter is a circular muscle at the opening of the stomach leading from the esophagus that controls contents entering the stomach.

18.3 What is the function of parietal cells?

Parietal cells secrete hydrochloric acid.

18.4 What is the function of chief cells?

Chief cells secrete proenzyme pepsinogen (pepsin).

Vomiting and Nausea

18.5 How does vomiting occur?

Vomiting is the result of stimulating the chemoreceptor trigger zone (CTZ) vomiting center in the cerebrum. When stimulated, the chemoreceptor trigger zone sends impulses to motor neurons to contract the diaphragm, anterior abdominal muscles, and stomach. This results in closing the glottis as the abdominal wall moves upward, forcing the stomach contents up into the esophagus.

18.6 What does dopamine transmit?

Dopamine transmits impulses from medication, toxins, and the vestibular center in the ear to the CTZ, resulting in a vomiting response.

18.7 What does acetylcholine transmit?

Acetylcholine transmits impulses from odor, smell, taste, and gastric mucosal irritation to the CTZ, resulting in a vomiting response.

18.8 Name three nonpharmacological ways to treat vomiting.

Three nonpharmacological ways to treat vomiting are to drink weak tea, eat gelatin, and eat crackers.

18.9 How do dopamine antagonists work?

Dopamine antagonists block dopamine receptors in the CTZ, preventing nausea and vomiting.

18.10 What is the function of emetics?

Emetics induce vomiting.

Diarrhea

18.11 What are critical to replace in a patient who has diarrhea?

Diarrhea can cause dehydration and electrolyte imbalance because intestinal fluids are rich in water, sodium, potassium, and bicarbonate. To rehydrate and restore electrolyte imbalance, patients are administered Gatorade, Pedialyte, Ricelyte, and electrolytes given IV.

18.12 How does antidiarrheal medication work?

Antidiarrheal medication decreases the hypermotility (increased peristalsis) that stimulates frequent bowel movements.

18.13 What are the side effects of opiate antidiarrheal medication?

Side effects of opiates are constipation and CNS depression when combined with tranquilizers, alcohol, and sedatives.

18.14 How does adsorbent antidiarrheal medication work?

Adsorbents coat the GI tract, adsorbing the bacteria or toxins that cause diarrhea.

Constipation

18.15 What are the nonpharmacological methods of treating constipation?

Nonpharmacological methods of treating constipation are increased dietary fiber and exercise.

18.16 What is the difference between a laxative and cathartic?

Laxatives result in soft stools. Cathartics results in soft to watery stools and cramping called purgatives.

18.17 Name three conditions when laxatives should not be administered.

Three conditions when laxatives should not be administered are intestinal obstruction, severe abdominal pain, and ulcerative colitis.

18.18 How do osmotic laxatives work?

Osmotic laxatives (hyperosmolar) pull water into the colon and increase water in the feces to increase bulk, and stimulating peristalsis.

18.19 What should be monitored when administering osmotic laxatives?

Monitor serum electrolytes, because osmotic laxatives contain electrolytes.

18.20 How do stimulant laxatives work?

Stimulant laxatives increase peristalsis by irritating sensory nerve endings in the intestinal mucosa, causing defecation within 12 hours.

18.21 What is an advantage of using bulk-forming laxatives?

Bulk-forming laxatives are natural fiber that absorbs water into the intestine, increasing fecal bulk and peristalsis and resulting in large soft stools between 8 hours and 3 days. This type of laxative does not cause dependency.

Peptic Ulcer

18.22 How to tranquilizers treat peptic ulcers?

Tranquilizers reduce vagal stimulation and decrease anxiety.

18.23 How do antacids work?

Antacids neutralize hydrochloric acid and reduce pepsin activity.

18.24 How do histamine$_2$ blockers work?

Histamine$_2$ blockers obstruct the H_2 receptors of the parietal cells in the stomach, reducing gastric acid secretion and concentration.

18.25 How do pepsin inhibitors work?

Pepsin inhibitors combine with protein, forming a viscous, nonabsorbable cover for the ulcers.

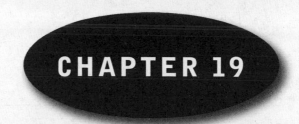

CHAPTER 19

Cardiac Circulatory Medications

19.1   The Cardiovascular System

The cardiovascular system consists of the heart, blood vessels, and blood. The pumping action of the heart circulates blood containing oxygen, nutrients, and hormones through a network of arteries into arterioles that connect to capillaries. Capillaries transport oxygenated blood to cells and absorb waster products such as CO_2, urea, creatinine, and ammonia. Capillaries connect to the network of veins via venules, which transport waste products to the lungs and kidneys.

19.2   The Heart

The myocardium (heart muscle) lies in a double-walled sac called the pericardium. The innermost layer of the heart is called the endocardium.

The heart is divided into four chambers. These are:

1. Right Atrium: Receives deoxygenated blood from the vena cava and coronary sinus and pumps blood into the right ventricle through the tricuspid valve
2. Right Ventricle: Pumps blood to the pulmonary artery through the pulmonary valve and pulmonary trunk to the lungs where CO_2 is exchanged for O_2
3. Left Atrium: Receives oxygenated blood from the pulmonary vein and pumps blood into the left ventricle through the bicuspid (mitral) valve
4. Left Ventricle: Pumps the blood into the aorta through aortic valve where blood enters circulation

Electrical impulses are generated first by the sinoatrial (SA) node and then moves to the atrioventricular (AV) node at 60 to 80 contractions per minute. Ventricles can contract independently at 30 to 40 contractions per minute. Contractions are influenced by the autonomic nervous system (see chapter 15) and medication.

19.3   Coronary Arteries

Coronary arteries provide blood-containing oxygen, nutrients, and hormones to the myocardium. Blockage of a coronary artery results in a myocardial infarction (heart attack). There are three major coronary arteries:

- Right coronary artery

- Left coronary artery
- Circumflex coronary artery

19.4 Blood Pressure

Blood pressure is resistance encountered when pumping blood throughout the circulatory system (systemic arterial pressure). The ventricles stretch when filled with blood. The force of this filling is called preload. When the ventricle contracts, the force of this contraction is called *afterload*. Afterload pushes against the pressure of the circulatory system. The average systemic blood pressure is 120/80 mmHg. The higher the resistance, the higher is the blood pressure.

Cardiac output is the total volume of blood expelled by the heart in a minute. The average cardiac output is 4 to 8 L/min. The stroke volume is the quantity of blood ejected from the left ventricle during each contraction. The average stroke volume is 70 ml/beat.

The workload of the heart is modified by using medication that increases or decreases preload and afterload, thereby adjusting stroke volume and cardiac output. Vasodilators decrease the preload and afterload, resulting in a decrease in blood pressure (arterial pressure) and cardiac output. Vasopressors increase the preload and afterload, causing in an increase in blood pressure cardiac output.

19.5 Circulation

There are two types of circulation.

- Pulmonary Circulation: Transports deoxygenated blood from the right ventricle through the pulmonary artery to the lungs. Oxygenated blood returns through the pulmonary vein to the left atrium.
- Systemic (Peripheral): Transports oxygenated blood from the left ventricle to the aorta and into the network of arteries. Nutrients and waste products in the blood are exchanged at capillary beds and returned to the heart by the network of veins.

19.6 Blood

Blood is composed of:

- Plasma: The fluid component of blood that consists of 55% of total blood volume is comprised mostly of water and a small percentage of solutes. Solutes are glucose, protein, lipids, amino acids, electrolytes, minerals, lactic and pyruvic acids, hormones, enzymes, oxygen, and carbon dioxide.
- Erythrocytes (red blood cells): Contain hemoglobin that binds with O_2 is exchange for CO_2
- Leukocytes (white blood cells): Provide cells for the immune system
- Thrombocytes (platelets): Cells that help form blood clots

19.7 Cardiac Medications

There are three groups of cardiac medications. These are Glycosides, Antianginals, and Antidysrhythmics. Cardiac medications regulate:

- Cardiac contraction

- Cardiac rate
- Cardiac rhythm
- Blood flow to the myocardium

19.8   Glycosides

Glycosides (digitalis) inhibit the sodium-potassium pump and increase intracellular calcium. Glycosides (digitalis) toxicity can develop. The antidote for glycosides toxicity is digoxin immune Fab (Ovine, Digibind). Glycosides:

- Increase cardiac contraction (positive inotropic action)
- Decrease heart rate (chronotropic action)
- Decrease conduction of the electrical stimulus (dromotropic action)
- Increase cardiac output
- Decrease preload (improves blood flow to kidneys and periphery)
- Decrease edema
- Increase fluid excretion
- Decrease fluid retention

CARDIAC GLYCOSIDE

Use	Prophylactic management and treatment of CHF; control of ventricular rate in patients with atrial fibrillation and flutter. Treatment and prevention of recurrent paroxysmal atrial tachycardia (PAT).	Half-life: 36–48 hours	Onset: PO: 1–5 hours IV: 5–30 minutes	Peaks: PO: 6–8 hours IV: 1–5 hours	Duration: PO: 2–4 days IV: 2–4 days
Example	Digoxin (Lanoxin)	Route: PO/IV	Pregnancy category: C		Pharmacokinetic: Readily absorbed from GI tract Widely distributed. PB; 30%. Metabolized in liver; Excreted in urine; minimally removed by hemodialysis.

How it works	• Direct action on cardiac muscle, conduction system. Decreases conduction rate through SA, AV node. Increases force, velocity of myocardial contraction.
Adult dose	• IV: 0.6–1 mg • PO: Initially, 0.5–0.75 mg, additional doses of 0.125–0.375 mg at 6–8 h intervals; range: 0.75–1.25 mg • Maintenance: PO/IV: 0.125–0.375 mg/day
Before administration	• Check the apical pulse before administering digoxin. Do not administer if pulse rate is less than 60 bpm (may be lower for elderly patients). • Check signs of peripheral and pulmonary edema, which indicate congestive heart failure (CHF). • Check serum digoxin level. The normal therapeutic drug range for digoxin is 0.5–2.0 ng/ml. • Check serum potassium level (normal range, 3.5–5.3 mEq/L) and report if hypokalemia • Blood samples are best taken 6–8 hours after dose or just before next dose • Obtain a drug history and report if a drug–drug interaction is possible. If the patient is taking a potassium-wasting diuretic or cortisone drug, hypokalemia might result, causing digitalis toxicity. • Assess for signs of digitalis toxicity which include: anorexia, nausea, vomiting, bradycardia, cardiac dysrhythmias, and visual disturbances. Report symptoms immediately.

(Continued)

(Continued from previous page)

CARDIAC GLYCOSIDE

Administration	PO
	• May give without regard to meals.
	• Tablets may be crushed.
	IV
	• May give undiluted or dilute with at least a fourfold volume of sterile water for injection of D5W (less than this may cause a precipitation). Use immediately. Give IV slowly over at least 5 minutes.
	• ECG monitoring should be done if dose is given intravenously.
After administration	• Monitor pulse for bradycardia.
	• Monitor ECG for arrhythmias for 1–2 hours After administration (excessive slowing of pulse may be a first clinical sign of toxicity).
	• Assess for gastrointestinal (GI) disturbances, neurologic abnormalities (signs of toxicity) q2–4 h during digitalization (daily during maintenance). Monitor serum potassium, magnesium levels.
Contraindications	• Ventricular fibrillation, ventricular tachycardia unrelated to CHF
	• *Cautions:* Impaired renal function, impaired hepatic function, hypokalemia, advanced cardiac disease, acute myocardial infarction, incomplete AV block cor pulmonale, hypothyroidism, pulmonary disease
Side effects/adverse reactions	• None significant; however, there is a very narrow margin of safety between a therapeutic and toxic result. Chronic therapy may produce mammary gland enlargement in women, but is reversible when the drug is withdrawn.
	Adverse/Toxic:
	• The most common early manifestations of toxicity are GI disturbances (anorexia, nausea, vomiting) and neurologic abnormalities (fatigue, headache, depression, weakness, drowsiness, confusion, nightmares). Facial pain, personality change, ocular disturbances (photophobia, light flashes, halos around bright objects, yellow or green color perception) may be noted.
Patient education	• Keep all follow-up appointments.
	• Take pulse (teach patient to take pulse correctly) and report pulse below 60/min (or as indicated by healthcare provider).
	• Learn and understand the signs of toxicity and the need to notify healthcare provider.
	• Wear/carry identification of digoxin therapy and inform dentist or other healthcare providers of taking digoxin.
	• Do not increase or skip doses.
	• Do not take over-the-counter (OTC) medications without consulting healthcare providers.
	• Report nausea, vomiting, or extremely slow pulse.

19.9 Antianginals

Angina pectoris is acute cardiac pain caused by inadequate blood flow (decreased oxygen) resulting from occlusion of coronary arteries or coronary artery spasm. Antianginals treat angina pectoris (Table 19.1) by:

- Increasing oxygen supply
- Decreasing oxygen demand of the heart

There are three types of angina. These are:

- Classic (stable): Triggered by stress and exertion and is relieved by rest
- Unstable (preinfarction): Progresses in severity and is not relieved by rest, often a sign of an impending heart attack
- Variant (Prinzmetal, vasospastic): Occurs at rest because of vasospasm

There are three types of antianginals. These are:

1. Nitrates: Nitrates decrease cardiac workload by vasodilatation. Commonly prescribed nitrates are:
   a. Nitroglycerin
   b. Isosorbide Dinitrate (Isordil, Sorbitrate): Administered sublingually, chewable tablets, immediate release tablets, sustained-released tablets, capsules
   c. Isosorbide Mononitrate (Monoket, Imdur): Immediate-release tablets, sustained-released tablets
2. Beta-blockers: Beta-blockers (see chapter 15) decrease cardiac workload and decrease cardiac oxygen demands. Commonly prescribed beta-blockers are:
   a. Atenolol (Tenormin)
   b. Metoprolol tartrate (Lopressor)
   c. Nadolol (Corgard)
   d. Propranolol HCl (Inderal)
3. Calcium Channel Blockers: Calcium channel blockers decrease cardiac workload and decrease the cardiac oxygen demands. Commonly prescribed calcium channel blockers are:
   a. Amlodipine (Norvasc)
   b. Bepridil HCl (Vascor)
   c. Diltiazem HCl (Cardizem)
   d. Felodipine (Plendil)
   e. Verapamil HCl (Calan, Isoptin)

TABLE 19.1 Effects of Antianginal Drugs on Angina

DRUG GROUP	VARIANT (VASOSPASTIC) ANGINA	CLASSIC (STABLE) ANGINA
Nitrates	Relaxation of coronary arteries, which decreases vasospasms and increases oxygen supply	Dilation of veins, which decreases preload and decreases oxygen demands
Beta-blockers	Not effective	Decreases heart rate and contractility, which decreases oxygen demand
Calcium channel blockers	Relaxation of coronary arteries, which decreases vasospasms and increases oxygen supply	Dilation of arterioles, which decreases after load and decreases oxygen demand. Verapamil and diltiazem ecrease heart rate and contractility.

NITRATES

Use	Lingual/sublingual/buccal dose used for acute relief of angina pectoris. Extended-release, topical forms used for prophylaxis, long-term angina management. IV form used in treatment of CHF associated with acute myocardial infarction (MI).	Half-life: 1–4 minutes	Onset: SL: 2–5 minutes Transmucosal tablet: 4–10 minutes Extended-release: 20–45 minutes Topical: 15–60 minutes Patch 20–60 minutes IV 1–2 minutes	Peaks: 4–8 minutes 4–10 minutes — 0.5–2 hours 1–3 hours	Duration: 30–60 minutes 3–5 hours 3–8 hours 3–8 hours 8–12 hours 3–5 hours

(Continued)

(Continued from previous page)

NITRATES

Example	Nitroglycerin	Route: SL/PO/ Topical/IV	Pregnancy category: B	Pharmacokinetic: Well absorbed after PO, sublingual, topical administration. Undergoes extensive first-pass metabolism in liver; excreted in urine; not removed by dialysis

How it works
- Decreases myocardial oxygen demand; reduces left ventricular preload and afterload; dilates coronary arteries, improves collateral blood flow to ischemic areas within myocardium. IV: Produces peripheral vasodilation.

Adult dose

Acute angina, acute prophylaxis
- Lingual spray: 1 spray onto or under tongue q3–5 min until relief is noted (no more than three sprays in 15-min period).
- SL: 0.4 mg q5 min until relief is noted (no more than 3 doses in 15 min); use prophylactically 5–10 min before activities that may cause an acute attack

Long-term prophylaxis of angina
- PO: 2.5–9 mg q8–12 h
- Topical: Initially, 1/2 inch q8h. Increase by 1/2 inch with each application; Range: 1–2 inches q8h up to 4–5 inches q4h
- Transdermal patch: Initially 0.2–0.4 mg/h; Maintenance: 0.4–0.8 mg/h; Consider patch on 12–14 h. Patch off 10–12 hours (prevents tolerance)

Usual parenteral dose
- IV: Initially 5 mcg/min via infusion pump. Increase in 5 mcg/min increments at 3- to 5-min intervals until B/P response is noted or until dosage reaches 20 mcg/min; then increase as needed by 10 mcg/min. Dosage may be further titrated according to patient's therapeutic response up to 200 mcg/min.

Before administration
- Record onset type (sharp, dull, squeezing), radiation, location, intensity, and duration of anginal pain, and precipitating factors (exertion, emotional stress).
- Assess B/P and apical pulse before administration and periodically after dose.
- Patient must have continuous ECG monitoring for IV administration.

Administration
- PO: Do not chew extended-release form.
- Spray: Do not shake oral aerosol canister before lingual spraying.
- Sublingual: Do not swallow; dissolve under the tongue; administer while seated; slight burning sensation under tongue may be lessened by placing tablet in buccal pouch; keep sublingual tablets in original container.
- Topical: Spread thin layer on clean/dry/hairless skin of upper arm or body (not below knee or elbow); using applicator or dose-measuring paper. Do not use fingers. Do not rub or massage into skin.
- Transdermal: Apply patch on clean/dry hairless skin of upper arm or body (not below knee or elbow).
- IV: Rate of administration: Use microdrop or infusion pump.

After administration
- Assess for facial/neck flushing.
- The cardioverter/defibrillator must not be discharged through paddle electrode overlying nitroglycerin system (may cause burns to patient or damage to paddle via arcing).
- Monitor VS. Hypotension is a common side effect.
- Monitor effects; report angina that persists.

Contraindications
- Hypersensitivity to nitrates, severe anemia, closed-angle glaucoma, postural hypotension, head trauma, increased intracranial pressure
- Sublingual: Early MI
- Transdermal: allergy to adhesives
- Extended-release: GI hypermotility/malabsorption, severe anemia
- IV: Uncorrected hypovolemia, hypotension, inadequate cerebral circulation, constrictive pericarditis, pericardial tamponade
- *Cautions:* Acute MI, hepatic, renal disease, glaucoma (contraindicated in closed-angle glaucoma), blood volume depletion from diuretic therapy, systolic B/P below 90 mmHg

Side effects/adverse reactions	• Frequent: Headache (may be severe) occurs mostly in early therapy, diminishes rapidly in intensity, usually disappears during continued treatment; transient flushing of face and neck, dizziness (esp. if patient is standing immobile or is in a warm environment), weakness, postural hypotension • Sublingual: Burning, tingling sensation at oral point of dissolution • Ointment: Erythema, pruritus • Occasional: GI upset. Transdermal: contact dermatitis Adverse/toxic • Drug should be discontinued if blurred vision, dry mouth, occurs. • Severe postural hypotension manifested by fainting, pulselessness, cold/clammy skin, profuse sweating. • Tolerance may occur with repeated, prolonged therapy (minor tolerance with intermittent use of sublingual tablets). High dose tends to produce severe headache.
Patient education	• Rise slowly from lying to sitting position and dangle legs momentarily before standing. • Take oral form on empty stomach (however, if headache occurs during therapy, take medication with meals). • Use inhalants only when lying down. • Dissolve sublingual tablet under tongue. Do not swallow. • Take at first sign of angina; if not relieved within 5 minutes dissolve second tablet under tongue. Repeat if no relief in another 5 minutes. If pain continues, contact healthcare provider or go to emergency department. • Do not change brands. • Keep container away from heat and moisture. • Do not inhale lingual aerosol, but spray onto or under tongue (avoid swallowing after spray is administered). Expel from mouth any remaining lingual/sublingual/intrabuccal tablet after pain is completely relieved. Place transmucosal tablets under upper lip or buccal pouch (between cheek and gum). Do not chew or swallow tablet. • Avoid alcohol (intensifies hypotensive effect). If alcohol is ingested soon after taking nitroglycerin, possible acute hypotensive episode (marked drop in B/P, vertigo, pallor) may occur.

CALCIUM CHANNEL BLOCKER

Use	PO: Treatment of angina due to coronary artery spasm (Prinzmetal's variant angina), chronic stable angina (effort-associated angina). Extended release: Treatment of essential hypertension and angina. Parenteral: Temporary control of rapid ventricular rate in atrial fibrillation/flutter. Rapid conversion of PSVT to normal sinus rhythm.	Half-life: 3–8 hours	Onset: PO: 30–60 minutes IV: Immediate	Peaks: 6–12 h	Duration: 24 hours
Example	Diltiazem hydrochloride (Cardizem)	Route: PO/IV	Pregnancy category: C	Pharmacokinetic: Well absorbed from GI tract. PB: 70%–80%; Undergoes first-pass metabolism in liver. Metabolized in liver; excreted in urine; not removed by hemodialysis	
How it works	• Inhibits calcium movement across cell membranes of cardiac and vascular smooth muscle (dilates coronary arteries, peripheral arteries/arterioles): decreases heart rate, myocardial contractility, slows SA and AV conduction. Decreases total peripheral vascular resistance by vasodilation				
Adult dose	Angina • PO: Initially 30 mg four times/day; increase up to 180–360 mg/day in three to four divided doses at 1- to 2-day intervals; (CD capsules): Initially 120–180 mg/day; titrate over 7–14 days; range: up to 480 mg/day				

Essential hypertension
- PO (extended-release): Initially 60–120 mg two times/day; (CD capsules): Initially 180–240 mg/day; Range: 240–360 mg/day; Range: 180–480 mg/day; (Dilacor XR): Initially, 180–240 mg/day; Range; 180–480 mg/day

Usual parenteral dosage
- IV Push: Initially 0.25 mg/kg actual body weight over 2 min; may repeat in 15 min at dose of 0.35 mg/kg actual body weight; subsequent doses individualized
- IV Infusion: After initial bolus injection 5–10 mg/h may increase at 5 mg/h up to 15 mg/h. Maintain over 24 h. *Note:* Refer to manufacturer's information for dose concentration/infusion rate.

Before administration	• Concurrent therapy of sublingual nitroglycerin may be used for relief of anginal pain. • Record onset, type (sharp, dull, squeezing), radiation, location, intensity, and duration of anginal pain, and precipitating factors (exertion, emotional stress). • Assess baseline renal/liver function tests. • Assess B/P; apical pulse immediately before drug is administered.
Administration	• PO: Give before meals and at bedtime; tablets may be crushed; do not crush sustained-release capsules. • IV: Infuse per dilution/rate chart provided by manufacturer.
After administration	• Monitor vital signs; pulse rate for bradycardia. • Assist with ambulation if dizziness occurs. • Assess for peripheral edema behind medial malleolus or the sacral area in bedridden patients. • Assess for asthenia or headache.
Contraindications	• Sick sinus syndrome/second- or third-degree AV block (except in presence of pacemaker), severe hypotension (less than 90 mmHg systolic), acute MI, pulmonary congestion • *Cautions:* Impaired renal/hepatic function, CHF
Side effects/adverse reactions	• Frequent: Peripheral edema, dizziness, lightheadedness, headache, bradycardia, asthenia (loss of strength, weakness) • Occasional: Nausea, constipation, flushing, altered ECG • Rare: Rash, micturition disorder (polyuria, nocturia, dysuria, frequency of urination), abdominal discomfort, somnolence Adverse/Toxic • Abrupt withdrawal may increase frequency/duration of angina; CHF, second- and third-degree AV block occur rarely. • Overdose produces nausea, drowsiness, confusion, slurred-speech, and profound bradycardia.
Patient education	• Do not abruptly discontinue medication. • Compliance with therapeutic regimen is essential to control anginal pain. • To avoid hypotensive effect rise slowly from lying to sitting position, wait momentarily before standing. • Avoid tasks that require alertness, motor skills until response to drug is established. • Contact healthcare provider if irregular heartbeat, shortness of breath, pronounced dizziness, nausea, or constipation occurs.

19.10   Antidysrhythmics

Antidysrhythmics restore normal cardiac rhythm in cardiac dysrhythmias. Cardiac dysrhythmia (arrhythmia) is deviation from the cardiac rate. These deviations are:

- Irregular heart rate
- Bradycardia (slow heart rate)
- Tachycardia (fast heart rate)

Table 19.2 lists the actions of Antidysthythmics and Table 19.3 describes classes of Antidysthythmics. There are four classes of Antidysrhythmics. These are:

1. Fast (sodium) channel blockers: 1A (I) (quinidine and procainamide), 1B (II) (lidocaine), and IC (III) (encainide, flecainide)
2. Beta-blockers: (see 19.9 Antianginals)
3. Prolong repolarization: Medications that extend the time when the electrical impulse returns to normal and is ready to fire again. Commonly prescribed prolonged repolarizations are:
   a. Bretylium (Bretylol)
   b. Amiodarone (Cordarone)
4. Slow (calcium) channel blockers (see 19.9 Antianginals)

TABLE 19.2 Antidysrhythmic Actions

MECHANISMS OF ACTION
Block adrenergic stimulation of the heart
Depress myocardial excitability and contractility
Decrease conduction velocity in cardiac tissue
Increase recovery time (repolarization) of the myocardium
Suppress automaticity (spontaneous depolarization to initiate beats)

TABLE 19.3 Classes and Actions of Antidysrhythmic Drugs

CLASSES	ACTIONS	EXAMPLES/SIDE EFFECTS
Class I Sodium channel blockers		
IA	Slows conduction; prolongs repolarization	Procainamide (Pronestyl, Procan) (less cardiac depression than quinidine, abdominal pain/cramping, nausea, diarrhea, vomiting, flushing, rash, pruritus, lupus-like syndrome with rash). Quinidine sulfate, polygalactorate, gluconate (Quinidex, Cardioquin) (nausea, vomiting, diarrhea, confusion, and hypotension).
IB	Slows conduction and shortens repolarization	Lidocaine (Xylocaine) (cardiovascular depression, bradycardia, and hypotension; dizziness, lightheadedness, and confusion)
IC	Prolongs conduction with little to no effect on repolarization	Flecainide (Tambocor) (nausea, vomiting, diarrhea, confusion)
Class II Beta blockers	Reduces calcium entry; decreases conduction velocity, automaticity, and recovery time (refractory period)	Esmolol (Brevibloc) (generally well tolerated, with transient and mild side effects) Propranolol HCl (Inderal) (Decreased sexual ability, drowsiness, difficulty sleeping, unusual tiredness/weakness)
Class III Prolong repolarization	Prolongs repolarization during ventricular dysrhythmias Prolongs action potential duration	Adenosine (Adenocard) (Facial flushing, shortness of breath,/dyspnea) Amiodarone HCl (Cordarone) (Corneal microdeposits are noted in almost all patients treated for greater than 6 months [can lead to blurry vision], hypotension, nausea, fever, bradycardia,

(Continued)

(Continued from previous page)

CLASSES	ACTIONS	EXAMPLES/SIDE EFFECTS
		constipation, headache, decreased appetite, nausea, vomiting, numbness of fingers/toes, photosensitivity, lack of muscular coordination); Bretylium tosylate (Bretylol) (Transitory hypertension followed by postural and supine hypotension in 50% of patients observed as dizziness, lightheadedness, faintness, vertigo)
Class IV Calcium channel lockers	Blocks calcium influx; slows conduction velocity, decreases myocardial contractility (negative inotropic), and increases refraction in the AV node	Verapamil HCl (Calan) (Constipation, dizziness, lightheadedness, headache, asthenia [loss of strength, energy]) Diltiazem (Cardizem) (Peripheral edema, dizziness, lightheadedness, headache, bradycardia, asthenia [loss of strength, weakness], nausea, constipation, flushing, altered ECG)

FAST (SODIUM) CHANNEL BLOCKER

Use	Prophylactic therapy to maintain normal sinus rhythm after conversion of atrial fibrillation and/or flutter. Treatment of premature ventricular contractions, paroxysmal atrial tachycardia, atrial fibrillation, ventricular tachycardia. Conversion/management of atrial fibrillation and PAT.	Half-life: 2.5–4.5 h	Onset: PO: 30 minutes IV: minutes	Peaks: PO: 1–1.5 h IV: 25–60 min	Duration: PO: 3–4 h (SR: 8H) IV: 3–4 h
Example	Procainamide (Pronestyl, Procan)	Route: PO/IV	Pregnancy category: C	Pharmacokinetic: Rapidly, completely absorbed from GI tract. PB: 15%–20%. Widely distributed; metabolized in liver; excreted in urine; removed by hemodialysis.	

How it works
- Prolongs refractory period by direct effect, decreasing myocardial excitability and conduction velocity. Depresses myocardial contractility.

Adult dose
Arrhythmias:
- IV 50–100 mg/dose; may repeat q5–10 min or 15–18 mg/kg; Maximum: 1–1.5 g then maintenance infusion of 3–4 mg/min; Range: 1–6 mg/min
- PO: Immediate-release: 250–500 mg q3–6 h; Sustained-release: 0.5–1 g q6 h; Procanbid: 1–2 g q12h

Before administration
- Check B/P and pulse for 1 full min (unless patient is on continuous monitor) before giving medication.
- Check drug and medical history.

Administration
- PO: Do not crush or break sustained-release tablets.
- IM/IV: May give by IM, IV push, or IV infusion
- For IV push, with patient in supine position, administer at rate not exceeding 25–60 mg/min; initial loading infusion, infuse 1 ml/min for up to 25–30 min; for IV infusion infused at 1–3 ml/min; check BP during infusion; if fall exceeds 15 mm Hg discontinue drug; contact prescriber
- B/P, ECG should be monitored continuously during IV administration and rate of infusion adjusted to eliminate arrhythmias.

After administration	• Monitor ECG for cardiac changes, particularly widening of QRS, prolongation of PR and QT interval. Notify provider of significant interval changes.
	• Assess pulse for strength/weakness, irregular rate.
	• Monitor intake and output.
	• Monitor electrolyte serum level (potassium, chloride, sodium).
	• Assess for complaints of GI upset, headache, dizziness, joint pain.
	• Monitor pattern of daily bowel activity, stool consistency.
	• Assess for dizziness.
	• Monitor B/P for hypotension.
	• Assess skin for evidence of hypersensitivity reaction (especially those on high dose therapy).
	• Monitor for therapeutic serum level (3–10 mcg/ml); therapeutic level 4–8 mcg/ml; toxic blood serum level greater than 10 mcg/ml
Contraindications	• Complete AV block; second- and third-degree AV block without pacemaker, abnormal impulses/rhythms because of escape mechanism
	• *Cautions:* Ventricular tachycardia during coronary occlusion, renal/hepatic disease, incomplete AV nodal block, digitalis intoxication, CHF, pre-existing hypotension
Side effects/adverse reactions	• Frequent: PO: Abdominal pain/ cramping nausea, diarrhea, vomiting
	• Occasional: Dizziness, giddiness, weakness, hypersensitivity reaction (rash, urticaria, pruritus, flushing)
	• Infrequent: IV: Transient but at times marked hypotension
	• Rare: Confusion, mental depression, psychosis
	Adverse/Toxic
	• Paradoxical, extremely rapid ventricular rate may occur during treatment of atrial fibrillation/flutter
	• Systemic lupus erythematosus-like syndrome (fever, joint pain, pleuritic chest pain) with prolonged therapy
	• Cardiotoxic effects occur most commonly with IV administration, observed as conduction changes (50% widening of QRS complex, frequent ventricular premature contractions, ventricular tachycardia, complete AV block)
	• Prolonged PR and QT intervals, flattened T waves occur less frequently (discontinue drug immediately)
Patient education	• Take medication at evenly spaced doses around the clock.
	• Contact provider if fever, joint pain/stiffness, or signs of upper respiratory infection occur.
	• Do not abruptly discontinue medication.
	• Compliance with therapy regimen is essential to control arrhythmias.
	• Do not use nasal decongestants or OTC cold preparations (stimulants) without prescriber approval.
	• Restrict salt and alcohol intake.

19.11 Heart Failure Medication

Heart failure is any structural or functional disorder that prevents the heart from filling with blood or pumping blood sufficiently. Heart failure is treated with:

- Vasodilators:
  - Increase cardiac output by reducing cardiac afterload.
  - Dilate the arterioles in the kidneys improving renal perfusion and increase fluid loss.
  - Improve circulation to the skeletal muscles.
- Angiotensin-converting enzyme (ACE) inhibitors: Decrease the release of aldosterone, reducing sodium retention and resulting in improved renal blood flow and decreased fluid volume by dilating dilate venules and arterioles.
- Diuretics: (see 19.17 Diuretics) Reduce fluid volume

19.12   Hypertension

Hypertension is increased blood pressure of systolic pressure greater than 140 mmHg and diastolic pressure greater than 90 mmHg. There are two types of hypertension. These are:

- Essential hypertension: Caused by conditions other than related to renal and endocrine disorders
- Secondary hypertension: Caused by renal and endocrine disorders

There are three stages of hypertension. These are:

- Pre-hypertension: 120–129/80–89 mmHg
- Stage 1 hypertension: 140–159/90–99 mmHg
- Stage 2 hypertension: at or greater than 160–179/100–109 mmHg

19.13   Blood Pressure and Kidneys

Blood pressure is maintained by the kidneys using the rennin-angiotensin system, which increases blood pressure by retaining sodium and water. Blood pressure is monitored by baroreceptors in the aorta and carotid sinus. If blood pressure is too high, then the baroreceptors signal the vasomotor center in the medulla to signal the rennin-angiotensin system to excrete sodium and water, thereby lowering the blood pressure. If blood pressure is too low, then the baroreceptors signal the vasomotor center in the medulla to signal the rennin-angiotensin system to retain sodium and water, thereby increasing the blood pressure.

19.14   Antihypertensives

Antihypertensives are used to treat hypertension in a stepped-care treatment after nonpharmacological treatment (lose weight, reduce sodium, limit alcohol consumption, stop smoking, exercise) has not achieved the desired results. The stepped-care treatment follows these steps. Treatment progresses to the next step if blood pressure remains elevated.

1. Diuretics or beta-blockers
2. Increase dose of diuretics, beta blockers, calcium blocker, ACE inhibitor, A-II blocker, or a combination
3. Diuretic with beta-blocker, added calcium blocker, ACE inhibitor or alpha blocker, or centrally acting sympatholytic
4. Administer two or three additional medications such as alpha blockers, direct-acting vasodilators, or adrenergic neuron blockers.

19.15   Combining Antihypertensive Drugs

There are five categories of antihypertensives.

Diuretics

Diuretics (see 19.17 Diuretics) are prescribed for hypertension that is not caused by renal-angiotensin-aldosterone involvement because diuretics increase rennin serum level. Diuretics promote sodium depletion decreasing extracellular fluid volume. Commonly prescribed diuretics are:

- Hydrochlorothiazide (Hydro DIURIL): Not used in renal insufficiency because it depresses renal flow. Combined with beta-blockers and angiotensin-converting enzyme to maintain serum potassium level.
- Furosemide (Lasix): Loop diuretic used for renal insufficiency because it does not depress renal flow.

Sympatholytics (Sympathetic Depressants)

There are five groups of sympatholytics (see chapter 15). These are:

1. Beta-Adrenergic Blockers: acebutolol HCl (Sectral), atenolol (Tenormin), metoprolol (Lopressor), Nadolol (Corgard), propranolol (Inderal)
2. Centrally Acting Sympatholytics (adrenergic blockers): clonidine HCl (Catapres), methyldopa (Aldomet)
3. Alpha-Adrenergic Blockers Phentolamine (Regitine); selective: Doxazosin mesylate (Cardura), terazosin HCl (Hytrin)
4. Adrenergic Neuron Blockers (peripherally acting sympatholytics): Guanethidine monosulfate (Ismelin), reserpine (Serpasil)
5. Alpha- and Beta-Adrenergic Blockers: Carteolol HCl (Cartrol, Ocupress)

Direct Arteriolar Vasodilators

Direct-acting arteriolar vasodilators relax the smooth muscles of the blood vessels, causing vasodilation, which results in an increase in blood flow to the brain and kidneys. Direct-acting arteriolar can be combined with diuretics to decrease the edema.

Angiotensin Antagonists

Angiotensin antagonists inhibit angiotensin-converting enzyme (ACE), resulting in inhibiting the formation of angiotensin II (vasoconstrictor) which blocks the release of aldosterone and causes lowered peripheral resistance.

Calcium Channel Blockers

Calcium channel blockers (see 19.9 Antianginals) dilate coronary arteries and arterioles, and decrease total peripheral vascular resistance.

DIRECT-ACTING ARTERIOLAR VASODILATORS

Use	Immediate reduction of B/P in hypertensive crisis. Produces controlled hypotension in surgical procedures to reduce bleeding. Treatment of acute CHF. Controls paroxysmal hypertension before/during surgery for pheochromocytoma; treatment adjunct for myocardial infarction, valvular regurgitation, peripheral vasospasm caused by ergot alkaloid overdose.	Half-life: 2 minutes	Onset: 1–2 minutes	Peaks: Dependent on infusion rate	Duration: Dissipates rapidly after stopping IV
Example	Sodium nitroprusside (Nitropride, Nitropress)	Route: IV	Pregnancy category: C	Pharmacokinetic: Reacts with hemoglobin in erythrocytes, producing cyanmethemoglobin, cyanide ions. Primarily excreted in urine.	
How it works	• Direct vasodilating action on arterial, venous smooth muscle. Decreases peripheral vascular resistance, preload, afterload, improves cardiac output. Dilates coronary arteries, decreases O_2 consumption, relieves persistent chest pain				
Adult dose	• IV: Initially 0.3 mcg/kg/min. Range: 0.5–10 mcg/kg/min. Do not exceed 10 mcg/kg/min (risk of precipitous drop in B/P).				

Before administration	• Patient must have continuous ECG monitoring and B/P monitoring. B/P is normally maintained about 30%–40% below pretreatment levels.
	• Assess medical and drug history.
Administration	• Protect solution from light; it should appear very faint brown in color; use only freshly prepared solution; once prepared do no keep or use longer than 24 hours; deterioration evidenced by color change from brown to blue, green, or dark red.
	• Discard unused portion.
	• Give by IV infusion only using infusion rate chart provided by manufacturer or protocol.
	• Administer using IV infusion pump or microdrip (60 gtt/min). Be alert for extravasation (produces severe pain, sloughing).
After administration	• Monitor rate of infusion frequently.
	• Monitor blood acid–base balance.
	• Medication should be discontinued if therapeutic response is not achieved within 10 minutes following IV infusion at 10 mcg/kg/min.
	• Monitor electrolytes, laboratory results.
	• Monitor intake and output
	• Assess for metabolic acidosis (weakness, disorientation, headache, nausea, hyperventilation, vomiting).
	• Monitor for potential rebound hypertension after infusion is discontinued.
Contraindications	• Compensatory hypertension (arteriovenous shunt or coarctation of aorta), inadequate cerebral circulation, moribund patients
	• *Cautions:* Severe hepatic, renal impairment, hypothyroidism, hyponatremia, elderly people
Side effects/adverse reactions	• Occasional: Flushing of skin, increased intracranial pressure, rash, pain/redness at injection site
	Adverse/Toxic
	• A too-rapid IV rate reduces B/P too quickly. Nausea, retching, diaphoresis (sweating), apprehension, headache, restlessness, muscle twitching, dizziness, palpitation retrosternal pain, and abdominal pain may occur. Symptoms disappear rapidly if rate of administration is slowed or temporarily discontinued.
	• Overdosage produces metabolic acidosis, tolerance to therapeutic effect.
Patient education	• Explain all procedures to patient and family.

19.16   Angiotensin Antagonists, ACE Inhibitors, and Angiotensin II

Angiotensin antagonists (Angiotensin-converting enzyme inhibitors) and ACE inhibitors lower blood pressure and are used to treat heart failure by causing the excretion of sodium and water. ACE inhibitors block the release of aldosterone. Aldosterone causes the retention of sodium. Cardiac output and heart rate remain unchanged. ACE inhibitors are administered to patients with elevated serum rennin levels. ACE inhibitors can cause angioedema in which the mouth, throat, lips, eyelids, hands, and feet swell.

Commonly prescribed ACE inhibitors are:

- Benazepril (Lotensin)
- Captopril (Capoten)
- Enalapril maleate (Vasotec)
- Enalaprilat (Vasotec IV)
- Lisinopril (Prinivil, Zestril)
- Ramipril (Altace)
- Losartan (Cozaar)
- Valsartan (Diovan)
- Irbesartan (Avapro)

ACE INHIBITORS

Use	Treatment of hypertension alone or in combination with other antihypertensives. Adjunctive therapy for CHF (in combination with cardiac glycosides, diuretics). Treatment of diabetic nephropathy, hypertension, or renal crisis in scleroderma.	Half-life: 11 hours	Onset: PO: 1 hour IV: 15 minutes	Peaks: PO: 4–6 hours IV: 1–4 hours	Duration: PO: 24 hours IV: 6 hours
Example	Enalapril maleate (Vasotec)	Route: PO/IV	Pregnancy category: D	Pharmacokinetic: Readily absorbed from GI tract (not affected by food). PB: 50%–60%; excreted in urine.	

How it works

- Suppresses rennin-angiotensin-aldosterone system (prevents conversion of angiotensin I to angiotensin II, a potent vasoconstrictor; may inhibit angiotensin II at local vascular, renal sites).
- Decreases plasma angiotensin II, increases plasma rennin activity, decreases aldosterone secretion.
- In hypertension, reduces peripheral arterial resistance.
- In CHF, increases cardiac output, decreases peripheral vascular resistance, B/P, pulmonary capillary wedge pressure, and heart rate.

Adult dose

Hypertension
- PO: Initially, 2.5–5 mg/day; Range: 10–40 mg/day in one to two divided doses.
- IV: 0.625–1.25 mg q6h up to 5 mg q6h

CHF:
- PO: Initially 2.5–5 mg/day; Range: 5–20 mg/day in two divided doses.

Before administration

- Obtain drug and medical history.
- Obtain B/P immediately before each dose (be alert to fluctuations).
- In patients with renal impairment, autoimmune disease, or taking drugs that affect leukocytes or immune response, CBC should be performed before therapy begins.

Administration

- Give without regard to food.
- Tablets may be crushed.
- For IV push, given undiluted over 5 minutes.
- For IV piggyback infuse over 10–15 minutes.

After administration

- Assist with ambulation if dizziness occurs.
- Monitor serum potassium, BUN, serum creatinine levels.
- Monitor pattern of daily bowel activity and stool consistency.
- Monitor for therapeutic response.

Contraindications

- History of angioedema with previous treatment with ACE inhibitors
- *Cautions:* Renal impairment, those with sodium depletion or on diuretic therapy, dialysis, hypovolemia, coronary/cerebrovascular insufficiency

Side effects/adverse reactions

- Frequent: Postural hypotension, headache, dizziness
- Occasional: Orthostatic hypotension, fatigue, diarrhea, cough, syncope
- Rare: Angina, abdominal pain, vomiting, nausea, rash, asthenia (loss of strength/energy), fainting

Adverse/Toxic
- Excessive hypotension ("first-dose" syncope) may occur in those with CHF, severely salt/volume depleted
- Angioedema (swelling of face, lips), hyperkalemia occurs rarely
- Agranulocytosis, neutropenia may be noted in patients with impaired renal function or collagen vascular disease (systemic lupus erythematosus, scleroderma)
- Nephrotic syndrome may be noted in those with history of renal disease

Patient education	• To reduce hypotensive effect, rise slowly from lying to sitting position and permit legs to dangle from bed momentarily before standing.
	• Several weeks may be needed for full therapeutic effect of B/P reduction.
	• Skipping doses or voluntarily discontinuing drug may produce severe, rebound hypertension.

19.17 Diuretics

Diuretics inhibit sodium and water reabsorption from the kidney tubules, resulting in diuresis (increase urine flow), lower blood pressure, and a decrease in peripheral and pulmonary edema. Diuretics influence one or more renal tubular segments, which is where most sodium and water is reabsorbed. Electrolytes, drugs, glucose, and waste products from protein metabolism are filtered in the glomeruli during this process. Every 1.5 hours, all extracellular fluid (ECF) is filtered by glomeruli (kidneys). Large products (protein and blood) remain in circulation and are not filtered by renal function.

Filtered sodium is reabsorbed at the proximal tubules, the Loop of Henle, distal tubules, or in the collecting tubules. Diuretics influence tubules closest to the glomeruli, causing natriuresis (sodium loss in the urine). Diuretics cause loss of other electrolytes (potassium, magnesium, chloride, bicarbonate). Diuretics that promote potassium excretion are called potassium-wasting diuretics or potassium-sparing diuretics.

19.18 Types of Diuretics

There are five categories of diuretics. These are:

- Thiazide and thiazide-like
- Loop or high-ceiling
- Osmotic
- Carbonic anhydrase inhibitor
- Potassium-sparing

19.19 Thiazide Diuretics

Thiazides cause sodium, chloride, potassium, magnesium, and water excretion (reabsorbs calcium) by affecting the distal convoluted renal tubule beyond the loop of Henle. Thiazides are not effective for immediate diuresis. When administering thiazides:

- Monitor electrolytes and glucose. Thiazides influence glucose tolerance and should not be administered to diabetics.
- Monitor kidney function. Do not administer thiazides to patients who have kidney disorders.
- Monitor for hyperuricemia (elevated serum uric acid level).
- Monitor for hyperlipidemia (elevated blood lipid levels).

Adverse effects of thiazides are:

- Dizziness
- Headaches
- Nausea
- Vomiting
- Constipation
- Urticaria (hives)
- Blood dyscrasias

THIAZIDE DIURETIC

Use	Adjunctive therapy in edema associated with CHF, hepatic cirrhosis, corticoid or estrogen therapy, renal impairment. In treatment of hypertension, may be used alone or with other antihypertensive agents. Treatment of diabetes insipidus; prevents calcium-containing renal stones.	Half-life: 5.6–14.8 hours	Onset: 2 hours	Peaks: 4–6 hours	Duration: 6–12 hours

Example	Hydrochlorothiazide (Hydro DIURIL, HCTZ)	Route: PO	Pregnancy category: D	Pharmacokinetic: Variably absorbed from GI tract; excreted in urine. Not removed by hemodialysis.

How it works
- Diuretic: Blocks reabsorption of water, electrolytes (sodium, potassium) at cortical diluting segment of distal tubule, promoting renal excretion
- Antihypertensive: Reduces plasma, extracellular fluid volume, decreases peripheral vascular resistance (PVR) by direct effect on blood vessels, reducing B/P

Adult dose
- 12.5–100 mg/day; Maximum: 200 mg/day

Before administration
- Check vital signs especially B/P for hypotension prior to administration.
- Assess baseline electrolytes; particularly check for low potassium.
- Evaluate edema, skin turgor, mucous membranes for hydration status.
- Assess muscle strength, mental status.
- Note skin temperature, moisture.
- Obtain baseline weight.
- Initiate intake and output.

Administration
- May give with food or milk if GI upset occurs, preferably with breakfast (may prevent nocturia).

After administration
- Continue to monitor B/P, vital signs, electrolytes, I&O, weight.
- Note extent of diuresis. Watch for changes from initial assessment (hypokalemia may result in weakness, tremor, muscle cramps, nausea, vomiting, change in mental status, tachycardia; hyponatremia may result in confusion, thirst, cold/clammy skin.? Be especially alert for potassium depletion in patients taking digoxin (cardiac arrhythmias).
- Potassium supplements are frequently ordered.
- Check for constipation (may occur with excessive diuresis).

Contraindications
- History of hypersensitivity to sulfonamides or thiazide diuretics, renal decompensation, anuria.
- *Cautions:* Severe renal disease, impaired hepatic function, diabetes mellitus, elderly/debilitated, thyroid disorders.

Side effects/ adverse reactions
- Expected: Increase in urine frequency/volume
- Frequent: Potassium depletion
- Occasional: Postural hypotension, headache, GI disturbances, photosensitivity reaction

Adverse/Toxic
- Vigorous diuresis may lead to profound water loss and electrolyte depletion, resulting in hypokalemia, hyponatremia, dehydration.
- Acute hypotensive episodes may occur.
- Hyperglycemia may be noted during prolonged therapy.
- GI upset, pancreatitis, dizziness, paresthesias, headache, blood dyscrasias, pulmonary edema, allergic pneumonitis, dermatologic reactions occur rarely. Overdosage can lead to lethargy, coma without changes in electrolytes or hydration.

Patient education
- Expect increased frequency and volume of urination.
- To reduce hypotensive effect, rise slowly from lying to sitting position and permit legs to dangle momentarily before standing.

- Eat foods high in potassium such as whole grains (cereals), legumes, meat, bananas, apricots, orange juice, potatoes (white, sweet), raisins.
- Protect skin from sun/ultraviolet rays (photosensitivity may occur).

19.20   Loop or High-Ceiling Diuretics

Loop or high-ceiling diuretics inhibit the transport of sodium in the ascending Loop of Henle and result in the excretion of sodium and water, potassium, calcium, and magnesium. Loop diuretics are more effective with inhibiting reabsorption of sodium than thiazides diuretics.

Loop diuretics cause vasodilation, increasing renal blood flow before diuresis and making it the prime choice in diuretics for patients who have decrease kidney function or end-stage renal disease. Side effects are:

- Hypokalemia
- Hyponatremia
- Hypocalcemia
- Hypomagnesemia
- Hypochloremia (leads to metabolic alkalosis)
- Orthostatic hypotension
- Thrombocytopenia
- Skin disturbances
- Transient deafness
- Thiamine deficiency (prolong use)
- Increased uric acid level

LOOP DIURETIC

Use	Treatment of edema associated with CHF, chronic renal failure, including nephritic syndrome, hepatic cirrhosis, acute pulmonary edema. Treats hypertension, either alone or in combination with other antihypertensives. Treatment of hypercalcemia.	Half-life: 30–90 minutes	Onset: PO: 30–60 minutes IM:—IV: 5 minutes	Peaks: 1–2 hours 30 minutes 20–60 minutes	Duration: 6–8 hours — 2 hours
Example	Furosemide (Lasix)	Route: PO/IM/IV	Pregnancy category: C	Pharmacokinetic: Well absorbed from GI tract. PB: 91%–97%; metabolized in liver; excreted in urine (in severe renal impairment, nonrenal clearance increases); not removed by hemodialysis.	
How it works	• Enhances excretion of sodium, chloride, potassium by direct action at ascending loop of Henle, producing diuretic effect				
Adult dose	• Edema/hypertension • PO: Initially 20–80 mg/dose; may increase by 20–40 mg/dose at 6- to 8-h intervals • IM/IV: 20–40 mg/dose may repeat in 1–2 h and increase by 20 mg/dose • IV Infusion: Bolus of 0.1 mg/kg, then 0.1 mg/kg/hr; may double q2 hours. Maximum: 0.4 mg/kg/h				
Before administration	• Check vital signs, especially B/P for hypotension before administration. • Assess baseline electrolytes; particularly check for low potassium. • Evaluate edema, skin turgor, mucous membranes for hydration status. • Assess muscle strength, mental status. • Note skin temperature, moisture.				

	• Obtain baseline weight.
	• Initiate intake and output.
Administration	• PO: Give with food to avoid GI upset, preferably with breakfast (may prevent nocturia).
	• IM: Temporary pain at injection site may be noted.
	• IV: May give undiluted but is compatible with D5W, 0.9% NS, or lactated Ringer's solutions; administer each 40 mg or fraction by IV push over 1–2 min. Do not exceed administration rate of 4 mg/min in those with renal impairment.
After administration	• Continue to monitor B/P, vital signs, electrolytes, I&O, weight.
	• Note extent of diuresis. Watch for changes from initial assessment. (Hypokalemia may result in weakness, tremor, muscle cramps, nausea, vomiting, change in mental status, tachycardia; hyponatremia may result in confusion, thirst, cold/clammy skin.)
	• Be especially alert for potassium depletion in patients taking digoxin (cardiac arrhythmias).
	• Potassium supplements are frequently ordered.
	• Check for constipation (may occur with excessive diuresis).
Contraindications	• Anuria, hepatic coma, severe electrolyte depletion
	• *Cautions:* Acute MI, oliguria, hepatic cirrhosis, history of gout, diabetes, systemic lupus erythematosus, pancreatitis
Side effects/ adverse reactions	• Expected: Increase in urinary frequency volume
	• Frequent: Nausea, gastric upset with cramping, diarrhea, or constipation, electrolyte disturbances
	• Occasional: Dizziness, lightheadedness, headache, blurred vision, paresthesia, photosensitivity, rash, weakness, urinary frequency/bladder spasm, restlessness, diaphoresis
	• Rare: Flank pain, loin pain
	Adverse/Toxic
	• Vigorous diuresis may lead to profound water loss and electrolyte depletion, resulting in hypokalemia, hyponatremia, dehydration. Sudden volume depletion may result in increased risk of thrombosis, circulatory collapse, sudden death. Acute hypotensive episodes may also occur, sometimes several days after beginning therapy.
	• Ototoxicity manifested as deafness, vertigo, tinnitus (ringing/roaring in ears) may occur especially in those with severe renal impairment.
	• Can exacerbate diabetes mellitus, systemic lupus erythematosus, gout, and pancreatitis.
	• Blood dyscrasias have been reported.
Patient education	• Expect increased frequency and volume of urination.
	• Report irregular heartbeat, signs of electrolyte imbalances (noted in the preceding), hearing abnormalities (such as sense of fullness in ears, ringing/roaring in ears).
	• Eat foods high in potassium such as whole grains (cereals), legumes, meat, bananas, apricots, orange juice, potatoes (white, sweet), raisins.
	• Avoid sun and sunlamps.

19.21 Osmotic Diuretics

Osmotic diuretics increase the osmolality (concentration) of the plasma and fluid in the renal tubules resulting in excretion of sodium, chloride, potassium (lesser degree), and water. Osmotic diuretics:

- Prevent kidney failure
- Decrease intracranial pressure (ICP) (cerebral edema)
- Decrease intraocular pressure (IOP) (e.g., glaucoma)

The most commonly prescribed osmotic diuretic is mannitol. Mannitol:

- Treats emergency intraocular pressure
- Induces frank diuresis when given with cisplatin and carboplatin to decrease the side effect of chemotherapy
- Can cause fluid and electrolyte imbalance, pulmonary edema (rapid shift of fluids)
- Can cause nausea, vomiting, tachycardia (rapid shift of fluids)

19.22   Carbonic Anhydrase Inhibitors

Carbonic anhydrase inhibitors increase excretion of sodium, potassium, and bicarbonate by blocking carbonic anhydrase, which is an enzyme that maintains acid-base balance. Carbonic anhydrase inhibitors are contraindicated in the first trimester of pregnancy.

Carbonic anhydrase inhibitors:

- Decrease intraocular pressure in patients with open-angle (not narrow-angle or acute) glaucoma
- Manages epilepsy
- Treats high-altitude sickness
- Treats acute mountain sickness

Side effects are:

- Fluid and electrolyte imbalance
- Metabolic acidosis
- Nausea
- Vomiting
- Anorexia
- Confusion
- Orthostatic hypotension
- Crystalluria
- Hemolytic anemia
- Renal calculi

CARBONIC ANHYDRASE INHIBITORS

Use	Treatment of open-angle, secondary or angle closure glaucoma, adjunct in managing absence seizures (e.g., petit mal), tonic-clonic, simple partial and myoclonic seizures. Prophylaxis/treatment of altitude sickness. Lowers intraocular pressure in treatment of altitude sickness. Lowers intraocular pressure in treatment of malignant glaucoma, treatment of toxicity of weakly acidic medications, prevents uric acid/renal calculi by alkalinizing the urine.	Half-life: 1–2 hours	Onset: 30 minutes	Peaks: 2–4 hours	Duration: 4–6 hours
Example	Acetazolamide (Diamox)	Route: PO/IV	Pregnancy category: B	Pharmacokinetic: Well-absorbed PO; metabolized in liver; excreted in urine.	

How it works	• Reduces formation of hydrogen and bicarbonate ions from carbon dioxide and water by inhibiting, in proximal renal tubule, the enzyme carbonic anhydrase, thereby promoting renal excretion of sodium, potassium, bicarbonate, water. • Ocular: Reduces the rate of aqueous humor formation, lowers intraocular pressure. Diamox only: Increases CO_2 tension, retards neuronal conduction, producing anticonvulsant activity.
Adult dose	Glaucoma: • PO: 250 mg one to four times/day; Extended release: 50 mg two times/day • IV: 500 mg may repeat in 24 hours, then continue with oral therapy Epilepsy: • PO: 375–1000 mg/day in up to four divided dose

	Altitude sickness: • PO: 250 mg two to four times/day. If possible begin 24–48 hours before ascent; continue for at least 48 hours at high altitude as needed to control symptom
Before administration	Glaucoma: • Assess affected pupil for dilation, response to light. Epilepsy: • Obtain history of seizure disorder (length, intensity, duration of seizure, presence of aura, LOC).
Administration	• Give without regard for food.
After administration	• Monitor for acidosis (headache, lethargy progressing to drowsiness, CNS depression, Kussmaul's respiration).
Contraindications	• Hypersensitivity to sulfonamides, severe renal disease, adrenal insufficiency, hypochloremic acidosis • *Cautions:* History of hypercalcemia, diabetes mellitus, gout, digitalized patients, obstructive pulmonary disease
Side effects/ adverse reactions	• Frequent: Unusually tired/weak, diarrhea, increased urination/frequency, decreased appetite/weight, altered taste (metallic), nausea, vomiting, numbness in extremities, lips, mouth • Occasional: Depression, drowsiness • Rare: Headache, photosensitivity, confusion, tinnitus, severe muscle weakness, loss of taste Adverse/Toxic • Long-term therapy may result in acidotic state. • Nephrotoxicity/hepatotoxicity occurs occasionally, manifested as dark urine/stools, pain in lower back, jaundice, dysuria, crystalluria, renal colic/calculi. • Bone marrow depression may be manifested as aplastic anemia, thrombocytopenia, thrombocytopenic purpura, leucopenia, agranulocytosis, hemolytic anemia.
Patient education	• Report presence of tingling or tremor in hands or feet, unusual bleeding/bruising, unexplained fever, sore throat, flank pain.

19.23   Potassium-Sparing Diuretics

Potassium-sparing diuretics excrete sodium and water and retain potassium by interfering with the sodium-potassium pump in the collecting distal duct renal tubules. Potassium-sparing diuretics do not require potassium supplements, which are needed with potassium-wasting diuretics. The diuretic effect is intensified with the combined use of potassium-sparing diuretics and potassium-wasting diuretic.

When administering potassium-sparing diuretics:

- Urine output must be at least 600 ml per day.
- Avoid potassium supplements.
- Monitor for hyperkalemia if taken along with ACE inhibitors.
- Monitor for anorexia, nausea, vomiting, and diarrhea.

POTASSIUM-SPARING DIURETIC

Use		Half-life:	Onset:	Peaks:	Duration:
	Treatment of excessive aldosterone production, essential hypertension, edema due to CHF; CHF, cirrhosis of liver/nephritic syndrome. Adjunct to potassium-losing diuretics or to potentiate action of other diuretics. Diagnosis of hyperaldosteronism. Treatment of polycystic ovary syndrome, female hirsutism.	0–24 hours	24–48 hours	48–72 hours	48–72 hours

| Example | Spironolactone (Aldactone) | Route: PO | Pregnancy category: D | Pharmacokinetic: Well absorbed from GI tract (increased with food). PB: 91%–98%; metabolized in liver; excreted in urine; unknown if removed by hemodialysis |

How it works
- Competitively inhibits action of aldosterone. Interferes with sodium reabsorption in distal tubule, increasing potassium retention while promoting sodium and water excretion.

Adult dose

Diuretic/hypertension
- PO: 25–200 mg/day in one to two divided doses

CHF:
- PO: 25 mg/day

Diagnosis of primary aldosteronism:
- PO: 100–400 mg/day in one to two divided doses

Before administration
- Weigh patient.
- Initiate intake and output.
- Evaluate hydration status by assessing mucous membranes, skin turgor.
- Obtain baseline electrolytes, renal/hepatic functions, and urinalysis.
- Assess for edema; note location and extent.
- Check baseline vital signs, and note pulse rate/regularity.

Administration

PO
- Oral suspension containing crushed tablets in cherry syrup is stable for up to 30 days if refrigerated.
- Drug absorption enhanced if taken with food; scored tablets may be crushed; do not crush or break film-coated tablets.

After administration
- Monitor electrolyte values, especially for increased potassium.
- Monitor B/P levels.
- Monitor for hyponatremia, mental confusion, thirst, cold/clammy skin, drowsiness, dry mouth.
- Monitor for hyperkalemia: colic, diarrhea, muscle twitching followed by weakness/paralysis and arrhythmias.
- Obtain daily weight.
- Note changes in edema, skin turgor.

Contraindications
- Acute renal insufficiency/impairment, anuria, BUN/creatinine over twice normal values levels, hyperkalemia;
- *Cautions:* Hepatic/renal impairment.

Side effects/ adverse reactions
- Frequent: Hyperkalemia for those on potassium supplements or those with renal insufficiency; dehydration, hyponatremia, lethargy
- Occasional: Nausea, vomiting, anorexia, cramping diarrhea, headache, ataxia, drowsiness, confusion, fever
- Male: Gynecomastia, impotence, decreased libido
- Female: Menstrual irregularities/amenorrhea, postmenopausal bleeding, breast tenderness
- Rare: Rash, urticaria, hirsutism

Adverse/Toxic
- Severe hyperkalemia may produce arrhythmias, bradycardia, tented T waves, widening QRS, ST depression. These can proceed to cardiac standstill or ventricular fibrillation.
- Cirrhosis patients are at risk for hepatic decompensation if dehydration/hyponatremia occurs.
- Those with primary aldosteronism may experience rapid weight loss, severe fatigue during high-dose therapy.

Patient education
- Expect increase in volume, frequency of urination.
- Therapeutic effect takes several days to begin and can last for several days when drug is discontinued.
- This may not apply if patient is on a potassium-losing drug concomitantly (diet and use of supplements should be established by prescriber).

- Notify provider for irregular/slow pulse, electrolyte imbalance (signs noted in the preceding).
- Avoid food high in potassium such as whole grains (cereals), legumes, meat, bananas, apricots, orange juice, potatoes (white, sweet), and raisins.

19.24 Circulatory Medication

Circulatory medication treats impaired blood flow by either restoring or preventing disruption of blood flow. There are four groups of circulatory medication. These are:

- Anticoagulants and antiplatelets (antithrombotics): Prevent platelets from aggregating, reducing risk for a blood clot.
- Thrombolytics (clot busters): Dissolve blood clots.
- Antilipemics: Decrease concentrations of blood lipids.
- Peripheral vasodilators: Dilate blood vessels.

19.25 Anticoagulants and Antiplatelets

Blood stasis (decreased circulation) results in formation of a thrombus (blood clot). Anticoagulants inhibit formation of a thrombus by combining with antithrombin III and inactivating thrombin to prevent formation of a fibrin clot. Anticoagulants have no effect on existing thrombi. Anticoagulants are given subcutaneously or intravenously.

Anticoagulants are prescribed for patients who:

- Are at risk for deep vein thrombosis
- Are at risk for pulmonary embolism
- Had myocardial infarction
- Have an artificial heart valve
- Had cerebrovascular accident

Commonly prescribed anticoagulants are:

- Heparin (antidote is protamine sulfate given IV)
- Warfarin (Coumadin) (antidote Vitamin K (phytonadione) (AquaMEPHYTON))
- Low molecular weight heparins (LMWHs) (antidote is protamine sulfate given IV)
- Enoxaparin sodium (Lovenox)
- Dalteparin sodium (Fragmin)

Antiplatelet medication prevents the aggregation of platelets that results in thrombi. Commonly prescribed antiplatelet medications are:

- Aspirin
- Dipyridamole (Persantine)
- Sulfinpyrazone (Anturane)

Adverse effects of Anticoagulants are:

- Increased risk of bleeding due to prolonged clotting time. Must monitor clotting time using PTT for heparin and PT for warfarin (Coumadin)
- Risk for thrombocytopenia due to decreased platelet count
- Thrombocytopenia, caused the decreased platelet count that results from Anticoagulants

- Petechiae
- Ecchymosis
- Tarry stools
- Hematemesis (indicative of occult bleeding)

ANTICOAGULANT LOW MOLECULAR WEIGHT

Use	Prevention of postop deep vein thrombosis (DVT) following hip or knee replacement surgery, abdominal surgery. Long-term DVT prevention following hip replacement surgery, nonsurgical acute illness. Treatment of unstable angina, non–Q-wave myocardial infarction, acute DVT (with warfarin). Prevents DVT after general surgical procedures.	Half-life: 4.5 hours	Onset: 2 hours	Peaks: 3–5 hours	Duration: 12 hours
Example	Enoxaparin sodium (Lovenox)	Route: SC	Pregnancy category: B	Pharmacokinetic: Well absorbed after SC administration. Eliminated in urine; not removed by hemodialysis.	

How it works
- Antithrombin, in presence of low molecular weight heparin, produces anticoagulation by inhibition of factor Xa. Enoxaparin causes less inactivation of thrombin, inhibition of platelets, and bleeding than standard heparin. Does not significantly influence bleeding time, prothrombin time (PT), activated partial thromboplastin time (APTT).

Adult dose
- Prevention of DVT (hip, knee surgery): 30 mg twice daily generally for 7–10 days
- Prevention of DVT (abdominal surgery): 40 mg daily for 7–10 days
- Prevention of long-term DVT (nonsurgical acute illness): 40 mg once daily for 3 weeks
- Angina, myocardial infarction: 1 mg/kg q12 h or 1.5 mg/kg once daily

Before administration
- Assess CBC, including platelet count.
- Obtain history of abnormal clotting or health problems that affect clotting such as severe alcoholism or severe liver or renal disease.
- Obtain drug history, especially antiplatelet medications such as aspirin.
- Obtain baseline PT or INR.

Administration
- Inject between left and right anterolateral and left and right posterolateral abdominal wall.
- Do not mix with other injections or infusions. Do not give IM.
- Patient should lie down before injecting medication.

After administration
- Periodically monitor CBC, platelet count, stool for occult blood. No need for daily monitoring in patients with normal presurgical lab values.
- Assess for any sign of bleeding; bleeding at surgical site, hematuria, blood in stool, bleeding from gums, petechiae, bruising, bleeding from injection sites

Contraindications
- Active major bleeding, concurrent heparin therapy, thrombocytopenia associated with positive in vitro test for antiplatelet antibody, hypersensitivity to heparin or pork products
- *Cautions:* Conditions with increased risk of hemorrhage, history of heparin-induced thrombocytopenia, impaired renal function, elderly uncontrolled arterial hypertension, history of recent GI ulceration and hemorrhage

Side effects/ adverse reactions
- Occasional: Injection site hematoma, nausea, peripheral edema
Adverse/Toxic
- Accidental overdosage may lead to bleeding complications ranging from local ecchymoses to major hemorrhage. Antidote: Protamine sulfate should be equal to the dose of enoxaparin. A second dose of 0.5 mg/mg protamine sulfate may be given if APTT tested 2–4 h after the first infusion remains prolonged

Patient education

- Usual length of therapy is 7–10 days.
- Do not take any OTC medications (especially aspirin) without consulting healthcare provider.
- Have laboratory tests performed as ordered.
- Inform dentist when taking an anticoagulant.
- Use a soft toothbrush when on anticoagulant medication.
- Use an electric razor.
- Carry or wear a medical identification card or jewelry (Medic-Alert).
- Try not to smoke.
- Avoid alcohol.
- Report any signs of bleeding such as petechiae, ecchymosis, purpura, tarry stools, bleeding gums, epistaxis, or expectoration of blood.

19.26 Thrombolytics

An embolus is a thrombus that moves through a blood vessels that can cause a thromboembolism (blockage), resulting in an ischemia (narrowing) that can cause decreased oxygen supply to tissues leading to tissue necrosis (death). The natural fibrinolytic process causes the disintegration of the thromboembolism into fibrin in 2 weeks. Thrombolytics promote the fibrinolytic process if administered within 4 hours after the thromboembolism, thereby reducing the ischemia and enabling increased oxygenation to tissues and minimizing necrosis.

Commonly prescribed thrombolytics are:

- Streptokinase
- Urokinase
- Tissue plasminogen activator (t-PA, alteplase)
- Anisoylated plasminogen streptokinase activator complex (APSAC, anistreplase)
- Reteplase (Retavase)

Adverse side effects of thrombolytics are:

- Allergic reactions
- Anaphylaxis (when using streptokinase)
- Reperfusion dysrhythmia
- Hemorrhagic (antidote aminocaproic acid (Amicar) inhibits plasminogen)
- Formation of new thrombus (administer heparin)

THROMBOLYTIC

Use	Management of acute myocardial infarction (AMI) for improvement of ventricular function following AMI, reduction of incidence CHF and reduction of mortality associated with AMI.	Half-life: 13–16 minutes	Onset: Immediate	Peaks: Rapid	Duration: 4–12 hours
Example	Reteplase, recombinant	Route: IC	Pregnancy category: C	Pharmacokinetic: Rapidly cleared from plasma; eliminated by the liver and kidney.	
How it works	• Activates fibrinolytic system by directly cleaving plasminogen to generate plasmin, an enzyme that degrades the fibrin of the thrombus, exerting thrombolytic action				
Adult dose	• Acute MI: IV bolus: 10 units over 2 minutes, then repeat 10 units 30 minutes after initiation of first bolus injection				
Before administration	• Obtain baseline B/P, apical pulse • Evaluate 12-lead ECG, CPK, CPK-MB, and electrolytes.				

	• Assess hematocrit, platelet count, thrombin (TT), activated thromboplastin (APTT), prothrombin time (PT), plasminogen and fibrinogen level before therapy is instituted. • Type and hold blood. • Assess pain (location, type, intensity).
Administration	• Give through an IV line in which no other medications are being administered simultaneously. • Give as a 10-unit plus 10-unit double bolus with each IV bolus administered over a 2-min period. • Give the second bolus 30 minutes after the first bolus injection. • Do not add other medications to the bolus injection solution. • Do not give second bolus if serious bleeding occurs after the first IV bolus is given.
After administration	• Carefully monitor all needle puncture sites and catheter insertion sites for bleeding. • Continuously monitor ECG for arrhythmias, B/P, pulse, respirations. • Check peripheral pulses and lung sounds. • Monitor for chest pain relief. • Notify healthcare provider of continuation or recurrence of chest pain (note location, type, intensity). • Avoid any trauma that may increase risk of bleeding (injections, shaving).
Contraindications	• Active internal bleeding, history of CVA, recent intracranial or intraspinal surgery or trauma, intracranial neoplasm, arteriovenous malformation or aneurysm, bleeding diathesis or severe uncontrolled hypertension (increases risk of bleeding) • *Cautions:* Recent major surgery (Coronary artery bypass graft, OB delivery, organ biopsy), cerebrovascular disease, recent GI or GU bleeding, hypertension, mitral stenosis with atrial fibrillation, acute pericarditis, bacterial endocarditis, hepatic/renal impairment, diabetic retinopathy, ophthalmic hemorrhaging, septic thrombophlebitis, occluded AV cannula at an infected site, advanced age, those receiving oral anticoagulants
Side effects/ adverse reactions	• Frequent: Bleeding at superficial sites (venous injection sites, catheter insertion sites, venous cutdowns, arterial punctures, sites of recent surgical procedures) Adverse/Toxic • Bleeding at internal sites (intracranial, retroperitoneal GI, GU, or respiratory) occurs occasionally. Lysis or coronary thrombi may produce atrial or ventricular dysrhythmias, stroke.
Patient education	• Explain thrombolytic treatment to the patient and family. Be supportive.

19.27   Antilipemics

Antilipemics lower lipid levels (Table 19.4). Lipids are composed of cholesterol, triglycerides, and phospholipids, which are bound to lipoproteins (Table 19.5) that transport lipids throughout the body. There are three classifications of lipoproteins:

1. Chylomicrons: Transport dietary lipids from the intestine to tissues throughout the body
2. Low-density lipoproteins (LDL): Transport cholesterol and triglycerides from the liver to peripheral tissues and regulate the synthesis of cholesterol; contribute to atherosclerotic plaque
3. High-density lipoproteins (HDL): Remove cholesterol from the blood stream and deliver cholesterol to the liver

Antilipemics are administered when non-pharmacological treatments to reduce lipids fail. These are lower dietary cholesterol and saturated fats. Commonly prescribed antilipemics are:

• Cholestyramine (Questran): Causes constipation and peptic ulcer
• Colestipol (Colestid): Not for longer term treatment can cause dysrhythmias, angina, thromboembolism, and gallstones
• Clofibrate (Atromid-S)
• Gemfibrozil (Lopid)

- Nicotinic acid or niacin (vitamin B$_2$): Many adverse effects
- Probucol: Poorly absorbed, causes diarrhea, contraindicated for cardiac dysrhythmias
- Bisphenol
- Statins: Inhibit cholesterol synthesis in the liver and decrease LDL by inhibiting HMG CoA reductase in cholesterol biosynthesis, resulting in reduction of LDL after 2 weeks.

Commonly prescribed statins are:

- Atorvastatin calcium (Lipitor)
- Cerivastatin (Baycol)
- Fluvastatin (Lescol)
- Lovastatin (Mevacor)
- Pravastatin sodium (Pravachol)
- Simvastatin (Zocor)

ANTIHYPERLIDEMIC HMG-COA REDUCTASE INHIBITOR

Use	Adjunct to diet therapy to decrease elevated total and LDL cholesterol concentrations in those with primary hypercholesterolemia (types IIa and IIb) and in those with combined hypercholesterolemia and hypertriglyceridemia	Half-life: 14 hours	Onset: 2 weeks	Peaks: — Duration: —
Example	Atorvastatin (Lipitor)	Route: PO	Pregnancy category: X	Pharmacokinetic: Poorly absorbed from GI tract; PB: 98%; metabolized in liver; minimally eliminated in urine; plasma levels markedly increased with chronic alcoholic liver disease; unaffected by renal disease

How it works	• Inhibits HMG-Co-A reductase, the enzyme that catalyzes the early step in cholesterol synthesis. Decreases LDL cholesterol, VLDL cholesterol, and plasma triglycerides, increases HDL cholesterol.
Adult dose	• PO: Initially 10 mg/day given as a single daily dose; Range: increase at 2- to 4-week intervals up to maximum of 80 mg/day.
Before administration	• Question for possibility of pregnancy before initiating therapy. • Assess baseline lab results: cholesterol, triglycerides, liver function tests.
Administration	• May be given without regard to meals. • Do not break film-coated tablets.
After administration	• Monitor for headache. • Assess for rash, pruritus, and malaise. • Monitor cholesterol and triglyceride lab results for therapeutic response.
Contraindications	• Active liver disease, unexplained elevated liver function tests • Pregnancy and lactation • *Cautions:* Anticoagulant therapy, history of liver disease, substantial alcohol consumption, major surgery, severe acute infection, trauma, hypotension, severe metabolic, endocrine, or electrolyte disorders, uncontrolled seizures
Side effects/ adverse reactions	• Generally well tolerated. Side effects usually mid and transient • Frequent: Headache

  • Occasional: Myalgia, rash/pruritus, allergy
  • Rare: Flatulence, dyspepsia

  Adverse/Toxic
  • Potential for cataracts and photosensitivity

Patient education • Follow special diet.
  • Periodic lab tests are essential.
  • Do not take other medications without healthcare provider's knowledge.

TABLE 19.4 Serum Lipid Values

LIPIDS	NORMAL VALUE (MG/DL)	LOW RISK (MG/DL)	LEVEL OF RISK FOR CAD MODERATE RISK	LEVEL OF RISK FOR CAD HIGH RISK (MG/DL)
Cholesterol	150–240	<200	200–240	>240
Triglycerides	40–190	Values vary with age	>190	
Lipoproteins LDL	60–160	<130	130–159	>160
Lipoproteins HDL	29–77	>60	35–50	<35

TABLE 19.5 Hyperlipidemia: Lipoprotein Phenotype Types II and IV Commonly Associated with Coronary Artery Disease

TYPE	MAJOR LIPIDS
I	Increased chylomicrons and increased triglycerides. Uncommon.
IIA	Increased low-density lipoprotein (LDL) and increased cholesterol.
IIB	Increased very low-density lipoprotein (VLDL), increased LDL, increased cholesterol and triglycerides. Very common.
III	Moderately increased cholesterol and triglycerides. Uncommon.
IV	Increased VLDL and markedly increased triglycerides. Very common.
V	Increased chylomicrons, VLDL, and triglycerides. Uncommon.

19.28 Peripheral Vascular Disease

Peripheral vascular disease is hyperlipemia form atherosclerosis and arteriosclerosis resulting in decreased circulation to the extremities and is characterized by:

  • Numbness of the extremities
  • Coolness of the extremities
  • Intermittent claudication

Peripheral vasodilators treat peripheral vascular disease by increasing blood flow to the extremities. Commonly prescribed vasodilators are:

  • Tolazoline (Priscoline) (see chapter 15)

- Isoxsuprine (Vasodilan)
- Nylidrin (Aplidin)
- Beta-adrenergic agonists (see chapter 15)
- Cyclandelate (Cyclan)
- Nicotinyl alcohol
- Papaverine (Cerespan, Genabid)
- Alpha-blocker prazosin (Minipress)
- Calcium channel blockers nifedipine (Procardia) (see 19.9 Antianginals)

VASODILATOR

Use	To increase circulation due to peripheral vascular disease (Raynaud's disease, arteriosclerosis obliterans) and cerebrovascular insufficiency	Half-life: 1.25–1.5 hours	Onset: 0.5 hour	Peaks: 1 hour	Duration: 3 hours
Example	Isoxsuprine HCl (Vasodilan)	Route: PO	Pregnancy category: C	Pharmacokinetic: Readily absorbed and excreted in urine; PB: UK	

How it works	• Acts directly on vascular smooth muscle
Adult dose	• 10–20 mg tid to QID
Before administration	• Obtain baseline vital signs. • Assess for signs of inadequate blood flow to the extremities: pallor, coldness of extremity, and pain. • Obtain drug and medical history.
Administration	• Take with meals to reduce GI disturbances. • Do not ingest alcohol with a vasodilator because it may cause a hypotensive reaction.
After administration	• Monitor VS, especially B/P and heart rate. Tachycardia and orthostatic hypotension can be problematic with peripheral vasodilator.
Contraindications	• Arterial bleeding, severe hypotension, postpartum, tachycardia
Side effects/ adverse reactions	• Nausea, vomiting, dizziness, syncope, weakness, tremors, rash, flushing, abdominal distention, chest pain Adverse/Toxic • Hypotension, tachycardia, palpitations
Patient education	• A desired response may take 1.5 to 3 months. • Do not smoke as it increases vasospasm. • Use aspirin or aspirin-like compounds only with healthcare provider approval. • Salicylates help in preventing platelet aggregation. • Change position slowly but frequently to avoid orthostatic hypotension, which is common when taking high doses of a vasodilator. • Report side effects such as flushing, headaches, and dizziness.

Solved Problems

Cardiovascular

19.1   What is afterload?

    The force of a ventricular contraction is called afterload. Afterload pushes against the pressure of the circulatory system.

19.2   What is preload?

The ventricles stretch when filled with blood. The force of this filling is called preload.

19.3   What is cardiac output?

Cardiac output is the total volume of blood expelled by the heart in a minute.

19.4   What is stroke volume?

The stroke volume is the quantity of blood ejected from the left ventricle during each contraction.

19.5   What is the function of a vasopressor?

Vasopressors increase the preload and afterload, resulting in an increase in blood pressure cardiac output.

Cardiac Medication

19.6   How do glycosides work?

Glycosides (digitalis) inhibit the sodium-potassium pump and increase intracellular calcium.

19.7   What is the function of glycosides?

Glycosides increase cardiac contraction, decrease heart rate, decrease conduction of the electrical stimulus, decrease preload, decrease edema, increase fluid excretion, decrease fluid retention, and increase cardiac output

19.8   What is angina pectoris?

Angina pectoris is acute cardiac pain caused by inadequate blood flow (decreased oxygen) because of occlusion of coronary arteries or from coronary artery spasm.

19.9   How do antianginals work?

Antianginals increase oxygen supply to the heart and decrease the oxygen demand of the heart.

19.10   What is a variant angina?

A variant angina occurs at rest due to vasospasm.

19.11   What is the function of nitrates?

Nitrates decrease cardiac workload by vasodilation.

19.12   How is isosorbide dinitrate administered?

Isosorbide dinitrate is administered sublingually, in chewable tablets, in immediate release tablets, in sustained-released tablets, or in capsules.

19.13   What is arrhythmia?

Cardiac dysrhythmia (arrhythmia) is deviation from the cardiac rate, including irregular heart rate, bradycardia, and tachycardia.

19.14   What is heart failure?

Heart failure is any structural or functional disorder that prevents the heart from filling with blood or pumping blood sufficiently.

19.15   How do vasodilators treat heart failure?

Vasodilators increase cardiac output by reducing cardiac afterload, dilating arterioles in the kidneys, improving renal perfusion, increasing fluid loss, and improving circulation to skeletal muscles.

19.16   How do ACE inhibitors work?

ACE inhibitors decrease the release of aldosterone, reducing sodium retention, resulting in improve renal blood flow, and decreasing fluid volume by dilating dilate venules and arterioles.

19.17   What maintains blood pressure?

Blood pressure is maintained by the kidneys using the rennin-angiotensin system, which increases blood pressure by retaining sodium and water.

19.18   What monitors blood pressure?

Blood pressure is monitored by baroreceptors in the aorta and carotid sinus.

19.19   What happens when blood pressure is high?

If blood pressure is too high, then the baroreceptors signal the vasomotor center in the medulla to signal the rennin-angiotensin system to excrete sodium and water, thereby lowering the blood pressure.

19.20   What happens when blood pressure is low?

If blood pressure is too low, then the baroreceptors signal the vasomotor center in the medulla to signal the rennin-angiotensin system to retain sodium and water, thereby increasing the blood pressure.

19.21   What is the first treatment of high blood pressure?

The first treatment of high blood pressure is nonpharmacological treatment (lose weight, reduce sodium, limit alcohol consumption, stop smoking, and exercise).

19.22   What is the second treatment of high blood pressure?

The second treatment of high blood pressure is to administer diuretics or beta-blockers.

19.23   How to ACE inhibitors work?

ACE inhibitors lower blood pressure and are used to treat heart failure by causing the excretion of sodium and water. ACE inhibitors block the release of aldosterone. Aldosterone causes the retention of sodium.

19.24   What are diuretics?

Diuretics inhibit sodium and water reabsorption from the kidney tubules, resulting in diuresis (increased urine flow), lower blood pressure, and a decrease in peripheral and pulmonary edema.

19.25   What are potassium-wasting diuretics?

Potassium-wasting diuretics are diuretics that promote the excretion of potassium.

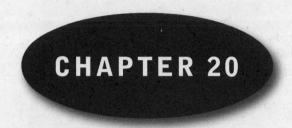

CHAPTER 20

Skin Disorders

20.1   The Skin

Skin has three major layers:

1. Epidermis: The epidermis is the outer layer and has five layers. Epidermal cells migrate from the stratum basal layer to the stratum corneum layer where they die. Their cytoplasm converts to keratin, which forms keratinocytes, a hard rough texture of the skin. Cells then stratum dysjunction (shed) and new cells take their place.

    a. *Stratum corneum*: The outer layer of the epidermis; comprised of dead cells that are replaced by new cells. These cells contain keratin, which prevents water evaporation, helps keep skin hydrated, and absorbs water.

    b. *Stratum lucidum*: A clear thin layer of dead cells between the stratum corneum and the stratum granulosum. This is called the barrier layer because of its waterproof properties.

    c. *Stratum granulosum:* Between the stratum spinosum and stratum lucidum. It provides waterproofing and keeps nutrients within the lower layers. This is the highest layer of epidermis where living cells are found.

    d. *Stratum spinosum:* Above the basal layer; provides structural support and resists skin abrasions.

    e. *Stratum basale:* At the base of the epidermis above the dermis. Cells in the basal layer replenish skin lost by stratum dysjunction (shedding) and provide melanin (pigmentation).

2. Dermis: The dermis, below the epidermis, contains two layers. The dermis has connective tissue that cushions stress and strains. It contains nerve endings, which provide the sense of touch and heat, and blood vessels, which nourish the skin.

    a. *Papillary layer:* Below the epidermis; regulates temperature and supplies nutrients by expanding and constricting blood flow according to temperature.

    b. *Reticular layer:* Contains collagen fibers and elastic fibers that give strength and elasticity to the skin. The dermal layer also contains sweat glands, hair follicles, sebaceous glands, blood vessels, and sensory nerve terminals.

3. Subcutis (hypodermis): The subcutis is the lowest layer of skin consisting of fatty tissue, blood and lymphatic vessels, nerve fibers, and elastic fibers.

20.2   Skin Disorders

Skin disorder is the disruption of the skin caused by inflammation, abnormal skin growth, allergic reactions, viral, bacteria or fungal infections, or trauma. Lesions (tissue damage) also disrupt the skin. Common lesions are:

- Macules: Flat with color changes
- Papules: Small elevated solid
- Vesicles: Small elevation containing fluid
- Pustules: Elevation containing pus (dead neutrophils)
- Plaques: Rough hard elevated, flat top

20.3 Acne Vulgaris

Acne vulgaris (acne) occurs when keratin plugs at the base of the pilosebaceous oil glands near the hair follicles become inflamed, resulting in papules, nodules, and cysts on the face, neck, shoulders, and back. Pilosebaceous glands produce oil for hair. Acne vulgaris is influenced by age, heredity, stress, hormonal changes and onset of puberty—all of which are beyond the patient's control. During adolescence there is an increased production of androgen, which increases sebum product (an oily skin lubricant). Sebum combines with keratin to form a keratin plug, which can become inflamed. Acne vulgaris is associated with testosterone level and the ingestion of food containing trans-fatty acids (TFA) (greasy foods). The patient has little control over developing acne vulgaris other than to eat a nutritional diet and practice good hygiene.

Treat acne vuglaris by gently applying a cleansing agent to the skin several times a day. Administer anti-acne medication, which dissolves keratin. Commonly prescribed antiacne medications are:

- Keratolytics
- Resorcinol
- Salicylic acid

Systemic treatment (Table 20.1) given for acne vulgaris may result in scarring, persistent hyperpigmentation, or failed topical treatment.

TABLE 20.1 Medication for Systemic Therapy for Acne Vulgaris

NONHORMONAL TREATMENT	HORMONAL TREATMENT
Antibiotics, oral	Corticosteroids
Tetracycline	Anti-inflammatory actions: high dose
Erythromycin	Androgen suppressant action: low dose
Minocycline	Sex hormones (for women only)
Trimethoprim-sulfamethoxazole	Estrogen (oral contraceptive medication)
Isotretinoin, oral	Antiandrogens

ACNE VULGARIS (SYSTEMIC PREPARATION)					
Use	Treatment of severe, recalcitrant cystic acne that is unresponsive to conventional acne therapies. Treatment of g-negative folliculitis, severe rosacea, correcting severe keratinization disorders	Half-life: 10–20 hours	Onset: UK	Peaks: UK	Duration: 5.3 hours
Example	Isotretinoin (Accutane)	Route: PO	Pregnancy category: X	Pharmacokinetic: Absorption enhanced when taken with a high-fat meal. It binds to plasma proteins (albumin), metabolized in the liver and excreted in feces and urine.	

How it works	• Exact mechanism of action is unknown. Reduces sebaceous gland size, inhibiting its activity. Produces anti-keratinizing, anti-inflammatory effects.
Adult dose	• Initially 0.5–2/mg/kg/day divided in two doses for 15–20 weeks. May repeat after at least 2 months of therapy.
Before administration	• Assess baselines for blood lipids and glucose. • Assess medical and drug history. • Obtain pregnancy test and determine birth control method being used for female patients.
Administration	• No known interactions with food
After administration	• Assess for decreased cysts. • Evaluate skin and mucous membranes for excessive dryness. • Monitor blood glucose and lipids.
Contraindications	• Women who are or may become pregnant while undergoing treatment; extremely high risk of major deformities in fetus while taking any amounts even for short periods of time • Hypersensitivity to isotretinoin or parabens (component of capsules) • *Cautions:* Renal, hepatic dysfunction
Side effects/ adverse reactions	• Frequent: Cheilitis (inflammation of lips); skin/mucous membrane dryness; skin fragility, pruritus, epistaxis, dry nose/mouth; conjunctivitis; hypertriglyceridemia; nausea, vomiting, abdominal pain • Occasional: Musculoskeletal symptoms including bone or joint pain, arthralgia, generalized muscle, aches; photosensitivity • Rare: Decreased night vision, depression Adverse/Toxic • Inflammatory bowel disease and pseudotumor cerebri (benign intracranial hypertension) have been associated with isotretinoin therapy.
Patient education	• A transient exacerbation of acne may occur during initial period. • May have decreased tolerance to contact lenses during and after therapy. • Do not take vitamin A because of additive effects. • Notify physician immediately of onset of abdominal pain, severe diarrhea, rectal bleeding (possible inflammatory bowel disease), or headache, nausea and vomiting, visual disturbances (possible pseudotumor cerebri). • Decreased night vision may occur suddenly; take caution with night driving. • Avoid prolonged exposure to sunlight; use sunscreens, protective clothing. • Do not donate blood during or for 1 month after treatment. Women: • Explain the serious risk to fetus if pregnancy occurs (both oral and written warnings are given, with patient acknowledging in writing that she understands the warnings and consents to treatment). • Must have a negative serum pregnancy test within 2 weeks before starting therapy; therapy will begin on the second or third day of the next normal menstrual period. • Effective contraception (using two reliable forms of contraception simultaneously) must be used for at least 1 month before, during, and at least 1 month after therapy.

20.4 Psoriasis

Psoriasis is a chronic skin disorder caused by accelerated growth of epidermal cells, resulting in erythematous papules and plaques covered with silvery scales appearing on the scalp, elbows, palms of the hands knees, and soles of the feet.

Antipsoriatic medication treats psoriasis. Commonly prescribed antipsoriatics are:

- Keratolytics (salicylic acid, sulfur): Loosens psoriasis scales
- Anthralin (Anthra-Derm, Lasan): Loosens psoriasis scales; can stain skin, clothing, hair, and erythema
- Coal tar (Estar, PsoriGel): Loosens psoriasis scales; available in shampoos, lotions, and creams; has unpleasant odor; causes burning and stings
- Calcipotriene (Dovonex): Synthetic vitamin D_3 derivative; suppresses cell growth, causes local irritation, monitor for hypercalciuria and hypercalcemia
- Methotrexate: Suppresses cell growth; for severe psoriasis
- Etretinate (Tegison): Treats pustular psoriasis; suppresses cell growth; used when other medications fail
- Ultraviolet A (UVA): Suppresses cell growth
- Photochemotherapy: Combines ultraviolet radiation with methoxsalen to suppress cell growth

---

ANTIPSORIATIC

Use	Treatment of mild to moderate plaque psoriasis. Solution: Treatment of chronic, moderately severe scalp psoriasis.	Half-life: UK	Onset: UK	Peaks: UK	Duration: UK
Example	Calcipotriene (Dovonex)	Route: Topical	Pregnancy category: C	Pharmacokinetic: PB: UK	

How it works	• A synthetic vitamin D_3 analogue. Regulates cell (keratinocyte) production and development; preventing abnormal growth and production of psoriasis (abnormal keratinocyte growth)
Adult dose	• Topical: Apply thin layer to affected skin twice daily (morning and evening); rub in gently and completely • Solution: Apply to lesions after combing hair
Before administration	• Establish baseline electrolytes, particularly serum and urine calcium. • Obtain history of the onset of skin lesions; note whether there is a family history of lesions. • Assess the psychological effects of skin lesions and changes in body image. • Obtain a culture of purulent draining skin lesions. • Obtain baseline vital signs; report any elevation in temperature.
Administration	• Rub ointment in gently and completely. • Use aseptic technique.
After administration	• Assess skin for irritation, erythema, worsening of psoriasis. • If irritation of lesions or surrounding uninvolved skin develops or if serum calcium level increases outside normal range, medication should be discontinued.
Contraindications	• Hypercalcemia or evidence or vitamin D toxicity or use on the face • *Caution:* History of nephrolithiasis
Side effects/ adverse reactions	• Frequent: Burning, itching, skin irritation • Occasional: Erythema, dry skin, peeling, rash, worsening of psoriasis, dermatitis • Rare: Skin atrophy, hyperpigmentation, folliculitis Adverse/Toxic • Potential for hypercalcemia (abdominal pain, depression, easy fatigability, high B/P, anorexia, nausea, thirst) may occur
Patient education	• Avoid contact with face or eyes. • Do not use harsh cleansers on the skin. Keep skin clean. • Apply using a clean technique. • Wash hands after application. • Report signs of local reaction. • Notify healthcare provider of any alternative treatments used to treat psoriasis. • Improvement noted usually beginning after 2 weeks of therapy. • Marked improvement after 8 weeks of therapy.

20.5   Warts

A wart is a benign hard, horny nodule lesion that typically appears on hands and feet. Commonly prescribed medications to remove warts are:

- Salicylic acid: Promotes desquamation. Risk for salicylism (toxicity), because it is absorbed through the skin.
- Podophyllum resin: Removes venereal warts. Not effective against common warts. Monitor for peripheral neuropathy, blood dyscrasias, and kidney impairment. Do not administer to pregnant women (teratogenic effect).
- Cantharidin (Cantharone, Verr-Canth): Removes common wart. Harmful to normal skin. Apply topically. Allow to dry. Cover with a nonporous tape for 24 hours. Repeat treatment in 1 week.

20.6   Dermatitis

Dermatitis is a skin eruption. There are two types of dermatitis:

Drug-Inducted Dermatitis

The patient is sensitized to the medication, causing a hypersensitive reaction (rash, urticaria, papules, or vesicles) or erythema multiforme and Stevens-Johnson syndrome, which is life threatening. Reaction can take minutes, hours, or a day. Medications known to cause dermatitis are:

- Penicillin
- Hydralazine hydrochloride (Apresoline)
- Isoniazid (INH)
- Phenothiazines
- Procainamide (Pronestyl)

Contact Dermatitis (Exogenous Dermatitis)

This is caused by a chemical agent in touch with the skin, resulting in skin rash with itching, swelling, blistering, oozing, or scaling. Chemical agents known to cause dermatitis are:

- Cosmetics
- Cleansing products
- Perfume, clothing
- Dyes
- Plants (poison ivy, oak, or sumac)

Dermatitis is prevented by avoiding the underlying cause. Medications used to treat dermatitis are:

- Burow's solution (aluminum acetate)
- Calamine lotion
- Antihistamine
- Antipruritics: Stops itching. Do not use on open wound or near eyes or genitals.
  - Diphenhydramine (Benadryl)
  - Cyproheptadine hydrochloride (Periactin)
  - Trimeprazine tartrate (Temaril)

- ○ Oatmeal of Alpha-Keri (bath)
- ○ Potassium permanganate
- ○ Aluminum subacetate
- ○ Normal saline
- ○ Glucocorticoids: (Table 20.2) ointments, creams, or gels. Absorption greater at face, scalp, eyelids, neck, axilla, and genitals. Prolonged use causes thinning of the skin with atrophy of the epidermis and dermis, and purpura from small-vessel eruptions.

TABLE 20.2 Topical Glucocorticoids

POTENCY	DRUG NAME	DRUG FORM
High	Amcinonide 0.1% (Cyclocort)	Cream, ointment
	Betamethasone dipropionate 0.05% (Diprosone)	Cream, ointment, lotion
	Desoximetasone 0.25% (Topicort)	Cream, ointment
	Desoximetasone 0.05%	Gel
	Diflorasone diacetate 0.05% (Florone)	Cream, ointment
	Halcinonide 0.1% (Halog)	Cream, ointment
	Triamcinolone acetonide 0.5% (Aristocort A, Kenalog)	Cream, ointment
Moderate	Betamethasone benzoate 0.025% (Benisone)	Cream, ointment
	Betamethasone valerate 0.1% (Valisone)	Cream, ointment, lotion
	Desoximetasone 0.05% (Topicort LP)	Cream, gel
	Fluocinolone acetonide 0.025% (Fluonid)	Cream, ointment
	Flurandrenolide 0.025% (Cordran, Cordran SP)	Cream, ointment, lotion
	Halcinonide 0.025% (Halog)	Cream, ointment
	Hydrocortisone valerate 0.2% (Westcort)	Cream, ointment
	Mometasone furoate 0.1% (Elocon)	Cream, ointment, lotion
	Triamcinolone acetonide (0.025%–0.1% (Aristocort A, Kenalog)	Cream, ointment, lotion
Low	Dexamethasone 0.1% (Decadron)	Cream
	Desonide 0.05% (Tridesilon)	Cream
	Fluocinolone acetonide 0.02% (Fluonid)	Solution
	Hydrocortisone 0.25%, 0.5%, 1.0%, 2.5% (Cortef, Hytone)	Cream, ointment
	Methylprednisolone acetate 0.25%, 1.0% (Medrol)	Ointment

20.7 Alopecia

Alopecia (male pattern baldness) occurs when hair follicles cannot regenerate because the hair shaft is lost as a result of aging or familial history. Temporary alopecia occurs by the following medications and returns once the patient stops taking the medication:

- Anticancer (antineoplastic) agents
- Gold salts
- Sulfonamides
- Anticonvulsants
- Aminoglycosides
- Nonsteroidal anti-inflammatory drugs (NSAIDs)

Alopecia is treated with minoxidil (Rogaine). Minoxidil causes vasodilation, increasing cutaneous blood flow, which stimulates hair follicle growth. Alopecia returns in 4 months after the patient stops taking minoxidil.

20.8 Burns

A burn breaks down skin, exposing underlying tissues and risking infection. Burns are classified by degree based on the depth of the burn. There are three burn classifications:

1. *Superficial (first-degree burn):* The epidermis is red, painful, dry, and no blisters (i.e., sun burn). Superficial burns are treated by removing clothing at the burn site and placing a cold wet compress on the burn site to constrict blood vessels, reducing swelling and pain. Superficial burns should be treated with antibiotics such as Bacitracin with polymyxin B (Polysporin) and similar over-the-counter (OTC) antibiotics.
2. *Partial-thickness (second-degree burn):* The epidermis is broken, red, blistered, swollen, and painful. Part of the dermis is exposed. There is a risk of infection. Partial-thickness burns are treated by removing clothing at the burn site, cleaning the burn with a non-abrasive solution, and then administering antibiotic ointment such as silver sulfadiazine (Silvadene) and an analgesic (see chapter 16) for pain. Cover the treated burn side with a nonstick dressing.
3. *Full-thickness (third-degree burn):* The epidermis is broken, exposing the dermis, nerves, muscles, tendons, and bone. The burn appears charred without pain (nerve endings destroyed). There is a risk for infection. Full-thickness burns are treated by administering analgesic (see chapter 16) to minimize the pain of cleaning and treating the burn. (Patients typically have a mixture of partial-thickness and full-thickness burns. There will be pain.) Remove clothing at the burn site and remove eschar (charred skin). Clean the burn with sterile saline and antiseptic (povidone-iodine; Betadine). Administer antibiotics (mafenide acetate; Sulfamylon), silver sulfadiazine (Silvadene), and silver nitrate (0.5% solution, nitrofurazone; Furacin) to prevent infection. Monitor and treat for fluid and electrolyte imbalance (see chapter 10). Monitor and treat for stress ulcers (see chapter 18). Monitor for smoke inhalation and treat with respiratory medications (see chapter 14).

ANTI-INFECTIVE

Use	Prevention, treatment of infection in second-and third-degree burns, protection against conversion from partial- to full-thickness wounds (infection causes extended tissue destruction). Treatment of minor bacterial skin infection and dermal ulcer.	Half-life: UK	Onset: on contact	Peaks: 2–4 hours	Duration: as long as applied
Example	Silver sulfadiazine (Silvadene)	Route: Topical	Pregnancy category: C	Pharmacokinetic: Some absorbed; PB: UK	
How it works	• Acts upon cell wall and cell membrane to produce bactericidal effect. Silver is released slowly in concentrations selectively toxic to bacteria.				
Adult dose	• Apply one to two times/day.				
Before administration	• Determine initial CBC, renal/hepatic function test results. • Assess burned tissue for infection; culture any wound drainage. • Assess fluid status. • Assess pain status. • Administer analgesics. • Cleanse wounds.				
Administration	• Apply to cleansed, débrided burns using sterile gloves. • Keep burn areas covered with silver sulfadiazine cream at all times; reapply to areas where removed by activity. • Apply dressings as necessary.				

After administration	• Evaluate fluid balance, renal function. • Maintain intake and output, renal function tests and report changes promptly. • Monitor vital signs. • Check serum sulfonamide concentrations carefully. • Assess burns, surrounding areas for pain, burning, itching, rash. (Antihistamines may provide relief.) • Silvadene therapy should continue unless reactions are severe. • Monitor CBC results.
Contraindication	• None significant. • *Cautions:* Impaired renal/hepatic function.
Side effects/ adverse reactions	• Side effects characteristic of all sulfonamides may occur when systemically absorbed, e.g., extensive burn areas (over 20% of body surface): anorexia, nausea, vomiting, headache, diarrhea, dizziness, photosensitivity, joint pain. • Frequent: Burning feeling at treatment site • Occasional: Brown-gray skin discoloration, rash, itching • Rare: Increased sensitivity of skin to sunlight Adverse/Toxic • If significant system absorption occurs, less often but serious are hemolytic anemia, hypoglycemia, diuresis, peripheral neuropathy, Stevens-Johnson syndrome, agranulocytosis, lupus erythematosus, anaphylaxis, hepatitis, toxic nephrosis. • Fungal superinfections may occur. Interstitial nephritis occurs rarely.
Patient education	• Therapy should continue until healing is satisfactory or the site is ready for grafting. • Notify healthcare provider of any side effects that indicate systemic absorption. • Administer pain medication as ordered. • Re-apply to areas that have been removed by activity. • Maintain dressings over wounds as necessary. • Keep all medical appointments. • Monitor for signs of infection (redness, heat, drainage [pus], increased pain).

20.9 Abrasions and Lacerations

Skin abrasion (scrape) and laceration (cut) expose the patient to the same risk for infection as burns. Abrasion and lacerations are treated by the following means.

Carefully cleanse the site with Betadine or hydrogen peroxide to prevent scarring. Administer antibiotics such as Neosporin and analgesics. A tetanus toxoid booster may be required for lacerations if the patient has not received it recently.

Monitor the site for redness, swelling, persistent pain, and purulent drainage (pus), as these are signs of infection.

Solved Problems

Skin

20.1 Where are nerve endings located in the skin?

Nerve endings are located in the dermis layer.

20.2 What are vesicles?

Vesicles are small elevations on the skin that contain fluid.

20.3 What do pustules contain?

Pustules contain dead neutrophils (pus).

Acne Vulgaris

20.4 How does acne vulgaris develop?

Acne vulgaris (acne) occurs when keratin plugs at the base of the pilosebaceous oil glands near the hair follicles become inflamed resulting in papules, nodules, and cysts on the face, neck, shoulders, and back.

20.5 Why do adolescents develop acne vulgaris?

During adolescence there is an increased production of androgen, which increases sebum product (an oily skin lubricant). Sebum combines with keratin to form a keratin plug, which can become inflamed.

20.6 What food is associated with acne vulgaris?

Acne vulgaris is associated with the ingestion of food containing trans-fatty acids (TFA; greasy foods).

20.7 What do keratolytics treat?

Keratolytics treat acne vulgaris and psoriasis.

Psoriasis

20.8 What is psoriasis?

Psoriasis is a chronic skin disorder caused by accelerated growth of epidermal cells, resulting in erythematous papules and plaques covered with silvery scales appearing on the scalp, elbows, palms of the hands, knees, and soles of the feet.

20.9 What are adverse side effects of coal tar?

Coal tar has an unpleasant odor, burns, and stings.

20.10 What is the therapeutic effect of calcipotriene?

Calcipotriene suppresses cell growth of skin.

Warts

20.11 What is the therapeutic effect of podophyllum resin?

Podophyllum resin removes venereal warts.

20.12 Who should not be treated with podophyllum resin?

Do not administer podophyllum resin to pregnant women (teratogenic effect).

20.13 What is the therapeutic effect of cantharidin?

Cantharidin removes common warts.

Dermatitis

20.14 What are two types of dermatitis?

Two types of dermatitis are drug-induced dermatitis and contact dermatitis.

20.15 What is drug-induced dermatitis?

The patient is sensitized to the medication, which causes a hypersensitive reaction (rash, urticaria, papules, or vesicles) or erythema multiforme and Stevens-Johnson syndrome, which is life threatening.

20.16   Name one medication that causes drug-induced dermatitis.

Penicillin causes drug-induced dermatitis.

20.17   What causes contact dermatitis?

Contact dermatitis is caused by a chemical agent in touch with the skin.

20.18   How is dermatitis prevented?

Dermatitis is prevented by avoiding the medication or chemical agent that causes dermatitis.

20.19   How does one stop itching caused by dermatitis?

Stop itching caused by dermatitis by administering antipruritics.

20.20   What is the adverse effect of administering glucocorticoid for prolonged periods for dermatitis?

Prolonged use causes thinning of the skin with atrophy of the epidermis and dermis, and purpura from small-vessel eruptions.

Burns

20.21   Why is there no pain in full-thickness burns?

There is no pain in full-thickness burns because nerve endings in the dermis are destroyed.

20.22   Describe a superficial burn.

The epidermis is red, painful, dry, and no blisters (sunburn).

20.23   What is the major difference between a superficial burn and a partial-thickness burn?

The skin is broken and blistered in a partial-thickness burn, but not in a superficial burn.

20.24   What are three major medications used treat full-thickness burns?

Three major medications used to treat full-thickness burns are antibiotics, analgesic, and fluids and electrolytes.

20.25   What medications are used to clean a burn?

Clean a burn with sterile saline and antiseptic (povidone-iodine; Betadine).

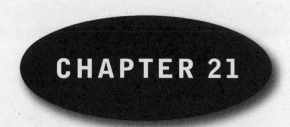

CHAPTER 21

Endocrine Medications

21.1   The Endocrine System

The endocrine system is composed of ductless glands that secrete hormones. Hormones are messengers distributed in circulating blood that influence cellular activities of other glands, tissues, and organs.

There are two types of hormones. These are:

- Proteins (small peptides)
- Steroids (secreted by the adrenal glands and the gonads)

Endocrine glands are described in Table 21.1

TABLE 21.1 Endocrine Glands and Their Secretions

GLAND	LOCATION	SECRETES
Pituitary (hypophysis) Anterior (adenohypophysis)	Base of the brain	Thyroid-stimulating hormone (TSH) Adrenocorticotropic hormone (ACTH)
		Gonadotropins (follicle-stimulating hormone; FSH) and luteinizing hormone (LH). Growth hormone (GH), prolactin, melanocyte-stimulating hormone (MSH).
Posterior (neurohypophysis)		Antidiuretic hormone (ADH), vasopressin, oxytocin
Thyroid gland	Anterior to the trachea (two lobes)	Thyroxine (T4) and triiodothyronine (T3)
Parathyroid gland	Lies on the dorsal surface of the thyroid gland (four glands, two pairs)	Parathyroid hormone (PTH)
Adrenal glands	Top of each kidney (two sections: Medulla is inner and cortex surrounds medulla)	Cortex secretes (glucosteroids and corticosteroids mineralocorticoids) Small amounts of androgen, estrogen, and progestin.

Pancreas	Left of and behind the stomach (exocrine and endocrine gland)	Exocrine secretes digestive enzymes into the duodenum; endocrine has cell clusters called islets of Langerhans; alpha islet cells produce glucagons; beta cells secrete insulin

21.2 Hormones

A hormone is a messenger that causes tissue, organ, and cellular activities to increase or decrease tissue equal to the amount of the hormones in the blood. Disease and aging cause inappropriate secretion of hormones, resulting in abnormal tissue, organ, and cellular activities. Hormonal therapy is used for hormones produced by the pituitary, thyroid, parathyroid, and adrenal glands and restores hormonal balance by either:

- Replacing hormone(s) if serum hormone(s) levels are low
- Inhibiting secretion if serum hormone(s) levels are high

21.3 The Pituitary Gland: Growth Hormone

The pituitary gland secretes growth hormone (GH) that influences growth.

Excess growth hormone: Hypersecretion of growth hormone is commonly caused by a pituitary tumor and results in:

- Gigantism: Abnormally excessive growth before and during puberty
- Acromegaly: Abnormally excessive growth after puberty

Insufficient growth hormone: Hyposecretion of growth hormone is referred to as GH deficiency and results in the patient not reaching a normal height.

Hypersecretion of growth hormone is treated by:

- Destroying the pituitary tumor with radiation
- Bromocriptine: Inhibits release of growth hormone from the pituitary
- Octreotide (Sandostatin): Suppresses release of the growth hormone; has GI side effects

Hyposecretion of growth hormone is treated by:

- Somatrem (Protropin): Growth hormone replacement
- Somatropin (Humatrope): Growth hormone replacement

ANTERIOR PITUITARY HORMONE

Use	Long-term treatment of children who have growth failure due to endogenous growth hormone deficiency or associated with chronic renal insufficiency (Nutropin only). Long-term therapy in adults with growthhhormone deficiency. Long-term treatment of short stature associated with Turner'ssyndrome; treatment of AIDS-wasting syndrome.	Half-life: 15–60 minutes	Onset: 1 hour	Peaks: 2 hour	Duration: 8 hours

| Example | Somatropin (Humatrope) | Route: SC/IM | Pregnancy category: D | Pharmacokinetic: Metabolized in the liver. |

How it works
- Acts directly on bone and tissue

Adult dose
Growth hormone deficiency
- IM/SC: (Humatrope): Up to 0.06 mg/kg three times/wk
- SC: (Nutropin): 0.3 mg/kg/wk
- SC: (Nutropin Depot): 1.5 mg/kg/mo or 0.75 mg/kg two times/mo
- SC: 0.04 mg/kg/wk in six to seven injections/wk. Maximum: 0.08 mg/kg/wk

Chronic renal insufficiency:
- SC: 0.375 mg/kg/wk divided into three to seven equal doses/wk

AIDS-wasting syndrome:
- SC: 4–6 mg at bedtime

Before administration
- Baseline assessment include thyroid function and blood glucose levels

Administration
- No interactions with food

After administration
- Monitor bone age, calcium, parathyroid, phosphorus, renal function, glucose, growth rate, thyroid function, decreased wasting in AIDS

Contraindication
- None significant
- *Cautions:* Diabetes mellitus, untreated hypothyroidism, malignancy

Side effects/adverse reactions
- Frequent: Development of persistent antibodies to growth hormone (generally does not cause failure to respond to somatropin); hypercalciuria during first 2–3 months of therapy
- Occasional: Headache, muscle pain, weakness, mild hyperglycemia, allergic reaction (rash, itching), pain, swelling at injection site, pain in hip/knee

Adverse/Toxic
- None significant

Patient education
- Correct procedure to reconstitute for IM/SC administration
- Safe handling and disposal of needles
- Need for regular follow-up with healthcare provider

21.4   The Pituitary Gland: Antidiuretic Hormone and Oxytocin

The posterior pituitary gland secretes:

- Antidiuretic hormone (ADH): A vasopressin and promotes water reabsorption from the renal tubules to maintain water balance in the body fluids
- Oxytocin: Starts labor contractions

Diabetes insipidus (DI) is a deficiency in antidiuretic hormone resulting from trauma to the hypothalamus and pituitary gland or brain tumor that causes the kidneys to excrete large amounts of water, leading to severe fluid volume deficit and electrolyte imbalances. Diabetes insipidus is treated by replacing the antidiuretic hormone with the administration of:

- Desmopressin acetate (DDAVP)
- Desmopressin (Stimate)
- Lypressin (Diapid)
- Vasopressin (aqueous) (Pitressin)
- Vasopressin tannate/oil (Pitressin Tannate)

POSTERIOR PITUITARY HORMONE

Use	Treatment of adult shock—refractory ventricular fibrillation (Class IIb). Prevents/controls polydipsia, polyuria, dehydration in patients with neurogenic diabetes insipidus. Stimulates peristalsis in the prevention or treatment of postop abdominal distention, intestinal paresis. Adjunct in treatment of acute, massive hemorrhage.	Half-life: 10–20 minutes	Onset: IM/SC:— IV: —	Peaks: —	Duration: 2–8 hours 0.5–1 hour

Example	Vasopressin (aqueous) (Pitressin)	Route: SC/IM/IV	Pregnancy category: B	Pharmacokinetic: Distributed throughout extracellular fluid. Metabolized in liver and kidneys. Excreted in urine.

How it works
- Increases reabsorption of water by the renal tubules resulting in decreased urinary flow rate, increased urine osmolality. Urea is also reabsorbed by the collecting ducts. Directly stimulates contraction of smooth muscle, preventing abdominal distention, intestinal paresis. Causes vasoconstriction with reduced blood flow in coronary, peripheral cerebral, and pulmonary vessels, but particularly in portal and splanchnic vessels. In large doses, may cause mild uterine contractions.

Adult Dose

Cardiac arrest
- IV: 40 units as a one-time dose

Diabetes insipidus
- Note: May administer intranasally on cotton pledgets, by nasal spray; individualize dosage.
- IM/SC: 5–10 units; two to four times/day. Range: 5–60 units/day
- IV infusion: 0.5 milliunits/kg/hr. May double dose q 30 min. Maximum: 10 milliunits/kg/h

Abdominal distention
- IM: Initially 5 units. Subsequent doses of 10 units q3–4 h

GI hemorrhage:
- IV infusion: Initially 0.2–0.4units/min progressively increased to 0.9 units/min

Before administration
- Establish baselines for weight, B/P, pulse, electrolytes, urine specific gravity

Administration
- Give with one to two glasses of water to reduce side effects
- IV: Dilute with D5W in water or 0.9% NaCl to concentration of 0.1–1 units/ml; give as IV infusions

After Administration
- Monitor intake and output.
- Restrict intake as necessary to prevent water intoxication.
- Weigh daily if indicated.
- Check B/P and pulse two times/day.
- Monitor electrolytes, urine, specific gravity.
- Evaluate injection site for erythema, pain, abscess.
- Report side effects to healthcare provider for dose reduction.
- Be alert for early signs of water intoxication (drowsiness, listlessness, headache).
- Hold medication and report immediately any chest pain/allergic symptoms.

Contraindications
- Chronic nephritis with nitrogen retention
- *Cautions:* Migraine, epilepsy, heart failure, asthma, or any condition in which rapid addition of extracellular water may be a risk
- *Extreme Caution:* Patients with vascular disease, especially coronary artery disease

Side effects/adverse reactions	• Frequent: Pain at injection site with vasopressin tannate
	• Occasional: Stomach cramps, nausea, vomiting diarrhea, dizziness, diaphoresis, paleness, circumoral pallor, trembling, "pounding" in head, eructation, flatulence
	• Rare: Chest pain, confusion. Allergic reaction: Rash or hives, pruritus, wheezing or difficulty breathing, swelling of mouth, face, feet, hands. Sterile abscess with vasopressin tannate
	Adverse/Toxic
	• Anaphylaxis, myocardial infarction, and water intoxication have occurred. Elderly and very young patients at higher risk for water intoxication.
Patient education	• Promptly report headaches, chest pain, shortness of breath or other symptoms.
	• Maintain a record of intake and output.

21.5   The Adrenal Gland

The adrenal glands are located at the top of each kidney and each is comprised of two parts.

Adrenal Cortex

The adrenal cortex produces corticosteroids that promote sodium retention and potassium excretion and are involved in stress response, immune response, inflammation regulation, carbohydrate metabolism, protein catabolism, electrolyte levels, and behavior. There are two corticosteroids:

- Glucocorticoids (cortisol): Glucocorticoids cause the kidneys to absorb sodium, resulting in water retention and increased blood pressure. Glucocorticoids are used to decrease inflammation, treat allergic reactions, and decrease stress. Glucocorticoids influence metabolism of carbohydrate, protein, and fat.
- Mineralocorticoids (aldosterone): Mineralocorticoids cause the kidneys to retain sodium and water, increasing fluid volume and increasing blood pressure. Blocking mineralocorticoid receptors by medication such as spironolactone decreases blood pressure.

Adrenal Medulla

The adrenal medulla produces catecholamines in response to stressors. These are epinephrine and norepinephrine. Catecholamines increase the supply of oxygen and glucose to the brain and muscles. Digestion decreases. Heart rate increases. Blood vessels and bronchioles dilate.

Secretion of hormones by the adrenal gland is controlled by the adrenocorticotropic hormone (ACTH), which is produced by the pituitary gland. Increased levels of adrenocorticotropic hormone result in increased secretions of hormones by the adrenal glands. Decreased levels of adrenocorticotropic hormone result in decreased secretions of hormones by the adrenal glands.

A deficiency in adrenal hormones can be caused by problems with the pituitary gland or problems with the adrenal gland. Healthcare providers determine the cause by administering corticotropin (Acthar), which is the adrenocorticotropic hormone. If after 60 minutes there are increased levels of glucocorticoids, there is a pituitary gland insufficiency. If no increase occurs, there is an adrenal gland insufficiency.

Hypersecretion of adrenal hormones is called Cushing's syndrome. Hyposecretion of adrenal hormones is called Addison's disease. Table 21.2 shows the effects hypersecretion and hyposecretion of the adrenal gland.

Glucocorticoid therapy involves administering glucocorticoids to reduce the effects of trauma, decrease infections, and reduce anxiety. Commonly prescribed medications for glucocorticoid therapy are:

- Beclomethasone dipropionate (Vanceril)
- Betamethasone (Celestone)
- Cortisone acetate (Cortone Acetate)
- Dexamethasone (Decadron)
- Fludrocortisone acetate (Florinef Acetate)

- Hydrocortisone (Hydrocortone)
- Methylprednisolone (Medrol, Solu-Medrol Depo-Medrol)
- Prednisolone
- Prednisone

TABLE 21.2 Effects of Adrenal Hyposecretion and Hypersecretion.

BODY SYSTEM	HYPOSECRETION	HYPERSECRETION
Metabolism		
Glucose	Hypoglycemia	Hyperglycemia
Protein Fat	Muscle weakness	Muscle wasting; thinning of the skin; fat accumulation in face, neck, and trunk (protruding abdomen, buffalo hump); hyperlipidemia; high cholesterol
Central nervous system	Apathy, depression, fatigue	Increased neural activity; mood elevation; irritability; seizures
Gastrointestinal	Nausea, vomiting, abdominal pain	Peptic ulcers
Cardiovascular	Tachycardia, hypotension, cardiovascular collapse	Hypertension; edema; heart failure
Eyes	None	Cataract formation
Fluids and electrolytes	Hypovolemia; hyponatremia; hyperkalemia	Hypervolemia; hypernatremia; hypokalemia
Blood cells	Anemia	Increased red blood cell count and neutrophils; impaired clotting

21.6 The Thyroid Gland

The thyroid gland, located in the neck and controlled by the hypothalamus and pituitary glands, controls metabolism and regulates protein synthesis. The hypothalamus gland releases the thyrotropin-releasing hormone (TRH) that stimulates the anterior pituitary gland to release thyroid-stimulating hormone (TSH), resulting in secretion of thyroid hormones by the thyroid gland.

The thyroid gland produces three hormones:

- Thyroxine (T4): Iodine is required for the production of thyroxine
- Triiodothyronine (T3)
- Calcitonin: Reduces serum level of calcium

21.7 Hypothyroidism

A deficiency in production of thyroxine and triiodothyronine is called hypothyroidism. There are two types of hypothyroidism:

- Primary hypothyroidism: The thyroid gland is unable to produce sufficient quantity of thyroxine and triiodothyronine, resulting in an increased serum level of thyrotropin-releasing hormone and thyroid-stimulating hormone.

- Secondary hypothyroidism: Either the hypothalamus is unable to release sufficient quantities of thyrotropin-releasing hormone or the anterior pituitary gland is unable to release sufficient thyroid-stimulating hormone.

Severe hypothyroidism is called myxedema, which results in:

- Lethargy
- Apathy
- Memory impairment
- Emotional changes
- Slow speech
- Deep coarse voice
- Edema of the eyelids and face
- Thick dry skin
- Cold intolerance
- Slow pulse
- Constipation
- Weight gain
- Abnormal menses

Hypothyroid is treated by administering:

- Levothyroxine sodium (Levothroid, Synthroid): Increases thyroxine and triiodothyronine for long-term treatment
- Liothyronine (Cytomel): Increases triiodothyronine for short-term treatment
- Liotrix (Euthyroid, Thyrolar): A mixture of levothyroxine sodium and liothyronine sodium
- Thyroid: Seldom used
- Thyroglobulin (Proloid): Seldom used

HYPOTHYROIDISM

Use	Replacement in decreased or absent thyroid function (partial or complete) absence of gland, primary atrophy, functional deficiency, effects of surgery, radiation or antithyroid agents, pituitary or hypothalamic hypothyroidism; management of simple (nontoxic) goiter and chronic lymphocytic thyroiditis; treatment of thyrotoxicosis (with antithyroid drugs) to prevent goitrogenesis and hypothyroidism. Management of thyroid cancer. Diagnostic in thyroid suppression tests.	Half-life: 6–7 d	Onset: PO: UK IV: 6–8 h	Peaks: 24 h–1 wk 24–48 h	Duration: 1–3 wk UK
Example	Levothyroxine (Synthroid)	Route: PO/IV	Pregnancy category: A	Pharmacokinetic: Variable incomplete absorption from GI tract. PB: greater than 99%; widely distributed; deiodinated in peripheral tissues, minimal metabolism in liver; eliminated by biliary excretion.	
How it works	• Involved in normal metabolism, growth, and development (especially CNS of infants). Possesses catabolic and anabolic effects. Increases basal metabolic rate, enhances gluconeogenesis, stimulates protein synthesis.				

Adult dose	Hypothyroidism:
	• PO: Initially 0.05 mg/day. Increase by 0.025 mg q2–3 wk. Maintenance: 0.1–0.2 mg/day
	Myxedema coma or stupor (medical emergency):
	• IV: Initially 0.4 mg. Follow with daily supplements at 0.2–0.2 mg. Maintenance: 0.05–0.1 mg/day
	Thyroid suppression therapy:
	• PO: 2–6 mcg/kg/day for 7–10 days
	TSH suppression in thyroid cancer, nodules, euthyroid goiters:
	• Use larger doses than that used for replacement therapy
	Congenital hypothyroidism:
	• Greater than 0.15 mg/day
	Usual parenteral dosage:
	IV: Initial dosage approximately one-half the previously established oral dosage
Before administration	• Question for hypersensitivity to tartrazine, aspirin, lactose.
	• Obtain baseline weight and vital signs.
	• Signs and symptoms of diabetes mellitus or diabetes insipidus, adrenal insufficiency, and hypopituitarism may become intensified.
	• Treat with adrenocortical steroids before thyroid therapy in coexisting hypothyroidism and hypoadrenalism.
Administration	• *Note:* Do not interchange brands because there have been problems with bioequivalence among manufacturers.
	• PO: Give at same time each day to maintain hormone levels.
	• Administer before breakfast to avoid insomnia.
	• Tablets may be crushed.
	• IV: Use immediately after reconstitution of 200 mcg or 500 mcg vial with 5 ml 0.9 NaCl to provide a concentration of 40 or 100 mcg/ml, respectively. Shake until clear. Use immediately and discard unused portion. Give each 100 mcg or less over 1 minute.
After administration	• Monitor pulse for rate, rhythm (report pulse of 100 or marked increase from baseline).
	• Assess for tremors and nervousness.
	• Check appetite and sleep pattern.
Contraindications	• Thyrotoxicosis and myocardial infarction uncomplicated by hypothyroidism, hypersensitivity to any component (with tablets: tartrazine, allergy to aspirin, lactose intolerance); treatment of obesity
	• *Caution:* Elderly persons, angina pectoris, hypertension or other cardiovascular disease
Side effects/adverse reactions	• Occasional: Children may have reversible hair loss upon initiation.
	• Rare: Dry skin, GI intolerance, skin rash, hives, pseudotumor cerebri (severe headache in children)
	Adverse/Toxic
	• Excessive dosage produces signs/symptoms of hyperthyroidism: weight loss, palpitations, increased appetite, tremors, nervousness, tachycardia, increased B/P, headache, insomnia, menstrual irregularities. Cardiac arrhythmias occur rarely.
Patient education	• Do not discontinue: Replacement for hypothyroidism is lifelong.
	• Follow up with healthcare visits and thyroid functions tests as ordered.
	• Take medication at the same time every day, preferably in the morning.
	• Monitor pulse, report marked increase, pulse of 100 or above, change of rhythm.
	• Do not change brands.
	• Notify provider promptly of chest pain, weight loss, nervousness or tremors, and insomnia.
	• Children may have reversible hair loss or increased aggressiveness during the first few months of therapy.
	• Full therapeutic effect may take 1–3 weeks.

21.8 Hyperthyroidism

An excess production of thyroxine and triiodothyronine is called hyperthyroidism.
There are two types of hyperthyroidism:

- Primary hyperthyroidism: The thyroid gland is hyperfunctioning, producing a high quantity of thyroxine and triiodothyronine, which results in an increased serum level of thyrotropin-releasing hormone and thyroid-stimulating hormone. This is called Graves' disease (exophthalmos, nervousness, irritability, weight loss).
- Secondary hyperthyroidism: Either the hypothalamus releases a high quantity of thyrotropin-releasing hormone or the anterior pituitary gland releases a high quantity of thyroid-stimulating hormone.

Hyperthyroidism is treated by administering antithyroid medication, which inhibits thyroxine and triiodothyronine production. These are:

- Propylthiouracil (PTU)
- Methylthiouracil (Tapazole)
- Methimazole: More potent and has a longer half-life than propylthiouracil
- Lugol's solution: Administer to patients having thyroidectomy
- Sodium iodide: Administer IV for thyroid crisis (thyroid storm), which is a severe symptom of hyperthyroidism

Caution: Prolonged use can cause goiter formation.

HYPERTHYROIDISM

Use 24 hours	Palliative treatment of hyperthyroidism; adjunct to ameliorate hyperthyroidism in preparation for surgical treatment or radioactive iodine therapy	Half-life: 1–2 hours	Onset: 1 hour	Peaks: 2.5 hours	Duration: 5 hours
Example	Propylthiouracil (PTU)	Route: PO	Pregnancy category: D	Pharmacokinetic: PB: 75%–80%; metabolized in liver, excreted in urine	

How it works	• In hyperthyroidism, inhibits synthesis of thyroid hormone. Diverts iodine from thyroid hormone synthesis.
Adult dose	• Initially; 300–400 mg/day. Maintenance: 100–150 mg/day.
Before administration	• Obtain baseline weight and pulse.
Administration	• Take without regard to meals.
After administration	• Monitor pulse and weight daily. • Check for skin eruptions, itching, swollen lymph glands. • Be alert to hepatitis (nausea, vomiting, drowsiness, jaundice). • Monitor hematology results for bone marrow suppression. • Check for signs of infection and bleeding.
Contraindications	• None significant • *Caution:* Patients greater than 40 years of age or in combination with other agranulocytosis-inducing drugs
Side effects/adverse reactions	• Frequent: Urticaria, rash, pruritus, nausea, skin pigmentation, hair loss, headache, paresthesia • Occasional: Drowsiness, lymphadenopathy, vertigo • Rare: Drug fever, lupuslike syndrome

Adverse/Toxic

- Agranulocytosis (may occur as long as 4 months after therapy), pancytopenia, fatal hepatitis.

Patient education
- Space evenly around the clock.
- Take resting pulse daily.
- Report as directed.
- Seafood and iodine products may be restricted.
- Report illness, unusual bleeding/bruising.
- Inform healthcare provider immediate of sudden/continuous weight gain, cold intolerance, or depression.

21.9   The Parathyroid Glands

The parathyroid glands secrete parathyroid hormone (PTH), which regulates serum calcium levels. Decreased serum calcium stimulates the parathyroid glands to secrete parathyroid hormone. Increased serum calcium inhibits secretion of parathyroid hormone.

Hypoparathyroidism is the deficiency in secretion of parathyroid hormone and is treated by administering parathyroid hormone. Hypoparathyroidism can cause hypocalcemia. Hyperparathyroidism is the oversecretion of parathyroid hormone caused by a parathyroid gland tumor or ectopic secretion of the parathyroid hormone as the result of lung cancer or prolonged immobility, causing loss of calcium from bone. Hyperparathyroidism is treated by administering calcitonin to decrease serum calcium and promote excretion of calcium by the kidneys or by treating the underlying cause.

21.10   The Pancreas

The pancreas secretes insulin, which metabolizes glucose. The body adjusts the amount of insulin based on the serum glucose level.

- Hyperglycemia: Serum glucose levels are high, stimulating the pancreas to secrete insulin to metabolize glucose.
- Hypoglycemia: Serum glucose levels are low, inhibiting the secretion of insulin and stimulating the intake of food and the production of glucose.

Chronic deficiency of insulin or the absence of insulin is called diabetes mellitus. There are three types of diabetes mellitus:

1. *Type I diabetes mellitus*: Type I diabetes mellitus is when the pancreas suddenly produces little or no insulin, requiring the patient to replace insulin daily via an injection. This is referred to as insulin-dependent diabetes mellitus (IDDM).
2. *Type II diabetes mellitus*: Type II diabetes mellitus (age-onset diabetes) is when the pancreas' ability to produced insulin is either diminished (age) or is insufficient to metabolize the excess serum glucose (overweight, lack of exercise). Insulin is produced but is not effective. The patient controls Type II diabetes mellitus by diet, exercise, and oral diabetes medication that stimulate insulin production in the pancreas and other organs. This is referred to as non–insulin-dependent diabetes (NIDDM).
3. *Gestations diabetes mellitus*: Gestations diabetes mellitus develops during the second or third trimester of pregnancy and resolves after delivery. During the pregnancy, this is treated with diet and insulin injections if necessary.

The signs and symptoms of diabetes are:

- Polyuria (increased urine output)
- Polydipsia (increased thirst)
- Polyphagia (increased hunger)

Medications can cause hyperglycemia. Once medication is discontinued serum glucose level returns to normal. These medications are:

- Glucocorticoids (cortisone, prednisone)
- Thiazide diuretics (hydrochlorothiazide [Hydro DIURIL])
- Epinephrine

21.11   Insulin

Insulin helps glucose to enter a cell. Inside the cell, glucose is used for cell metabolism. Glucose cannot enter the cell without insulin, resulting in the cell signaling the body to increase intake of glucose (food), thinking there is not any serum glucose.

Insulin is destroyed by GI secretions, which is why insulin cannot be administered orally. Insulin is injected subcutaneously in an insulin syringe (see chapter 6). The site and depth of the injection affect the absorption of insulin. Insulin can be delivered using an insulin pump, which is surgically implanted in the abdomen. The insulin pump delivers an infusion of insulin. A bolus of insulin is administered before meals either intraperitoneally or IV. Insulin can also be administered intranasally to provide a rapid-onset effect and a short duration (although this method is expensive and rarely used). Insulin injectors can be used to deliver insulin under high pressure through the skin into fatty tissue without a needle. This results in bruising, pain, and burning.

There are four types of insulin:

- Rapid-acting (regular or Lispro (Humalog) insulin): Onset 1/2 to 1 hour, peak 2 to 4 hours, and duration of 6 to 8 hours
- Intermediate-acting (NPH, Humulin N, Lente, and Humulin L insulin): Onset 1 to 2 hours, peak 6 to 12 hours, duration 18 to 24 hours
- Long-acting (Ultralente insulin): Onset 5 to 8 hours, peak 14 to 20 hours, duration 30 to 36 hours
- Combinations: Humulin 70/30 (NPH 70%, regular 30%); Humulin 50/50 (NPH 50%, regular 50%)

Unopened insulin vials must be temperature-controlled until needed. Once opened, the insulin vial can be kept at room temperature for 1 month or in the refrigerator for 3 months. Do not put an open insulin vial in the freezer. Do not place in direct sunlight or a high-temperature area.

Serum glucose level is usually taken before administering insulin. Healthcare providers prescribe insulin on a sliding scale based on the level of serum glucose. This assures that the correct dose of insulin is administered. If too much insulin is administered, the patient experiences hypoglycemic reaction (Table 21.3).

TABLE 21.3 Hypoglycemic Reactions and Diabetic Ketoacidosis

REACTION	SIGNS AND SYMPTOMS
Hypoglycemic reaction (insulin shock)	Headache, lightheadedness, nervousness, apprehension, tremor, excess perspiration; cold, clammy skin, tachycardia, slurred speech, memory lapse, confusion, seizures
	Blood sugar less than 60 mg/dl
Diabetic ketoacidosis (hyperglycemic reaction)	Extreme thirst, polyuria, fruity breath odor, Kussmaul breathing (deep, rapid, labored, distressing, dyspnea), rapid, thready pulse, dry mucous membranes, poor skin turgor
	Blood sugar level greater than 250 mg/dl

ANTIDIABETIC DRUGS

Use	Treatment of insulin-dependent type I diabetes mellitus; noninsulin-dependent type II diabetes mellitus when diet/weight control therapy has failed to maintain satisfactory blood glucose levels or in event of pregnancy, surgery, trauma, infection, fever, severe, renal, hepatic, or endocrine dysfunction. Regular insulin used in emergency treatment of ketoacidosis, to promote passage of glucose across cell membrane in hyperalimentation, to facilitate intracellular shift of K+ in hyperkalemia.	Half-life: 10 minutes –1 hour	Onset: 0.5–1 hour	Peaks: 2–4 hours	Duration: 6–8 hours

Example	Regular Insulin	Route: SC/IV	Pregnancy category: B	Pharmacokinetic: Well absorbed with all routes of administration. Metabolized by the liver and muscle and excreted in the urine. PB: UK.

How it works
- Facilitates passage of glucose, K., Mg across cellular membranes of skeletal and cardiac muscle, adipose tissue; controls storage and metabolism of carbohydrates, protein, fats. Promotes conversion of glucose to glycogen in liver.

Adult dose
- Dosage for insulin in individualized/monitored
- Usual dosage guidelines: Note; adjust dosage to achieve pre-meal and bedtime glucose level of 80–140 mg/dl
- SC: 0.5–1 unit/kg/day

Before administration
- Check blood glucose levels.
- Discuss lifestyle to determine extent of learning and emotional needs.
- Assess drug and medical history.
- Assess patient's knowledge of disease.
- Check vital signs.

Administration
- Administer SC as per guidelines, rotate injection sites.

After administration
- Assess for hypoglycemia (cook wet skin, tremors, dizziness, headache, anxiety, tachycardia, numbness in mouth, hunger, diplopia).
- Check sleeping patient for restlessness or diaphoresis.
- Check for hyperglycemia (polyuria, polyphagia, and polydipsia) nausea and vomiting, dim vision, fatigue, deep rapid breathing.
- Be alert to conditions altering glucose requirements such as fever, increased activity or stress, surgical procedures.

Contraindications
- Hypersensitivity or insulin resistance may require change of type or species source of insulin.

Side effects/adverse reactions
- Occasional: Local redness, swelling, itching (owing to improper injection technique or allergy to cleansing solution or insulin)
- Infrequent: Somogyi effect (rebound hyperglycemia) with chronically excessive insulin doses. Systemic allergic reaction (rash, angioedema, anaphylaxis), lipodystrophy (depression at injection site due to breakdown of adipose tissue), lipohypertrophy (accumulation of SC tissue at injection site rotation)
- Rare: Insulin resistance

Adverse/Toxic
- Severe hypoglycemia (owing to hyperinsulinism) may occur in overdose of insulin, decrease or delay of food intake, excessive exercise, or those with brittle diabetes. Diabetic ketoacidosis may result from stress, illness, omission of insulin dose, or long-term poor insulin control.

Patient education
- Prescribed diet is an essential part of therapy.
- Do not skip or delay meals.
- Carry candy, sugar packets, other sugar supplements for immediate response to hypoglycemia.
- Wear/carry medical alert identification.
- Check with provider when insulin demands are altered (e.g., fever, infection, trauma, stress, heavy physical activity).
- Do not take other medications without consulting provider.
- Weight control, exercise, hygiene (including foot care), and not smoking are integral parts of the therapy. Protect skin, and limit sun exposure.
- Inform dentist, physician, or surgeon of medication before any treatment is given.

21.12   Oral Antidiabetics

Oral antidiabetic medications are used to treat Type II diabetes mellitus by stimulating the secretion of insulin. These are:

- Sulfonylureas: There are two generations of sulfonylureas. These are:
  - First-generation sulfonylureas are:
    - Tolbutamide (Orinase)
    - Acetohexamide (Dymelor)
    - Tolazamide (Tolinase)
    - Chlorpropamide (Diabinese)
  - Second-generation sulfonylureas increase tissue response to insulin and decrease glucose production by the liver resulting in greater hypoglycemic potency at smaller doses. They have a longer duration and cause few side effects, but should not be used if the patient has liver or kidney dysfunction. Sulfonylureas are:
    - Glipizide (Glucotrol)
    - Glyburide nonmicronized (DiaBeta, Micronase)
    - Glimepiride (Amaryl)
- Nonsulfonylureas: Nonsulfonylureas decrease hepatic production of glucose from stored glycogen, resulting in reduced increase in serum glucose after a meal and limits the degree of postprandial (after a meal) hyperglycemia.
  - Metformin (Glucophage): Decreases the absorption of glucose from the small intestine and may increase insulin receptor sensitivity as well as peripheral glucose uptake at the cellular level. Does not produce hypoglycemia or hyperglycemia. Can cause GI disturbances.
- Alpha-glucosidase inhibitor: Inhibits alpha glucosidase, the digestive enzyme in the small intestine that is responsible for the release of glucose from the complex carbohydrates in the diet. Carbohydrates cannot be absorbed and instead pass into the large intestine. Does not cause a hypoglycemic reaction.
  - Acarbose (Precose)
- Thiazolidinediones: Decrease insulin resistance and help muscle cells to respond to insulin and use glucose more effectively.
  - Pioglitazone (Actos)
- Repaglinide (Prandin): Short-acting similar to sulfonylureas. Does not cause hypoglycemic reaction.

21.13   Medication That Increases Glucose

It is critical that the serum glucose level be restored in a patient who has hypoglycemia. The following medications are used to treat hypoglycemia.

Glucagon

Glucagon is a hyperglycemic hormone secreted by the alpha cells of the islets of Langerhans in the pancreas and increases blood sugar by stimulating glycogenolysis (glycogen breakdown) in the liver. Glucagon increases serum glucose levels 5 to 20 minutes after administration. It is given to patients who are semiconscious or unconscious and unable to ingest carbohydrates.

Oral Diazoxide (Proglycem)

Oral diazoxide (Proglycem) increases serum glucose level by inhibiting insulin release from the beta cells and stimulating release of epinephrine (Adrenalin) from the adrenal medulla. Oral diazoxide is used to treat chronic hypoglycemia caused by hyperinsulinism resulting from islet cell cancer or hyperplasia. It is not for hypoglycemic reactions.

ANTIDIABETIC: SECOND-GENERATION SULFONYLUREA

Use	Adjunct to diet/exercise in management of noninsulin-dependent diabetes mellitus (type 2, NIDDM). Use in combination with insulin or metformin in patients not controlled by diet/exercise in conjunction with oral hypoglycemic agent.	Half-life: 5–9.2 hours	Onset: —	Peaks: 2–3 hours	Duration: 24 hours
Example	Glimepiride (Amaryl)	Route: PO	Pregnancy category: C	\

Pharmacokinetic: Completely absorbed from GI tract. PB: greater than 99%. Metabolized in liver; excreted in urine and eliminated in feces. | |

How it works	• Promotes release of insulin from beta cells of pancreas, increases insulin sensitivity at peripheral sites, lowering blood glucose concentration.
Adult dose	• PO: Initially 1–2 mg once daily with breakfast or first main meal; Maintenance: 1–4 mg once daily. After dose of 2 mg is reached, dosage should be increased in increments of up to 2 mg q1–2 wk. Based on blood glucose response. Maximum 8 mg/day • Combination with insulin therapy: 8 mg once daily with breakfast or first main meal with low-dose insulin • Renal function impairment: PO: 1 mg/once day
Before administration	• Check blood glucose level. • Discuss lifestyle to determine extent of learning, emotional needs. • Assure follow-up instruction if patient/family do not thoroughly understand diabetes management or glucose-testing techniques.
Administration	• Give with breakfast or first main meal.
After administration	• Monitor blood glucose and food intake. • Assess for hypoglycemia (cool wet skin, tremors, dizziness, anxiety, headache, tachycardia, numbness in mouth, hunger, diplopia) or hyperglycemia (polyuria, polyphagia, polydipsia, nausea, vomiting, dim vision, fatigue, deep rapid breathing). • Be alert to conditions that alter glucose requirements fever, increased activity or stress, surgical procedures.
Contraindications	• Sole therapy for type I diabetes mellitus, diabetic complications (ketosis, acidosis, diabetic coma), stress situations (severe infection, trauma, surgery), severe renal or hepatic impairment. • *Cautions:* Severe diarrhea, intestinal obstruction, prolonged vomiting, liver disease, hyperthyroidism (not controlled), impaired renal function, adrenal insufficiency, debilitation, malnutrition, pituitary insufficiency

Side effects/adverse reactions	• Frequent: Altered taste sensation, dizziness, drowsiness, weight gain, constipation, diarrhea, heartburn, nausea, vomiting, stomach fullness, headache
	• Occasional: Increased sensitivity of skin to sunlight, peeling of skin, itching, rash
	Adverse/Toxic
	• Hypoglycemia may occur due to overdosage, insufficient food intake, especially with increased glucose demands. GI hemorrhage, cholestatic hepatic jaundice, leucopenia, thrombocytopenia, pancytopenia, agranulocytosis, and aplastic or hemolytic anemia occur rarely.
Patient education	• Prescribed diet is principal part of treatment. Do not skip or delay meals.
	• Carry candy, sugar packets, or other sugar supplements for immediate response to hypoglycemia.
	• Wear medical alert identification.
	• Check with healthcare provider when glucose demands are altered (e.g., fever, infection, trauma, stress, heavy physical exercise).

Solved Problems

Hormones

21.1 What are the two types of hormones?

The two types of hormones are proteins and steroids.

21.2 What is a hormone?

A hormone is a messenger that causes tissue, organ, and cellular activities to increase or decrease tissue equal to the amount of the hormones in the blood.

21.3 What is hormone therapy?

Hormone therapy replaces or inhibits secretion of hormones.

Pituitary Gland

21.4 What hormone is produced by the pituitary gland?

The pituitary gland secretes growth hormone (GH), antidiuretic hormone (ADH), and oxytocin.

21.5 What is acromegaly?

Acromegaly is abnormally excessive growth after puberty.

21.6 What happens if there is hyposecretion of growth hormone?

Hyposecretion of growth hormone is referred to as GH deficiency and results in the patient not reaching a normal height.

21.7 How is hypersecretion of growth hormone treated?

Hypersecretion of growth hormone is treated by destroying the pituitary tumor with radiation, administering Bromocriptine (inhibits release of growth hormone from the pituitary gland), and administering Octreotide (suppresses release of the growth hormone).

21.8 How is hyposecretion of growth hormone treated?

Hyposecretion of growth hormone is treated with Somatrem (growth hormone replacement) and Somatropin (growth hormone replacement).

21.9   What is the function of Antidiuretic hormone (ADH)?

Antidiuretic hormone is a vasopressin and promotes water reabsorption from the renal tubules to maintain water balance in the body fluids

21.10   What is diabetes insipidus (DI)?

Diabetes insipidus (DI) is a deficiency in antidiuretic hormone resulting from trauma to the hypothalamus and pituitary gland or a brain tumor that causes the kidneys to excrete large amounts of water, leading to severe fluid volume deficit and electrolyte imbalances.

21.11   What hormone is administered to start labor?

Oxytocin starts labor contractions.

21.12   How is diabetes insipidus treated?

Diabetes insipidus is treated by replacing the antidiuretic hormone by administering desmopressin acetate (DDAVP), desmopressin (Stimate), lypressin (Diapid), vasopressin (aqueous; Pitressin), and vasopressin tannate/oil (Pitressin Tannate).

Adrenal Gland

21.13   What controls the secretion of hormones by the adrenal gland?

The secretion of hormones by the adrenal gland is controlled by the adrenocorticotropic hormone (ACTH), which is produced by the pituitary gland.

21.14   How do healthcare providers determine the cause of decreased levels of adrenocorticotropic hormone?

Healthcare providers determine the cause of decreased levels of adrenocorticotropic hormone by administering corticotropin (Acthar), which is the adrenocorticotropic hormone. If after 60 minutes there are increased levels of glucocorticoids, then there is a pituitary gland insufficiency. If no increase occurs, then there is an adrenal gland insufficiency.

21.15   What is Cushing's syndrome?

Cushing's syndrome is the hypersecretion of adrenal hormones.

21.16   What is glucocorticoid therapy?

Glucocorticoid therapy involves administering glucocorticoids to reduce the effects of trauma, decrease infections, and reduce anxiety.

Thyroid Gland

21.17   What are the three possible causes of hypothyroidism?

Three possible causes of hypothyroidism are the decreased secretion of thyrotropin-releasing hormone (TRH) by the hypothalamus gland, decreased secretion of thyroid-stimulating hormone (TSH) by the pituitary gland, and decreased secretion of thyroid hormones by the thyroid gland.

21.18   How is the serum calcium level reduced?

The serum calcium level is reduced by administering calcitonin.

21.19   What is secondary hypothyroidism?

Secondary hypothyroidism is either the hypothalamus is unable to release sufficient quantities of thyrotropin-releasing hormone or the anterior pituitary gland is unable to release sufficient thyroid-stimulating hormone.

21.20 How is hypothyroidism treated?

Hypothyroid is treated by administering levothyroxine sodium (increases thyroxine and triiodothyronine for long-term treatment), Liothyronine (increases triiodothyronine for short-term treatment), Liotrix (a mixture of levothyroxine sodium and liothyronine sodium), thyroid (seldom used), or thyroglobulin (seldom used).

Pancreas

21.21 What medications cause hyperglycemia?

The medications that cause hyperglycemia are glucocorticoids, thiazide diuretics, and epinephrine.

21.22 What are four types of insulin?

Four types of insulin are rapid-acting, intermediate-acting, long-acting, and combinations.

21.23 How do oral antidiabetic medications treat Type II diabetes mellitus?

Oral antidiabetic medications are used to treat Type II diabetes mellitus by stimulating the secretion of insulin.

21.24 Can oral antidiabetic medications be used in place of insulin injections?

No. Insulin injections are administered when the pancreas is unable to product sufficient insulin. Oral antidiabetic medication stimulates insulin secretion.

21.25 How does metformin work?

Metformin decrease the absorption of glucose from the small intestine and may increase insulin receptor sensitivity as well as peripheral glucose uptake at the cellular level.

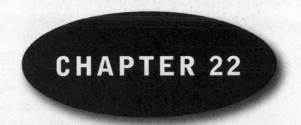

CHAPTER 22

Eye and Ear Disorders

22.1 Eye Disorders

There are three common disorders of the eye. These are:

1. Glaucoma: Increased intraocular pressure (IOP) that causes increased pressure on the optic nerve, resulting in decreased peripheral vision and eventually blindness. There are two types of glaucoma:
   a. Chronic open-angle glaucoma occurs when the open drainage angle of the eye is blocked, leading to gradually increased IOP that leads to optic nerve damage. Damage occurs gradually and painlessly.
   b. Angle-closure glaucoma occurs when the drainage angle of the eye narrows, becoming suddenly and completely blocked. IOP increases rapidly, causing severe eye pain, blurred vision, headache, rainbow haloes around lights, nausea and vomiting, which lead to blindness.
2. Conjunctivitis: Inflammation of the conjunctiva (white part of eye), resulting in the conjunctiva becoming pink or red and itchy. There are four types of conjunctivitis:
   a. Viral conjunctivitis affects one eye, causing excessive eye watering and a light discharge from the eye.
   b. Bacterial conjunctivitis affects both eyes, causing a heavy greenish discharge.
   c. Allergic conjunctivitis affects both eyes, causing itching and redness and excessive tearing. The patient may also experience an itchy and red nose.
   d. Giant papillary conjunctivitis (GPC) affects both eyes, causing contact lens intolerance, itching, heavy discharge, and tearing and red bumps on the underside of the eyelids.
3. Corneal abrasion: A cut or scratch on the cornea caused by rubbing eyes, contact lens, sand, dust, dirt, or for no apparent reason, resulting in pain and sensitized cornea (feels like something in eye) and photophobia. Corneal abrasions are identified by administering Fluorescein sodium and Fluress (fluorescein sodium and benoxinate HCl), which are dyes that cause corneal scratches to turn bright red, foreign bodies to become surrounded by green a ring, and loss of conjunctiva to appear orange-yellow.

22.2 Eye Medication

There are eight types of medications (Table 22–1) used to treat eye disorders. These are:

1. *Topical anesthetics:* Topical anesthetics are used to anesthetize the eye for eye examination and removal of foreign bodies from the eye. Onset is 1 minute and duration is 15 minutes. The blink reflex is temporarily lost and the corneal epithelium temporarily dries. Use a protective eye patch until the

effects of the drug wear off.

2. *Antiinfectives and antimicrobials:* Antiinfectives and antimicrobials (see chapters 12 and 13) are administered to treat eye infections and can cause local skin and eye irritation.

3. *Lubricants:* Lubricants alleviate discomfort associated with dry eyes and moisten contact lenses and artificial eyes. Lubricants moisten eyes during anesthesia and unconsciousness.

4. *Miotics:* Miotics lower IOP in open-angle glaucoma, increasing blood flow to the retina, which results in decreased retinal damage and prevention of vision loss. There are two types of miotics, direct-acting cholinergics and cholinesterase inhibitors. Adverse effects are headache, eye pain, decreased vision, brow pain, nausea, vomiting, diarrhea, frequent urination, precipitation of asthma attacks, increased salivation, diaphoresis, muscle weakness, and respiratory difficulty.

5. *Carbonic anhydrase inhibitors:* Carbonic anhydrase inhibitors are used for long-term treatment of open-angle glaucoma and interfere with the production of carbonic acid, resulting in decreased IOP. Adverse effects are lethargy, anorexia, drowsiness, paresthesia, depression, polyuria, nausea, vomiting, hypokalemia, and renal calculi. Do not administer in the first trimester of pregnancy or to patients who are allergic to sulfonamides.

6. *Osmotics:* Osmotics reduces IOP by decreasing vitreous humor volume. It is also used as a preoperative and postoperative medication and in the emergency treatment of closed-angle glaucoma. Adverse effects are headache, nausea, vomiting, and diarrhea. Elderly patients can become disoriented.

7. *Anticholinergic mydriatics:* Anticholinergic mydriatics (see chapter 15) dilate the pupils for diagnostic procedures and ophthalmic surgery. Adverse effects are tachycardia, photophobia, dryness of the mouth, edema, conjunctivitis, and dermatitis.

8. *Cycloplegics:* Cycloplegics paralyze eye muscles for diagnostic procedures and ophthalmic surgery. Adverse effects are tachycardia, photophobia, dryness of the mouth, edema, conjunctivitis, and dermatitis.

22.3   Eye Medication: Patient Education

When administering eye medication to a patient, be sure that the patient:

- Understands the therapeutic effect of the medication
- Has observed a demonstration of the proper technique to administer eye drops and ointment
- Understands the side effects of the medication
- Knows to administer the medication at bedtime because of possible temporary vision loss
- Knows to record each time the medication is administered
- Consults the healthcare provider before stopping the medication
- Wears a medical alert bracelet if taking glaucoma medications

---

DIRECT-ACTING MIOTIC

TABLE 22.1 Ophthalmic Medications

ANTIBACTERIALS	ANTIFUNGAL	ANTIVIRAL	ANTI-INFLAMMATORIES
Chloramphenicol (Chloromycetin Ophthalmic) Ciprofloxacin (Cipro) Erythromycin Gentamicin sulfate (Garamycin Ophthalmic) Norfloxacin (Chibroxin) Tobramycin (Nebcin, Tobrex)	Natamycin (Natacyn Ophthalmic	Idoxuridine (IDU) Trifluridine (Viroptic) Vidarabine monohydrate (Vira-A)	Dexamethasone Diclofenac Na (Voltaren) Suprofen Profenal) Ketorolac tromethamine (Acular) Olopatadine HCL Ophthalmic solution Medrysone (HMS Liquifilm) Prednisolone acetate Prednisolone Na phosphate Combination: TobraDex

Silver nitrate 1% (used in neonates to prevent ophthalmia neonatorum) Tetracycline HCL (Achromycin Ophthalmic)			(tobramycin 0.3% and dexamethasone 0.1%)
Miotics: Cholinergics and beta-adrenergic blockers	Indirect-acting cholinesterase inhibitors: Short acting	Beta-adrenergic blockers	Carbonic anhydrase Inhibitors
Acetylcholine Cl (Miochol) Carbachol intraocular (Miostat) Pilocarpine HCL (Isopto Carpine) Pilocarpine nitrate (Ocusert Pilo–20) Echothiophate iodide (Phospholine Iodide)	Physostigmine salicylate (Isopto Eserine)	Betaxolol HCl (Betoptic) Levobunolol HCl Timolol maleate (Timoptic)	Acetazolamide (Diamox) Brinzolamide ophthalmic sus. 1% Dichlorphenamide (Daranide) Dorzolamide (Trusopt) Methazolamide (Neptazane)
Osmotics	Mydriatics and cycloplegics		
Glycerin Isosorbide (Ismotic) Mannitol (Osmitrol) Urea (Ureaphil)	Atropine sulfate Cyclopentolate HCl Dipivefrin HCl Epinephrine HCl Epinephrine borate Homatropine hydrobromide (Isopto Homatropine) Scopolamine hydrobromide Tropicamide (Mydriacyl Ophthalmic)		

Use	To induce miosis; to decrease IOP in glaucoma	Half-life: UK	Onset: Ophthalmic: 45–60 minutes Ocusert: 2 hours Gel: 1 hour	Peaks: Ophthalmic: 75 minutes Ocusert: 1.5–2 hours Gel: 3–12 hours	Duration: Ophthalmic: 4–14 hours Ocusert: 1 hour Gel: 18–24 hours
Example	Pilocarpine (Isopto Carpine, Pilopine HS. Ocusert Pilo–20 and –40)	Route: Ophthalmic	Pregnancy category: C	Pharmacokinetic: Some systemic absorption; binds to ocular tissue; excretion: UK; PB: UK	
How it works	• Stimulation of papillary and ciliary sphincter muscles				
Adult dose	• Solution: 1%–2%, 1–2 gtt, TID/QID • Gel: Apply 0.5-in ribbon in lower eyelid at bedtime				

- Ocusert: Replaced q7d

Before administration	• Assess medical and drug history. • Check vital signs (baseline). • Assess level of anxiety; the possibility of diminished vision or blindness increases anxiety. • Assess patient's eye pigment; patients with dark, heavily pigmented eyes may benefit from a pilocarpine concentration greater than 4%.
Administration	• When administering drops, apply gentle pressure to the inner canthus to prevent or minimize system absorption.
After administration	• Monitor vital signs. Heart rate and blood pressure may decrease with large doses of cholinergics. • Monitor for side effects. • Monitor for postural hypotension. • Check breath sounds for rales and rhonchi. • Maintain oral hygiene with excessive salivation. • Have atropine available as antidote.
Contraindications	• Retinal detachment, adhesions between iris and lens, acute ocular inflammation, must avoid systemic absorption of drug with coronary artery disease, obstruction of GI/GU tract, epilepsy, asthma
Side effects/ adverse reactions	• Blurred vision, eye pain, headache, eye irritation, brow ache, stinging and burning, nausea, vomiting, diarrhea, increased salivation and sweating, muscle tremors, contact allergy; conjunctival irritation with Ocusert Adverse/Toxic • Dyspnea, hypertension, tachycardia, retinal detachment. Long-term: bronchospasm; corneal abrasion and visual impairment potential with Ocusert
Patient education	• Teach to administer eye drops and ointment correctly with return demonstrations. • Keep appointments and regular medical supervision. • Do not stop medication suddenly. • Report side or adverse effects. • Avoid driving or operating machinery while vision is impaired. • Avoid atropine-like drugs. Check labels on over-the-counter medications. Ocular Therapeutic Systems (Ocusert) • Store drugs in refrigerator. • Discard damaged or contaminated disks. • Myopia is minimized by bedtime insertion in the upper conjunctival sac. • If self-administering, follow instructions related to insertion and removal. • Check for presence of disk in conjunctival sac at bedtime and when arising. • Temporary stinging may occur. Notify healthcare provider if blurred vision or brow pain occurs. Cholinesterase Inhibitors • First dose should be administered by healthcare provider and followed by tonometry (measurement of IOP) reading. • Tightly cap tube because ointment is inactivated by water.

OSMOTIC (OSMOTIC DIURETIC, ANTIGLAUCOMA, ANTIHEMOLYTIC)

Use		Half-life:	Onset:	Peaks:	Duration:
Prevention, treatment of oliguric phase if acute renal failure (before evidence of permanent renal failure). Reduces increased intracranial pressure caused by cerebral edema, edema of injured spinal cord, intraocular pressure caused by acute glaucoma. Promotes urinary excretion of toxic substances (aspirin, bromides,		15–100 minutes	1–3 hours CIOP: 0.5–1 hour CSF pressure: 15 minutes	UK	IOP: 4–6 hours CSF: 3–8 hours

imipramine, barbiturates).

Example	Mannitol (Osmitrol)	Route: IV	Pregnancy category: C	Pharmacokinetic: Remains in extracellular fluid; primarily excreted in urine. Removed by hemodialysis.

How it works

- Elevates osmotic pressure of glomerular filtrate, increases flow of water into interstitial fluid and plasma, inhibiting renal tubular reabsorption of sodium, chloride, producing diuresis. Enhances flow of water from eye into plasma, reducing intraocular pressure (IOP)

Adult dose

- *Note:* Test dose of 12.5 g for adults over 3–5 min to produce a urine flow of at least 30–50 ml/h over 203 h
- Initially 0.5–1 g/kg, then 0.25–0.5 g/kg q4–6 h

Before administration

- Check B/P; pulse before giving medication.
- Assess skin turgor, mucous membranes, mental status, and muscle strength.
- Obtain baseline weight.
- Initiate intake and output monitoring.
- Check for eye pain and pressure.
- Assess IV site for patency before each dose. Extravasation is noted with pain and thrombosis.

Administration

- Administer IV infusion over 30–90 minutes.
- Rate of administration should be titrated to promote urinary output of 30–50 ml/h.
- Use filter for infusion of 20% or more concentration.
- Do not add KCl or NaCl to mannitol 20% or greater.
- Do not add to whole blood for transfusion.

After administration

- Monitor urinary output to ascertain therapeutic response.
- Monitor electrolyte, BUN, renal, hepatic, reports.
- Assess vital signs, skin turgor, mucous membranes.
- Weigh patient daily.
- Monitor for signs of hyponatremia (confusion, drowsiness, thirst, or dry mouth, cold/clammy skin).
- Monitor for signs of hypokalemia (changes in muscle strength, tremors, muscle cramps, changes in mental status, cardiac arrhythmias; hyperkalemia (colic, diarrhea, muscle twitching followed by weakness of paralysis, and cardiac arrhythmias).

Contraindications

- Increasing oliguria or anuria, CHF, pulmonary edema, organic CNS disease, severe dehydration, fluid overload, active intracranial bleeding (except during craniotomy), severe electrolyte depletion
- *Cautions:* Impaired renal, hepatic function

Side effects/ adverse reactions

- Frequent: Dry mouth, thirst
- Occasional: Blurred vision, increased urination, headache, arm pain, backache, nausea, vomiting, urticaria (hives), dizziness, hypotension, hypertension, tachycardia, fever, angina-like chest pain

Adverse/Toxic

- Fluid and electrolyte imbalance may occur because of rapid administration of large doses or inadequate urinary output, resulting in overexpansion of extracellular fluid. Circulatory overload may produce pulmonary edema or congestive heart failure. Excessive diuresis may produce hypokalemia or hyponatremia. Fluid loss in excess of electrolyte excretion may produce hypernatremia and hyperkalemia.

Patient education

- Expect increased frequency and volume of urination.
- Report side effects to healthcare provider.
- Use hard candy and tepid water to relieve dry mouth.

22.4 Ear Disorders

Common ear disorders follow.

Cerumen Impaction

Cerumen impaction occurs when cerumen, produced by glands in the outer ear canal, fails to wash away and becomes impacted. Cerumenolytics (hydrogen peroxide solution) are used to irrigate the ear canal. Cerumenex, Debrox, olive oil, or mineral oil is used to treat chronic cerumen impaction.

Otitis Externa and Otitis Media

Otitis externa and otitis media are infections of the external and middle ear respectively and are treated with analgesics (see chapter 16) and antibiotics (see chapter 13). Table 22–2 contains commonly prescribed antibiotics for ear infections.

Hint: Some ear infections are caused by a virus and are not treated with antibiotics.

TABLE 22.2 **Common Antibiotics Used to Treat Ear Infections**

EXTERNAL EAR	INTERNAL EAR
Acetic acid and aluminum acetate (Otic Domeboro)	Amoxicillin (Amoxil, Augmentin)
Boric acid (Ear-Dry), Carbamide peroxide (Debrox)	Ampicillin trihydrate (Polycillin)
Chloramphenicol (Chloromycetin Otic)	Cefaclor (Ceclor)
Polymyxin B	Erythromycin (E-Mycin)
Tetracycline (Achromycin)	Penicillin (Pentads, Pen-V)
Trolamine polypeptide oleate-condensate (Cerumenex)	Sulfonamides (Azulfidine, Bactrim)
	Clarithromycin (Biaxin)
	Amoxicillin and potassium clavulanate (Augmentin)
	Loracarbef (Lorabid)

Vestibular Disorders

Vestibular disorders are dizziness, unsteadiness, or imbalance when walking. Vertigo, nausea, headache, and muscular aches in the neck and back, motion sickness, and sensitivity to noise and bright lights may be mild (lasting minutes) or severe (resulting in total disability). Ménière's disease, labyrinthitis, and inner ear infections can cause vestibular disorders. Common causes of vestibular disorders follow:

- Ear pain: Self-resolves in 72 hours. Healthcare providers typically prescribe analgesics (acetaminophen or ibuprofen) to relieve the pain in the interim.
- Ear congestion: Caused by improper drainage of the eustachian tube and is relieved by administering antihistamine-decongestant medications (Actifed, Allerest, Dimetapp, Drixoral, Novafed, Ornade, Phenergan, and Triaminic).

22.5 Ear Medication: Patient Education

When administering ear medication to a patient, be sure that the patient:

- Understands not to place any foreign objects (Q-tips) into the ear canal
- Knows that cerumenolytics should be used to remove cerumen

- Places two drops of alcohol in the ear canal to keep it dry before swimming to prevent otitis externa (swimmer's ear)
- Knows to keep medication in a light-resistant container because many ear medications are sensitive to light
- Remembers to take antibiotics for the prescribed length of time (10–14 days)
- Understands that he or she should not stop taking antibiotics once the pain has subsided
- Knows to report any change in hearing

Solved Problems

Eye Disorders

22.1 What is glaucoma?

Glaucoma is increased intraocular pressure (IOP), causing increased pressure on the optic nerve that results in decreased peripheral vision and, eventually, blindness.

22.2 What is chronic open-angle glaucoma?

Chronic open-angle glaucoma occurs when the open drainage angle of the eye is blocked, leading to gradual increased IOP, which leads to optic nerve damage. Damage occurs gradually and painlessly.

22.3 What is conjunctivitis?

Conjunctivitis is inflammation of the conjunctiva (white part of eye), resulting in the conjunctiva becoming pink or red and itchy.

22.4 If one eye has viral conjunctivitis why would you not administer antibiotics?

Antibiotics treat bacterial, not viral, conjunctivitis.

22.5 Name the four types of conjunctivitis.

The four types of conjunctivitis are viral conjunctivitis, bacterial conjunctivitis, allergic conjunctivitis, and giant papillary conjunctivitis.

22.6 Why would Fluress be used for a suspected corneal abrasion?

Corneal abrasions are identified by administering Fluorescein sodium and Fluress (fluorescein sodium and benoxinate HCl), which are dyes.

22.7 What does it mean if there is a green ring on the cornea after administering Fluress?

A green ring appearing on the cornea after administering Fluress means that there are foreign antibodies present.

22.8 What is a corneal abrasion?

A corneal abrasion is a cut or scratch on the cornea caused by rubbing eyes, contact lens, sand, dust, dirt, or for no apparent reason, resulting in pain, sensitized cornea (feels like something in eye), and photophobia.

22.9 Why are topical anesthetics used in eye disorders?

Topical anesthetics are used to anesthetize the eye for examination and removal of foreign bodies.

22.10 What happens to the eye when topical anesthetics are applied?

The blink reflex is temporarily lost and the corneal epithelium temporarily dries.

22.11 How long does it take for topical anesthetics to take effect on the eye?

The onset for topical anesthetics is 1 minute and the duration is 15 minutes.

22.12   What precaution must be used when using topical anesthetics on the eye?

A protective eye patch must be used to cover the eye until the effects of the drug wear off.

22.13   How are eye infections treated?

Anti-infectives and antimicrobials are administered to treat eye infections.

22.14   What medication lowers IOP in open-angle glaucoma?

Miotics lower IOP in open-angle glaucoma.

22.15   When are eye lubricants prescribed?

Lubricants alleviate discomfort associated with dry eyes and moisten contact lenses and artificial eyes. Lubricants moisten eyes during anesthesia and unconsciousness.

22.16   What medication is used for emergency treatment of closed-angle glaucoma?

Osmotics are used for emergency treatment of closed-angle glaucoma.

22.17   What medication is used for long-term treatment of open-angle glaucoma?

Carbonic anhydrase inhibitors are used for long-term treatment of open-angle glaucoma, interfering with the production of carbonic acid, which results in decreased IOP.

22.18   What medication is used to dilate the pupils for diagnostic procedures and ophthalmic surgery?

The medication used to dilate the pupils for diagnostic procedures and ophthalmic surgery is anticholinergic mydriatics.

22.19   What medication is used to paralyze eye muscles for diagnostic procedures and ophthalmic surgery?

The medication used to paralyze eye muscles for diagnostic procedures and ophthalmic surgery is cycloplegics.

22.20   Why should most eye medication be taken at bedtime?

Eye medication should be taken at bedtime because of possible temporary vision loss.

Ear Disorders

22.21   How do you prevent otitis externa?

Place two drops of alcohol in the ear canal to keep it dry before swimming to prevent otitis externa (swimmer's ear).

22.22   What is the therapeutic effect of cerumenolytics?

Cerumenolytics (hydrogen peroxide solution) is used to irrigate the ear canal and loosen impacted cerumen.

22.23   How is otitis media treated?

Otitis media is treated with analgesics and antibiotics.

22.24   Why might antibiotics not be used for ear infection?

Some ear infections are caused by a virus and are not treated with antibiotics.

22.25   How is ear pain treated?

Ear pain self resolves in 72 hours. Healthcare providers typically prescribe analgesics (acetaminophen or ibuprofen) to relieve the pain in the interim.